MASSAGE
& AROMATHERAPY

MASSAGE
& AROMATHERAPY

**Simple Techniques
to Use at Home to Relieve Stress,
Promote Health, and Feel Great**

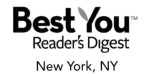

Best You™
Reader's Digest
New York, NY

Contents

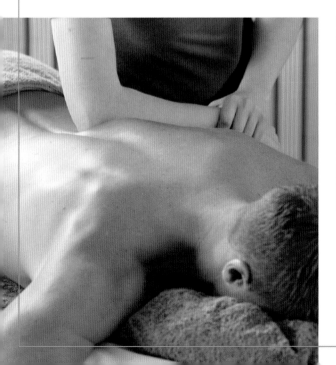
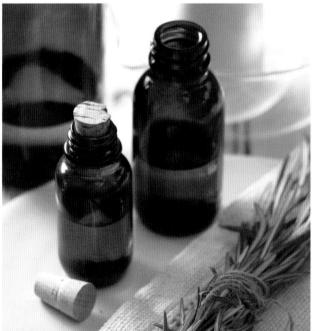
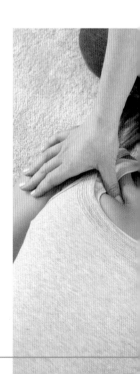

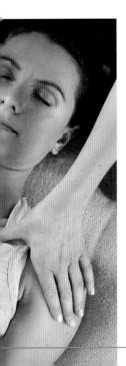
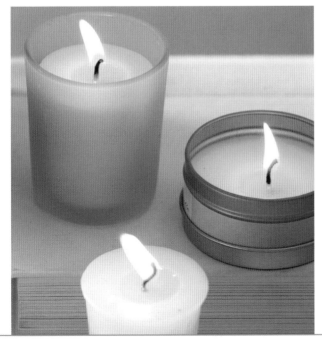
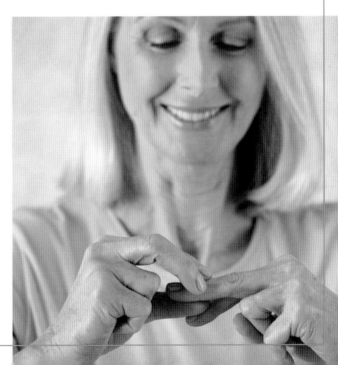

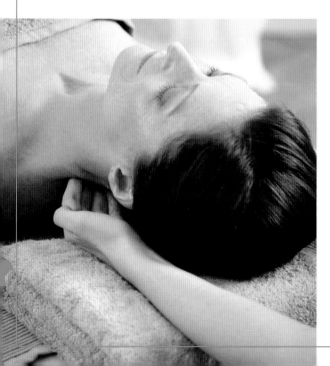
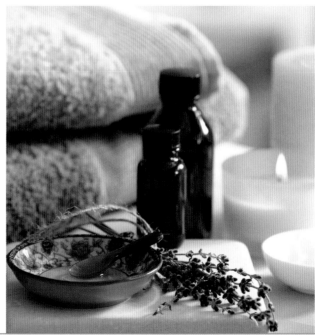
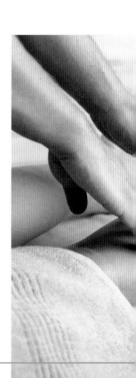

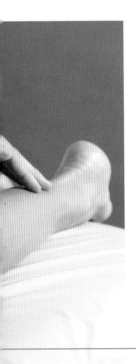

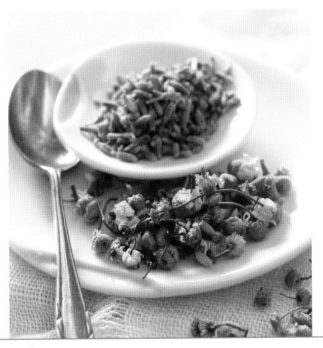

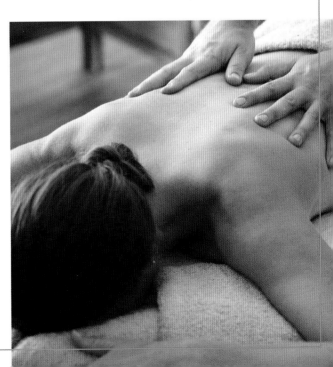

Introduction

The relaxing and sensuous pleasures of a massage with scented oils have been enjoyed for centuries, but it has only been in the last century or so that aromatherapy pioneers have established the healing credentials of essential oils, and that clinically controlled, scientific testing has begun to discover how they work.

Massage with essential oils is a supremely effective way of using them to best effect – not only are their aromas inhaled and absorbed via the lungs to relieve tension and improve relaxation, but also the nutrients from the oils are thought to be absorbed into the skin, and from there, into the bloodstream.

You can use aromatherapy and massage to restore vitality and to treat a truly remarkable variety of ailments, from muscular aches and pains, anxiety and depression, headaches, insomnia and digestive upsets to women's health problems, including a lacklustre libido, premenstrual syndrome and menopause symptoms. Not only do aromatherapy and massage represent one of the most practical and immediate methods of healing yourself and your family in the privacy of your own home, they are also highly pleasurable and affordable.

The use of aromatherapy continues to grow around the world. Essential oils are widely used by beauty therapists and remedial masseurs, as well as by other natural therapists who employ holistic healthcare techniques. Always consult your doctor before undertaking treatment for any serious or long-term health condition, and advise that practitioner of any at-home or professional complementary treatments you decide to use, including aromatherapy and massage.

THE EDITORS

Opposite The essential oils of rose, chamomile and rosemary can each be used with massage to treat a wide range of ailments and conditions.

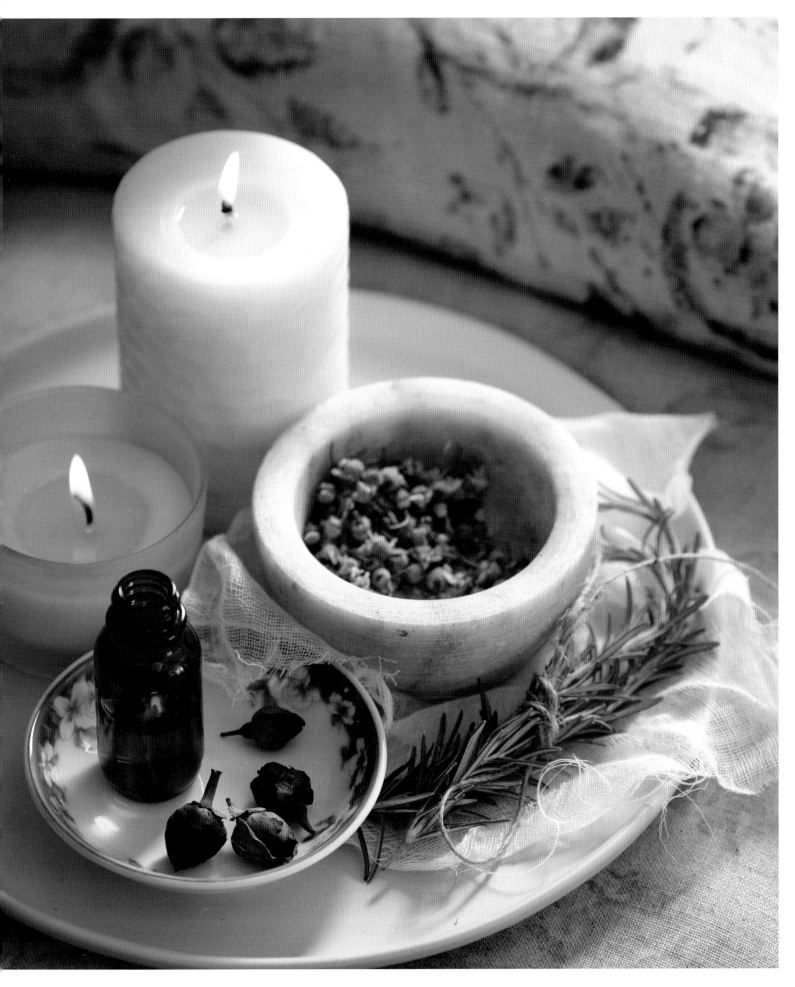

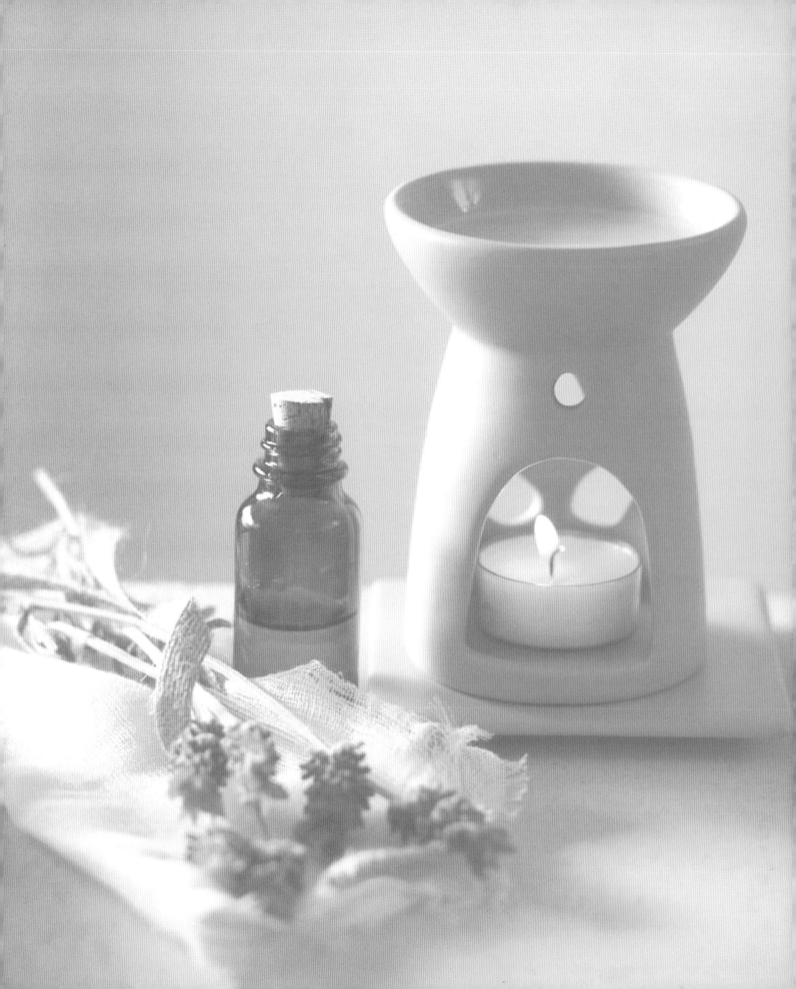

AROMATHERAPY
essentials

About essential oils

When using essential oils, it's important to buy quality organic products, store them correctly and use them carefully, especially when administering them to people with skin sensitivities, pregnant women, babies and children.

A powerful therapy

The use of essential oils to heal, inspire and soothe – or, as it is known today, aromatherapy – is a very ancient art. Early civilisations, notably the Egyptians and Greeks, recommended using aromatics – via inhalation, massage, baths and perfume – to ease the stresses and strains of daily life as well as enhance physical and mental health. Recently, the medicinal prowess of essential oils, especially their antibacterial and wound-healing benefits, has been documented.

But the most exciting new developments in aromatherapy lie in 'psychoneuroimmunology', an emerging field that covers a broad range of established and

For example, rosemary is both an antispasmodic and a digestive stimulant, and also has fumigant, insecticidal, decongestant, anti-inflammatory and pain-relieving properties, making it as necessary in a massage oil for arthritic pain or indigestion as in a steam inhalation for a chesty cold, or a room spray to repel flies.

Many essential oils – including tea tree, lemon, eucalyptus and pine – have some potent antiviral properties; others, such as ylang ylang and chamomile, are effective sedatives; still others, such as juniper and hyssop, help to stimulate the circulation of blood and lymph fluid, thus aiding the elimination of waste as well as relieving pain.

massage for healing and preventing disease as well as using aromatic essential oils such as camphor and sandalwood to purify the air in hospitals and disinfect patients' wounds.

Steam distillation

Basically, the steam distillation method entails placing plant material in a still (a large stainless steel container or vat). Pressurised steam is then passed through the plant material to release the essential oil from the plant fibres in a fragrant mist, which travels down a tube to a condenser. Here it is surrounded by cold water, which lowers the temperature and turns the steam back into aromatic water. The essential oil left floating on the surface of this water is then removed.

Other extraction methods

Two other methods of extraction include physical expression and solvent extraction. With the first, the essential oil is literally squeezed out of the plant material, a method commonly used with citrus fruits, such as bergamot, lemon, lime, mandarin and orange.

Solvent extraction entails the use of chemicals, which are usually derived from petroleum, to separate the fragrant essences from plant material. Essences extracted in this way are favoured by the perfume industry because of their high, nature-identical

During World War I, rosemary and tea tree essential oils were used in hospitals for their antiseptic effects.

experimental techniques that have the potential to enhance mental and emotional health, balance mood, encourage calm and harmony, relieve stress and improve memory. Science is also confirming what aromatherapy practitioners have long known – that individual essential oils can have a wide range of different therapeutic properties.

Production methods

It was during the first century CE that the Persian doctor Avicenna developed the art of steam distillation to produce aromatic oils similar to those we know and use today. So sophisticated was his method that it has remained largely unchanged for nearly 1000 years. Avicenna recommended daily aromatic quality; however, in aromatherapy there are concerns about the oils retaining solvent residues, which may provoke allergic reactions.

Quality supplies

Always buy quality essential oils from reputable suppliers, as the best quality oils will give the best possible results. Check that the essential oil is pure, and has not been mixed with a carrier oil, such as almond oil. The oil's price is the best indicator – for example, a concentrated, 100% essential oil of rose will be far more expensive than one labelled 'rose aromatic oil' or 'rose perfume oil' (the latter two varieties are usually a blend of 2–5% essential oil with carrier oil). On the upside, you will need much less of a pure essential oil and it will last much longer.

Also check that the oil is certified organic by a reputable certifying authority (refer to page 236). However, at the time of writing, the application of industry certification is not widespread. If in doubt, write to the manufacturer and ask them to provide information about their sourcing, testing and production methods.

Safe storage

The UV rays of sunlight can compromise the quality and efficacy of essential oils. Always buy oils in dark-coloured glass bottles with glass pipettes; never use plastic or rubber pipettes, as the essential oils will cause them to perish. Never store essential oils or essential oil blends in plastic or metal containers, as the oils may react with the plastic or metal – instead, use dark-coloured glass or china bottles and jars, with non-metallic caps.

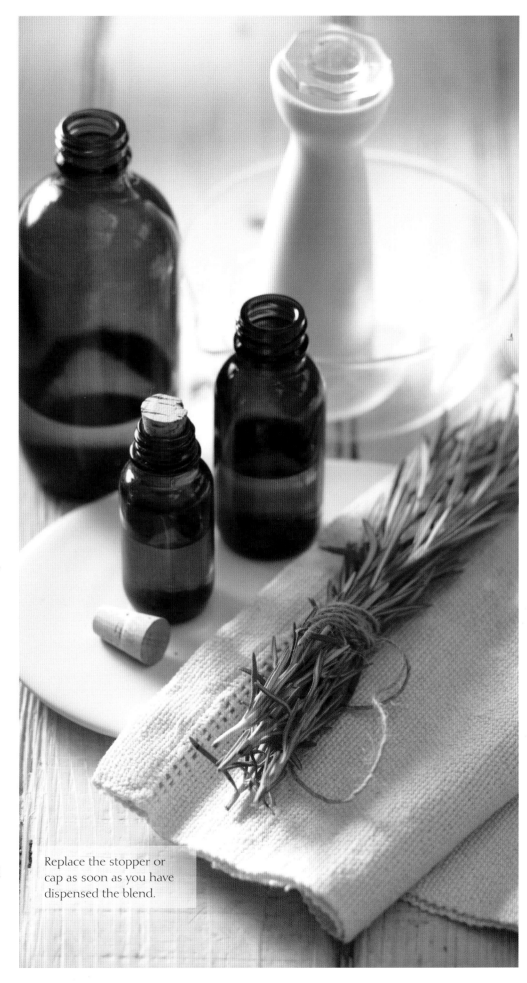

Replace the stopper or cap as soon as you have dispensed the blend.

The aromatic water is collected and sold as, for example, orange-flower water, rosewater and lavender water for health, beauty and food-flavouring purposes.

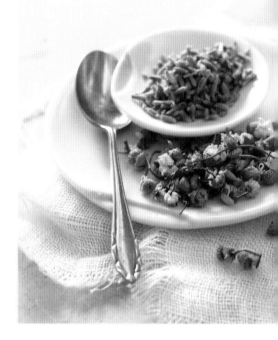

Do not store essential oils where they will be exposed to heat or moisture (such as in a bathroom or kitchen); instead keep them in a cool (c. 15°C), dry, dark place. If you need to store them in a refrigerator, keep them in a tightly sealed box to prevent the oils' fragrance from entering the food. Essential oils are highly volatile, so cap the bottles immediately after use or the contents will begin to oxidise and may eventually evaporate.

Refrigeration may turn several essential oils cloudy, but they should clear at room temperature. Similarly, it is normal for some of the resinous essential oils, such as myrrh, to become thicker with age. To make it more liquid again, just place the bottle in warm water for 15 minutes.

When you open an essential oil, write the date on its label so you can keep track of how long you have had it. After the 'use by' or 'best before' date, use any remaining oil in a potpourri, but not in any topical blends, such as massage oils, as it is likely to have lost its therapeutic benefits. Out-of-date essential oils are also more likely to provoke a skin reaction.

If an essential oil begins to take on a discoloured appearance, becomes sticky or starts to smell 'off', it will be past its best. In this case, discard the oil.

Never use or store essential oils near or on varnished surfaces, as they may discolour them or dissolve the coating. (See also the information on page 61.)

With any home-made aromatherapy blends, label the jars or bottles clearly and store them well out of reach of children. Note that blends that have been mixed with carrier oils will have a much shorter shelf life than either the essential oils or the unfragranced carrier oils themselves; therefore, discard remaining blends after a maximum of two months.

Safety

Essential oils are natural and they have many health benefits, but you should be aware that several are also potentially hazardous if they're not used correctly.

For example, several essential oils may be phototoxic or photosensitising in some people – that is, they can cause skin pigmentation when they are applied to the skin before exposure to sunlight; these include – but are not limited to – bergamot, grapefruit, mandarin, tangerine, lemon, lime, orange, lovage and angelica essential oils.

If you plan to use any of these essential oils in a massage blend, do so at least 12 hours prior to exposure to sunlight, as this will allow sufficient time for your skin to process the oils.

Both anise and fennel essential oils may closely resemble female hormones in their physiological effects, so avoid using them if you have a history of hormone-related cancer, such as breast cancer.

Some experts recommend that people with epilepsy also avoid fennel, along with rosemary, hyssop and sage essential oils, as they may provoke convulsions.

Do not let essential oils get into the eyes or mouth, never ingest them, and do not take them internally by other means – for example, vaginally or rectally.

During pregnancy

Several essential oils are contraindicated during pregnancy, and the aromatherapy blends suggested in this book for treating ailments of pregnancy, such as stretch marks, are only appropriate for women in their third trimester (that is, from 7 to 9 months). They are also presented here in the lowest possible concentration. However,

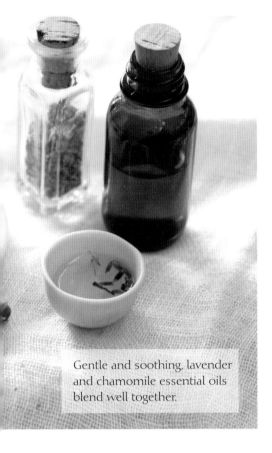

Gentle and soothing, lavender and chamomile essential oils blend well together.

To patch-test all the blends in this book, massage a very small amount in the crook of the elbow or inside of the wrist, cover with a small adhesive bandage and leave for 24 hours.

If no irritation results, you may assume the blend is safe to use. But if there is a reaction, wash off the blend immediately with soap and water and apply an unscented carrier oil, such as sweet almond oil. Do not apply neat essential oils to the skin, unless you're using a drop of lavender or tea tree for a minor burn or insect bite, or acne lesion or pimple, provided it does not come in contact with the unaffected surrounding skin.

slightly higher concentrations may be recommended in blends for particular health ailments, such as arthritis or muscular tension. If you are pregnant, consult a qualified midwife, doctor or aromatherapist first.

Some essential oils also have an emmenagogue action (that is, they stimulate menstruation and hormonal activity), and must be avoided during pregnancy. These oils include – but are not limited to – angelica, cinnamon, clary sage, ginger, jasmine, juniper and marjoram. Other essential oils that are generally regarded as being too strong and pungent for use during pregnancy – a time when a woman's sense of smell is heightened – include rosemary and myrrh.

However, a massage of the back, shoulders and legs can be wonderfully soothing for a mother-to-be. Always use either an unscented carrier oil, such as sweet almond, with no added essential oils, or a blend that contains half the amount of essential oils recommended in the recipe – but only after the first six months of pregnancy.

Skin sensitivities
Although most essential oils are regarded as being non-irritating to the skin, any substance applied to it can cause a reaction. If you have highly sensitive skin, be particularly cautious with black pepper, basil, cedarwood, clary sage, chamomile, ginger, juniper, lemon, tea tree and thyme, as they can irritate the skin and mucous membranes unless used in very low dilution.

Babies and children
Breastfeeding mothers should avoid the use of essential oils altogether: the aromas stimulate the baby and possibly disrupt his sleeping and eating patterns, and it's also possible for trace amounts of substances from the oils to enter the mother's blood-stream and, ultimately, her breast milk, with unknown results for the baby.

Some practitioners advocate never using essential oils on babies younger than 12 months, while others approve of using them in very small amounts. Or you can use an unscented carrier oil, such as sweet almond oil, to massage a baby or toddler.

As a general rule, for older children stick to the gentle, soothing essential oils, such as chamomile and lavender, and only use them in a much greater dilution than for adult application – no more than 4–5 drops of essential oil to 3 tablespoons of carrier oil.

Citrus essential oils tend to have the shortest life span, while oils with a spicy or woody fragrance, such as frankincense, last longer, and may even improve with age.

CAUTIONS Always keep essential oils out of reach of children. If ingested, many are toxic, even fatal. If you suspect that a child has ingested an essential oil, go directly to a hospital for medical treatment; do not attempt to induce vomiting at home, as treatment should not be delayed.

Using aromatherapy with massage

Although the pleasures of an aromatherapy massage have been known for centuries, it has only been in the last century that aromatherapy pioneers and scientific testing have begun to establish its healing credentials.

The pioneers

The aromatherapy pioneers include French perfumer René-Maurice Gattefossé and Austrian beautician Marguerite Maury who, in the 1960s, was the first to start documenting and comparing the mind–body effects of different oils. Maury studied the different forms of massage, including pressure-point therapy and traditional Tibetan techniques, in order to determine which ones delivered the best results.

Maury also introduced the idea of creating specific blends of essential oils to suit both the patient's personality and their emotional and physical health requirements. In other words, she went beyond simply using the oils for their beautiful fragrances and investigated their special effects on the body's chemistry.

Maury recorded her findings and was intrigued to discover that her clients – mainly women seeking skin rejuvenation and beauty enhancement – also reported that the aromatherapy massage treatments resulted in improved mood, relief of pain and insomnia, and even an increased libido.

The first book on aromatherapy was written by Robert Tisserand in the 1970s.

How essential oils work

Massage with essential oils is a supremely effective way of using them to best effect – not only are their aromas inhaled and absorbed via the lungs to relieve tension and improve relaxation, but also, due to their microscopic molecular structure, nutrients from the oils are thought to be absorbed into the skin, and from there, to the bloodstream.

Together, aromatherapy and massage may be used for a truly remarkable and wide variety of ailments, from anxiety and depression to women's health problems – including lacklustre libido, premenstrual syndrome and undesirable menopause symptoms, such as hot flushes, headaches, muscular aches and pains, insomnia and various digestive upsets.

Aromatherapy and massage represent one of the most down-to-earth, practical and immediate methods of healing yourself and your family in the privacy of your home. It is also highly pleasurable and affordable, and may even lead you to embark on a new career (see box, opposite).

Essential oils are widely used by beauty therapists and remedial massage therapists, as well as by other natural therapists who employ holistic healthcare

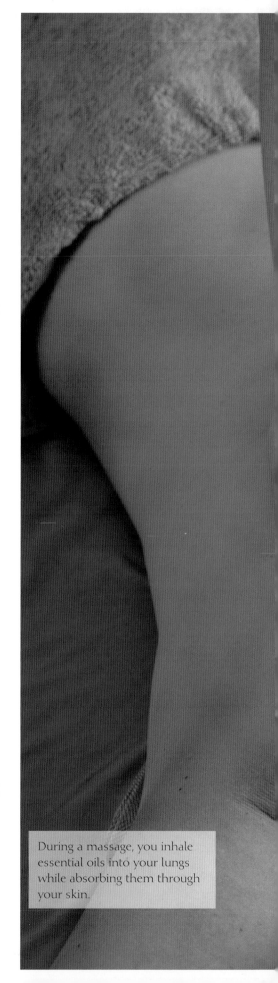

During a massage, you inhale essential oils into your lungs while absorbing them through your skin.

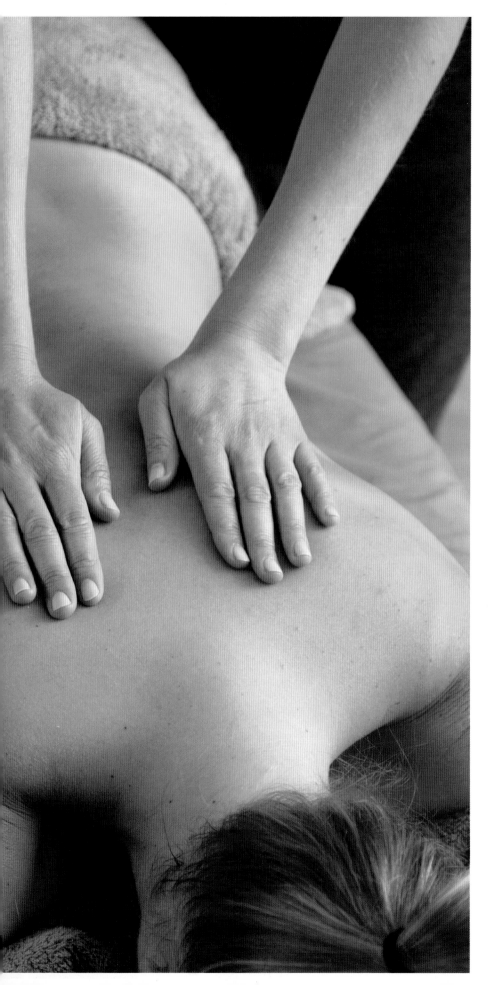

If you wish to develop your interest in aromatherapy and massage into a career, there are a number of colleges offering courses, either in face-to-face tutorials or via distance education. Some schools also offer introductory evenings and weekend workshops so you can 'sample' the work before committing to a full study program.

As a general rule, the longer the course, the more extensive the training will be. For example, a two-year diploma course would cover physiology, anatomy and the relevant basics of diet and lifestyle.

techniques. Regulations regarding the training of therapists vary from country to country. To find a qualified therapist, contact a professional association (refer to the list of websites in 'To find a qualified therapist' on page 236).

CAUTIONS Always consult with a doctor before undertaking treatment of any serious or long-term health condition, and advise him or her of any professional or at-home complementary treatments you decide to use, including aromatherapy and massage. In particular, some homoeopaths consider that the strong odours of some essential oils, notably eucalyptus and other camphoraceous scents, can interfere with the action of homoeopathic preparations. Always advise your homoeopath if you are using essential oils as well as their prescribed medicines.

Vaporisers, diffusers and burners

You can use vaporisers, diffusers and burners to release the aroma of essential oils into the atmosphere and create a calm, positive, energised mood, or to provide specific qualities that will help heal emotional and physical disorders.

Diffusing the scent

Using vaporisers, diffusers or burners is a simple way to bring the healing power of essential oils into your life on a daily basis.

Your sense of smell is directly connected to the limbic system, the part of the brain that affects your emotions, so one of these devices can instantly create a special atmosphere for a party, set the scene for a relaxing evening at home, or settle your mind and body before meditation. They also make a useful adjunct to other healing treatments using aromatherapy, such as massage, compresses, inhalations, footbaths and cosmetics.

Vaporisers

These devices work by gently heating essential oils with an electrical element so they release a gentle steam of aromatic micro-droplets into the air. There are several different types available. With some, the oils are added, usually neat, to a dish or bowl, and then heated. Others feature a replaceable pad or sponge onto which you drop the essential oils; a small fan then blows on the pad, spreading the molecules through the air.

Both the design and size of vaporisers also vary widely – some are small enough to plug directly into a power socket, but others are larger and heavier. They pose less of a fire risk than a burner, so a vaporiser may be a good choice for a sick room, where it can be left on overnight.

Burners

By far the most common method of disseminating aromatherapy fragrances is the burner. Add a few drops of essential oil and a little water to the dish or bowl, which sits above a shelf or tray holding a tea-light candle. Burners come in a great variety of shapes, sizes and materials, including glazed clay, ceramic, glass and stainless steel.

Avoid using burners with trays made of any metal other than stainless steel, as they will react with the essential oils. Choose a model that has a dish with a non-porous surface so it can be washed, making it less likely for the aromas to permanently impregnate the dish. Never leave a burner unattended in a room, especially if children are present.

Diffusers

A ceramic diffuser, or light bulb ring, is an easy way to release the aroma of essential oils into a room. Simply add a few drops of the oils, according to the manufacturer's instructions (some may suggest adding a little water as well), and hang it around the light bulb with the well facing up. The room is filled with fragrance when the bulb heats up.

Note that after use the ring will be hot to touch, so refill it only when it is cold.

Some blends to try

These recipes are suitable for a vaporiser, burner or diffuser. For more recipes for aromatherapy blends, devised for specific conditions, see pages 64–81.

If using an electrical vaporiser in a sick room, check the manufacturer's instructions, and do not leave it on overnight or unattended.

Head-clearing blend

Ease congestion in a patient with a cold or sinusitis, encourage sleep and keep germs at bay.

3 drops tea tree essential oil
1 drop eucalyptus essential oil
1 drop pine essential oil

1 In a burner, place the oils with 2 tablespoons of water.
2 Place a tea-light candle on the shelf provided, and light it.

Time out blend

Create an uplifting atmosphere, so you can rest and also rejuvenate your spirit.

3 drops sandalwood essential oil
1 drop cedarwood essential oil
1 drop jasmine essential oil

Add the oils to the bowl or pad of a vaporiser. Note that requirements and sizes for individual vaporisers vary – check the manufacturer's instructions and adjust the quantities of the essential oils accordingly.

Sweet surrender

This blend of fragrances will evoke a warm, sensuous atmosphere conducive to romance and intimacy.

3 drops ylang ylang essential oil
1 drop patchouli essential oil
1 drop geranium essential oil

Insert oils in the well of a diffuser or light bulb ring. As with vaporisers, quantities required may vary, so always follow the manufacturer's instructions. For safety's sake, it is recommended that the rings only be used on low-wattage bulbs.

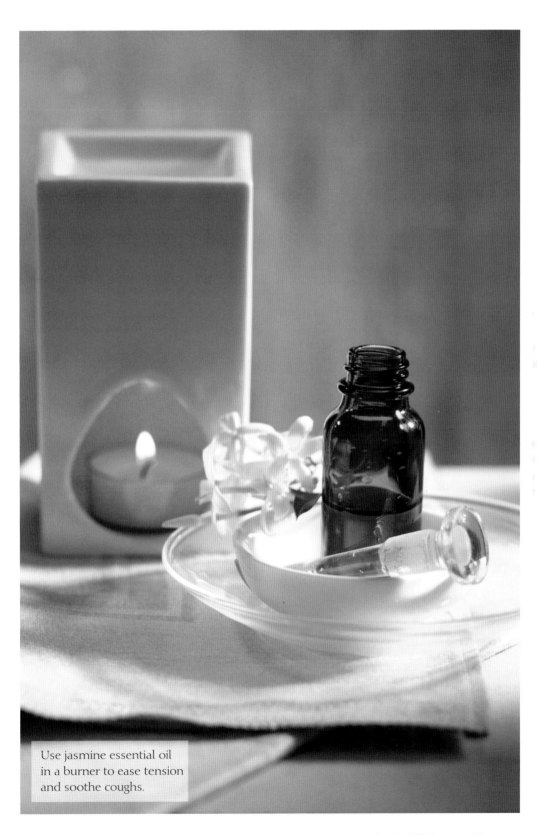

Use jasmine essential oil in a burner to ease tension and soothe coughs.

In the home

Add fragrance to every room in your home by using essential oils in vaporisers and light rings, and adding them to mixes for sachets and potpourri. They also help mask undesirable odours, such as pet smells and mildew.

Scented drawer liners

These lovely rectangular pouches for lining your drawers will protect and perfume your clothes.

 fine organdie or muslin (length
  depends on size and number
  of drawers)
 ½ cup dried lavender flowers
 ½ cup dried rose petals
 dried zest of 1 orange, crushed
 ½ teaspoon ground nutmeg
 pinch allspice
 1 tablespoon orris root powder
 5 drops rose essential oil
 5 drops lavender essential oil

1 Measure the base of your drawer, and make a paper pattern.
2 Pin the pattern to the doubled fabric, then cut out 2 rectangular pieces.
3 With the right sides facing, stitch around three sides, and turn the right way out.
4 Mix together the flowers and the other ingredients.
5 Fill the sachet sparingly with the fragrant mixture, and hand stitch the fourth seam shut.

Fragrant sleep pillow

The hops in this pillow not only give the mixture a slightly deeper, musky aroma but also encourage sleep.

 1 cup dried hops
 1 cup dried rose petals
 ½ cup dried lavender
 3 dried bay leaves, crumbled
 2 teaspoons cloves, crushed
 10 drops lavender essential oil
 small plain cotton cushion case
  (available from craft shops)

1 Crush all the herbs, then combine them with lavender essential oil in a bowl.
2 Spoon the mixture into the cushion case and stitch securely.
3 Tuck the sleep pillow between your pillow and its case, or slip it under your pillow, where the scent will linger all night long.

Coathanger sachets

For centuries lavender has been used to protect precious linen and clothing from moths.

 ½ cup dried lavender
 1 tablespoon dried marjoram
 1 tablespoon dried thyme
 4 crumbled bay leaves
 dried peel of 1 orange, crushed
 1 teaspoon ground nutmeg
 2 tablespoons orris root powder
 20 drops lavender essential oil
 small muslin or cotton bags
  (available from craft shops)

1 Mix the ingredients together.
2 Fill small muslin or cotton bags with this mix and tie them to your coathangers with ribbon.

Rose linen spray

Before ironing linen and clothes, mist them with this rose-scented water.

 10 drops rose essential oil
 3 tablespoons of rosewater

Combine the rose essential oil with the rosewater and enough water to make up 125 ml (½ cup). Store in a pump-spray bottle.

*'Let us stay awhile at that house,
for the linen is clean
and smells of lavender.'*

GEOFFREY CHAUCER (C. 1343–1400)

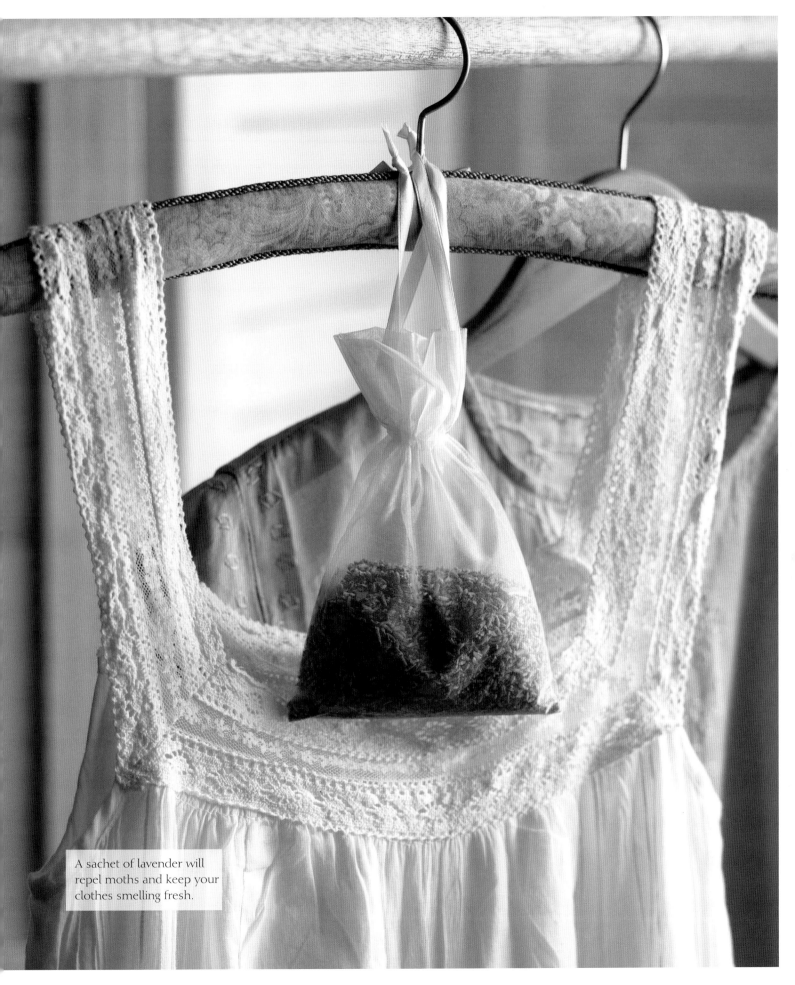

A sachet of lavender will repel moths and keep your clothes smelling fresh.

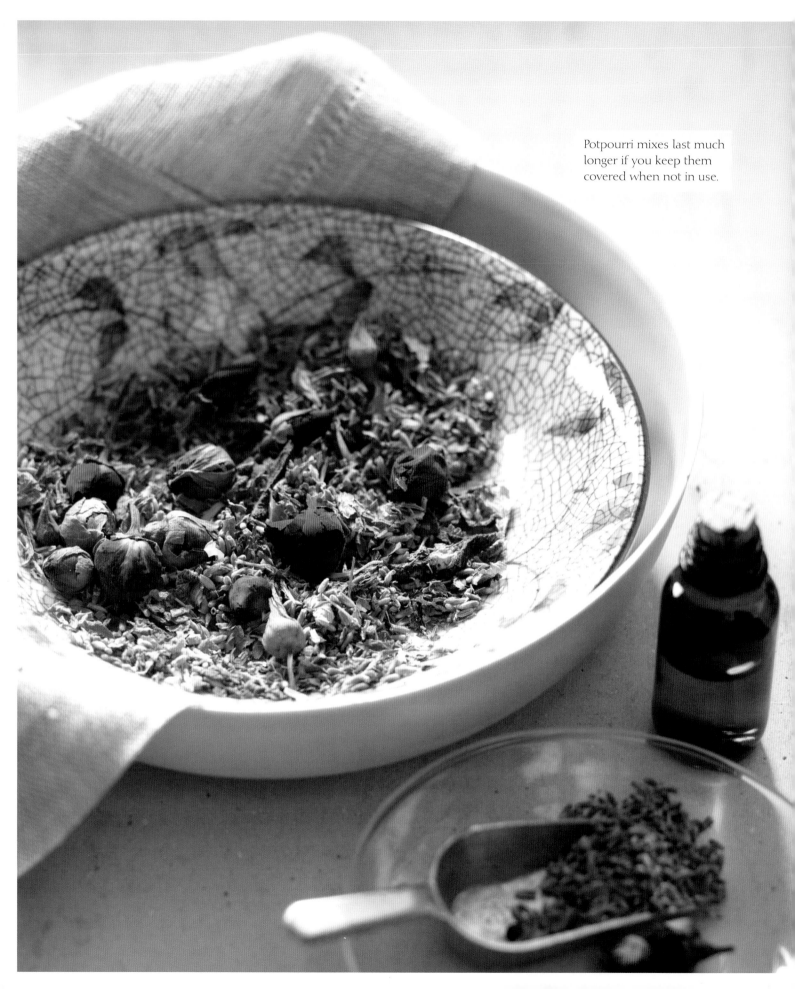

Potpourri mixes last much
longer if you keep them
covered when not in use.

Rose-scented candles

Fill your home with the sweet perfume of roses. If you buy a candle-making kit from a hobby or candle shop, follow the packet instructions for quantities.

350 g paraffin wax
35 g stearin (helps the wax to harden)
sachet pink candle dye powder
20 drops rose essential oil

1 Prepare the candle moulds according to the manufacturer's instructions.
2 Melt the wax in a double boiler over a low heat.
3 Melt the stearin and dye in a second double boiler, then add rose essential oil.
4 Stir in the stearin mixture.
5 Mould the candles and trim the wicks, according to the manufacturer's instructions.
6 Polish the hardened candles with cotton wool that has been dipped in rose essential oil.

Welcome home blend

This spicy citrus blend will fill your home with a refreshing fragrance.

2 drops bergamot essential oil
2 drops geranium essential oil
1 drop mandarin essential oil
1 drop black pepper essential oil

1 Place the essential oils in the dish of an aromatherapy vaporiser along with 2 tablespoons of water.
2 Light a tea-light candle and place it underneath the vaporiser so it heats the mixture, filling the room with fragrance.

Fresh mint room spray

This invigorating mint spray has citrus undertones. Just shake it thoroughly before using it as a room spray.

10 drops peppermint essential oil
5 drops lemon essential oil
5 drops orange essential oil
2 tablespoons of orange flower water

1 Combine the essential oils and orange flower water with enough water to make up 125 ml (½ cup).
2 Store in a pump-spray bottle.

Lemon verbena potpourri

Placed in a porcelain or silver bowl near the front door, this zesty mix is a wonderful way to welcome guests to your home.

1 cup dried lemon verbena
1 cup dried lavender
½ cup dried baby rosebuds
1 tablespoon dried marjoram
dried zest of 2 lemons, crushed
3 tablespoons orris root powder
15 drops lemon essential oil
5 drops lavender essential oil

1 Combine herbs and zest with orris root powder.
2 Add essential oils and mix well with your hands.

'Stuff your pillow with hops newly dried until you feel it comfortable to your head. Those who cannot catch their sleep will find such a pillow serviceable.'

SEVENTEENTH-CENTURY RECIPE

Beauty and health

These aromatherapy treatments will lift your spirits and rejuvenate your entire body. Essential oils help relax the nervous system, stimulate the circulation, restore skin tone and hydration, and relieve a host of minor ailments.

Creamy cleanser

An excellent skin food, packed with vitamins A and E and essential fatty acids, this cleanser will lubricate your skin and restore its elasticity.

> 1 tablespoon cocoa butter
> 1 teaspoon honey
> 1 tablespoon jojoba oil
> 1 tablespoon olive oil
> 2 drops sandalwood essential oil
> 1 drop frankincense essential oil

1 In a double boiler over low heat, melt cocoa butter, stirring.

2 Whisk in honey and jojoba, olive oil and essential oils. Cool, then store in a clean glass jar.

3 To use, apply to face and neck with fingertips, using light circular movements.

4 Rinse off with warm water and pat dry.

Chamomile lotion

This light lotion helps to moisturise, cleanse and gently bleach the skin, making it particularly good for reddened skin or age spots.

> ¼ cup strong chamomile tea, strained
> ¼ cup cream
> 1 tablespoon rosewater
> 1 teaspoon glycerine
> 3 drops chamomile essential oil

1 Place all the ingredients in a bowl and whisk thoroughly.

2 Store in a glass container in the fridge, and discard after 2 days.

3 To use, apply to face and neck with a cottonwool ball, massage lightly with fingertips, then rinse off.

Rose balm

Before applying moisturiser, use this gentle tonic to help close your pores and refine the texture of your skin.

> 50 ml rosewater
> 2 tablespoons witch hazel
> 1 teaspoon orange flower water
> 1 teaspoon glycerine
> 3 drops rose essential oil

1 Combine all ingredients in a glass bottle and shake well; cap securely.

2 To use, stroke over skin with a cottonwool ball after cleansing.

Peppermint aftershave

The witch hazel helps to heal and disinfect any shaving nicks, the vinegar balances your skin's pH and the peppermint stimulates your circulation.

> ½ cup peppermint leaves, bruised
> 1 tablespoon witch hazel
> 1 tablespoon apple cider vinegar
> 3 drops peppermint essential oil

1 Place the peppermint leaves in a bowl. Pour over 125 ml (½ cup) boiling water, cover and steep until cold.

2 Strain.

3 Add witch hazel, vinegar and oil, and pour into a bottle with a non-metallic cap. Shake before use. For an extra invigorating tingle, store in the refrigerator.

Citrus and honey scrub

This scrub brings a healthy glow to sallow skin – almond meal's soothing properties help heal any infection while the orange juice and essential oil act as an astringent.

> 1 tablespoon honey
> 1 tablespoon freshly squeezed orange juice, strained
> 3 tablespoons almond meal
> natural yogurt, sufficient to form a paste
> 1 drop orange essential oil

1 Melt honey over low heat and whisk in orange juice. Remove from heat and cool slightly.

2 Combine honey mixture with almond meal, adding enough yogurt to form a paste, then add the essential oil and stir well.

3 To use, massage into your face and neck with circular movements, avoiding your eye area and lips. Rinse off and pat dry.

Apricot nourishing serum

The combination of gentle apricot kernel oil and the restorative properties of rose essential oil make this blend invaluable for preventing fine wrinkles.

1 x 1000 IU vitamin E capsule
1 x 250 mg evening primrose oil capsule
1 tablespoon apricot kernel oil
1 tablespoon jojoba oil
1 teaspoon rosehip oil
2 drops rose essential oil

1 Pierce capsules and squeeze contents into a bowl.

2 Add other ingredients and stir. Store in a small, dark glass bottle, preferably one that has a dripper neck insert.

3 To use, warm a few drops between your fingers and pat gently under your eyes and around your lip line and throat.

Lavender antiseptic lotion

Lavender is a valuable herb for treating skin problems – it inhibits infection-causing bacteria while soothing your skin, helping to control the over-secretion of sebum and preventing scarring.

1 cup fresh lavender flowers
1 tablespoon witch hazel
pinch of salt
3 drops lavender essential oil
2 drops tea tree essential oil

1 Put lavender flowers in a bowl and pour over 250 ml (1 cup) boiling water. Cover and steep for 1 hour. Strain and measure out ¼ cup.

2 Combine all ingredients in a bowl, mix well and store in a small, dark glass bottle.

3 To use, apply to skin with a cottonwool ball.

Facial massage oil

Use this rich, smooth oil for a luxurious face and throat massage that will stimulate your circulation, relax your skin and relieve tension.

2 tablespoons sweet almond oil
1 teaspoon walnut oil
1 teaspoon jojoba oil
2 drops rose essential oil
1 drop clary sage essential oil

Combine all ingredients in a bowl, mix well, then follow the instructions in the 'Facial self-massage' box below.

Strengthening nail oil

Help to prevent splitting or flaking nails with this recipe.

5 x 100 mg lecithin capsules
1 tablespoon castor oil
1 tablespoon wheatgerm oil
3 drops lemon essential oil
2 drops rosemary essential oil

1 Pierce lecithin capsules and squeeze contents into a bowl.

2 Add the oils, and stir. Pour mixture into a small, dark glass jar.

3 To apply, massage a few drops into clean nails twice a day, then buff to improve circulation and add shine.

Facial self-massage

Make sure your hands, neck and face are clean, then rub your hands together with a little of the 'Facial massage oil', and close your eyes.

1 Place the fingers of both hands on your chin. With an upward sweep towards the temples, smooth the skin back to the cheekbones. Repeat 10 times.

2 Use your fingertips to gently make large circular motions at the temples. Repeat 10 times. Run your fingers outwards across your forehead, always moving away from an imaginary line down the middle of your face.

3 With quick, light movements, use the thumbs and pads of your fingertips to gently pick up small sections of your cheeks. Feel along the jawbone – near the point where it's joined to the upper jaw, there's a slight indentation. Massage this area for a count of 10.

4 Place your fingertips on your earlobes and gently lift up and forward in a circular motion. Repeat 10 times. Then with little fingers at the nose, index fingers at the temples and middle fingers at the bridge of the nose, gently lift up and around; repeat 10 times.

5 Spread your fingers through your hair and massage your scalp with small, circular movements. For a count of 10, use your thumbs to apply circular pressure to the hollows at the back of your neck where the spine and the skull join.

Beauty spa

Why not set aside a few hours for yourself next weekend, and indulge in a home spa treatment? Relax in a perfumed bath, or lift your mood in a citrus shower, then pamper yourself with aromatherapy facial and hair treatments.

Fragrant bath

This luxurious blend soothes nerves and aching limbs, and promotes sleep.

¼ cup almond oil
¼ cup grapeseed oil
1 tablespoon honey
1 tablespoon brandy
3 drops rose essential oil
2 drops jasmine essential oil
1 drop neroli essential oil
1 drop patchouli essential oil
1 drop ylang ylang essential oil

1 Combine in a bowl, and store in a small dark glass bottle.
2 Shake before use, and add up to 2 tablespoons of the blend to a warm bath.

Invigorating footbath

Ease sore or tired feet with this particularly invigorating footbath.

3 drops rosemary essential oil
3 drops pine essential oil
2 drops tea tree essential oil
2 drops peppermint essential oil

1 Pour 1 litre medium-hot water into a shallow broad tray or dish, large enough to hold both feet.
2 Add the essential oils, and mix together.
3 Soak feet for 15–20 minutes, then pat dry.

Zingy shower

Improve your mood, concentration and accuracy with this treatment.

5 drops lemon essential oil

1 Sprinkle the oil on a face washer and place it over the grating in the shower recess.
2 Run a warm shower (if you make it too hot, you'll feel lethargic afterwards, rather than invigorated) and step in. Steam from the warm water disperses the oil and spreads the aromatherapeutic benefits.

Soothing facial compress

Compresses enable a therapeutic liquid to be applied to the skin and are valuable in helping to clear up blemishes and soothe sunburn or rashes. The oatmeal helps shrink blood vessels, and can ease and prevent redness.

1 tablespoon finely ground oatmeal
2 drops chamomile essential oil
large square cottonwool, large enough to cover the face

1 Mix the oatmeal with 4 tablespoons warm water, and leave for 5 minutes to thicken slightly.
2 Add the chamomile essential oil and stir. Strain.
3 To assemble, see the box above on 'Making a compress'.

Making a compress

1 Cut out a cottonwool mask with two holes for the eyes and another for the mouth and nostrils.
2 Moisten the cottonwool in the infusion. Squeeze gently and flatten.
3 Apply to the face while lying down. Cover with a face washer and gently spread over the compress to stop drips.
4 After 5–10 minutes, remove the compress, rinse your skin and pat dry.

Pear hydrating mask

A wonderful treatment for sensitive skin, this mask combines cooling, emollient pear with cream that is rich in skin-nutritive fats.

1 tablespoon peeled and grated pear
1 tablespoon fresh double cream
5 drops rose essential oil
2 drops sandalwood essential oil
rice flour

1 Combine pear, cream and oils in a bowl. Mix in sufficient rice flour to thicken into a paste.
2 Smooth mask over face and neck, and leave for 10 minutes, then rinse off.

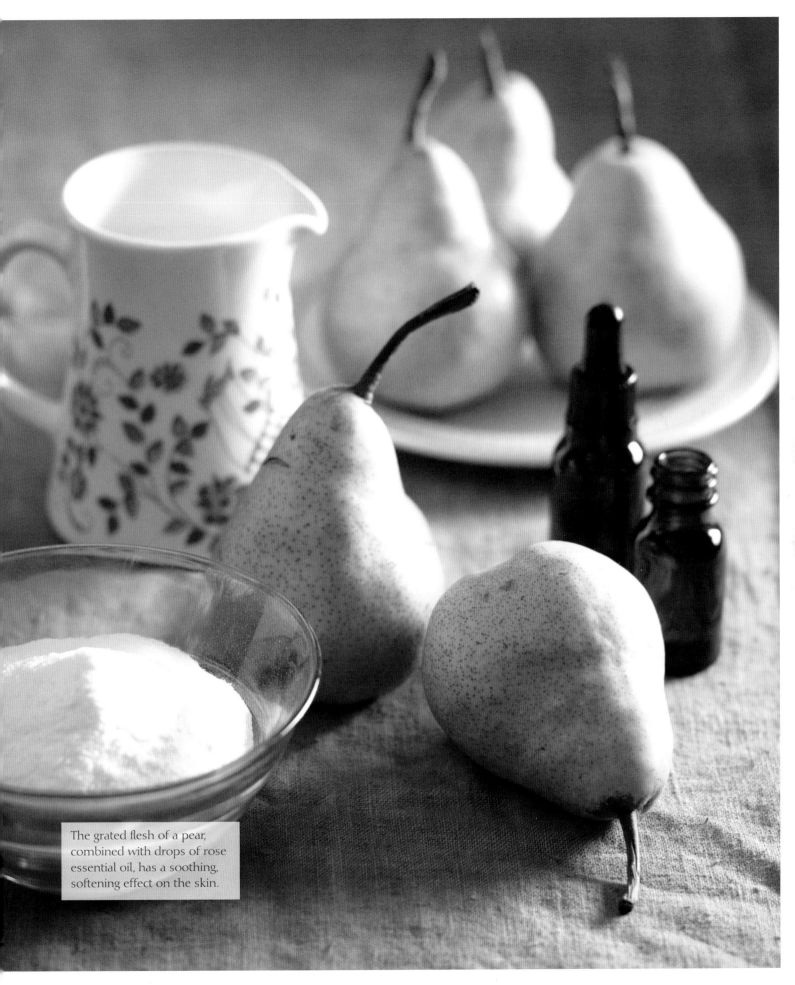

The grated flesh of a pear, combined with drops of rose essential oil, has a soothing, softening effect on the skin.

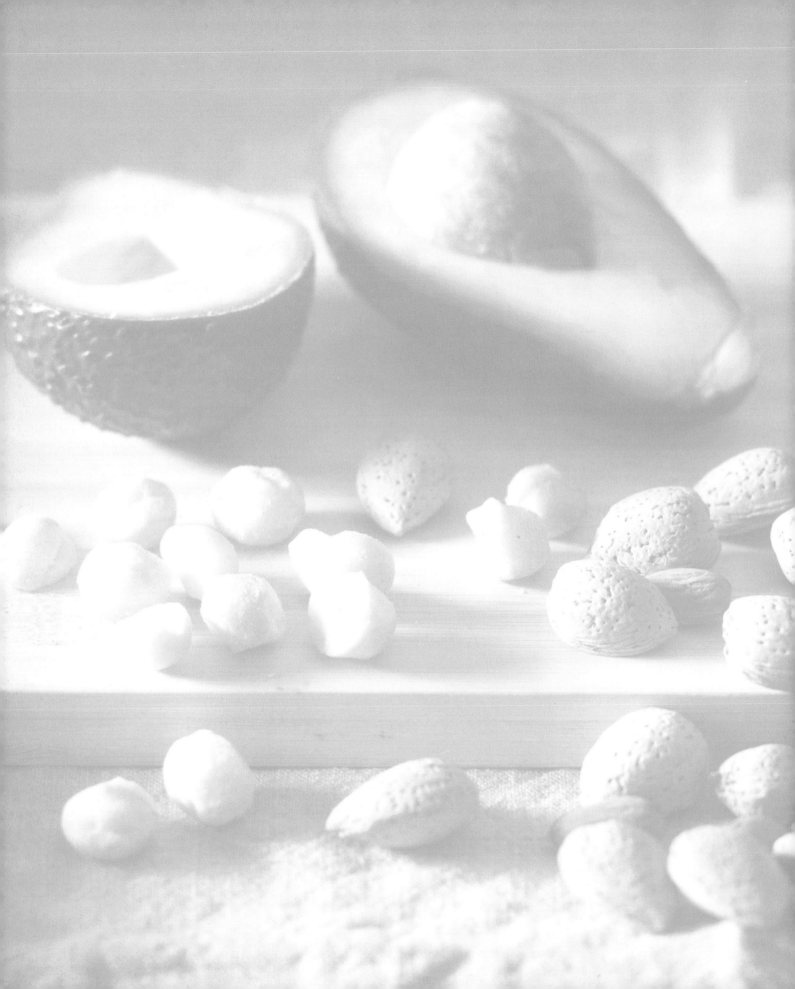

top 30
ESSENTIAL OILS

Basil

Ocimum basilicum

Nicknamed 'the herb of royalty', basil's Latin name comes from *basileum*, or 'king', possibly referring to its use in an oil for anointing kings at their coronation. Its fresh, warm, spicy scent makes it a favourite culinary herb, but it also has a long history of use in Asian and European medicine.

KEY PROPERTIES ● Antidepressant ● antispasmodic ● circulation-boosting ● digestive ● expectorant ● nervine ● tonic

ANTIOXIDANT POWERHOUSE

According to researchers, basil essential oil has significant antioxidant effects, and appears to be able to reduce the activity of free radicals, which are associated with an increased risk of health problems. Human studies may confirm this oil's potential in future treatments for fighting conditions such as heart disease.

PROFILE

Basil essential oil is obtained via steam distillation from the plant's highly aromatic green leaves and flowering tops, picked just before flowering when their scent is the strongest. Colourless to a pale yellow, basil has pungent, spicy and volatile active ingredients that give it its head-clearing, camphoraceous scent. It blends well with other spicy aromas, such as frankincense, and with sharp, clean scents, including lavender and citrus oils such as neroli and lemon.

APPLICATIONS & EFFECTS

For centuries basil has been used to heal the body, mainly to treat brain, respiratory and digestive problems. An inhalation may help treat allergies, sinus congestion, chest infections, headaches, migraines, asthma, croup, bronchitis, coughs, colds and flu as well as feverish conditions.

Using a basil-based massage blend on the belly may ease digestive problems such as nausea and flatulence, and also painful menstruation. When used as both a massage oil and bath additive, basil essential oil is recommended for treating muscle aches and pain. It is particularly good for stimulating circulation and easing stiffness and strain.

Minor uses for basil oil include healing insect bites and stings (mix 1 drop with 2 drops of tea tree essential oil and ½ teaspoon of sweet almond oil, then massage into the affected area); as a gargle (dilute with other oils, such as thyme); to stimulate hair growth (dilute with other oils, such as rosemary); and in a compress to reduce pain caused by injury, rheumatism or gout.

MIND & MOOD

The seventeenth-century herbalist John Gerard wrote that 'Basil expels the melancholy vapours from the heart', and it is indeed a valuable tonic for relieving mild anxiety, depression and stress; calming the nervous system; easing insomnia; and helping counter a wide range of nervous and emotional disorders, including premenstrual syndrome (PMS), hormonal mood swings, poor concentration, agitation and mental fatigue.

On a psycho-emotional level, basil's warming, uplifting effect is thought to put 'fire in the belly' – in other words, to boost confidence, heal grief, strengthen conviction, provide insight, focus an overactive mind and provide the energy and willpower required to overcome emotional insecurity in order to undertake new challenges.

CAUTIONS Avoid using during pregnancy. Basil is generally non-sensitising in low concentrations but can irritate sensitive skin. Patch-test before using if you have sensitive skin.

Feeling scattered? Burn basil essential oil to focus your mind and improve concentration.

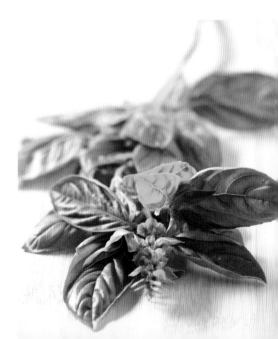

Bergamot

Citrus bergamia

A classic ingredient in eau-de-cologne and Earl Grey tea, bergamot takes its name from the Italian city of Bergamo. Long used in Italian folk medicine for treating ringworm, ulcers and snakebite, it is now used for easing anxiety as well as skin, respiratory and urinary tract infections.

KEY PROPERTIES ● Antibacterial ● antidepressant ● antiseptic ● antispasmodic ● deodorant ● detoxifying ● disinfectant

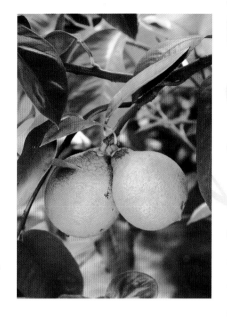

PROFILE

Bergamot essential oil is obtained by cold expression or steam distillation of the greenish yellow rind of the bergamot orange. Pale yellow to pale green, it has a delightfully uplifting, euphoric, refreshing scent with a hint of spice and balsam, which makes it rich and fruity rather than sharp and citrusy. It blends well with other citrus-type oils, such as grapefruit, orange and lemon; it also makes an interesting counterpoint to softer, milder scents, such as chamomile, and floral types, such as clary sage, rose, geranium, lavender and jasmine.

APPLICATIONS & EFFECTS

Thanks to its antiseptic, disinfectant and diuretic effects, this essential oil has a special affinity with healing urinary tract infections – use it as a preventive wash or in a sitz bath to help reduce itching and the spread of infection. As it is also thought that recurrent bouts of this condition may be associated with pent-up emotions, stress and frustration, the fragrance of bergamot essential oil may have a two-fold effect, helping to ease the anxiety that may trigger or worsen the condition in the first place.

Bergamot's properties earn it a place in topical skincare preparations, including compresses, skin creams or toners and massage oils, especially

Bergamot essential oil was a key ingredient in the ancient beauty remedy called Hungary Water.

those for treating acne, blemishes and skin infections, and it is a valuable inclusion in treatments for varicose veins, haemorrhoids and eczema.

As well as reducing infection and speeding healing, this essential oil has a subtle balancing and regulating effect, which may play a role where hormonal imbalances are involved. It can also be used to boost immunity; as a deodorant (both personal and in the home); as an insect repellent; and in countering mouth infections, notably cold sores.

MIND & MOOD

Bergamot is perhaps second only to lavender essential oil as a 'natural all-round balancer'. In the early twentieth century, the renowned aromatherapist Robert Tisserand described its aroma as 'harmonising'; much clinical and anecdotal study since then confirms its psycho-emotional benefits in a bath, massage blend or inhalation for treating depression, anxiety, tension, stress-related disorders, nervous tension, premenstrual syndrome (PMS), insomnia, apathy, listlessness,

burnout, loneliness, grief, appetite disorders where stress is involved, anger, frustration, bitterness and other problematic mental and emotional states.

BERGAMOT BREAKTHROUGHS

● *In an Italian study, researchers have found that bergamot essential oil increases mental activity, at least in animals.*

● *British research published in the* Journal of Applied Microbiology *has shown that the flavonoids in bergamot essential oil inhibit the growth of* Salmonella *bacteria.*

● *An in vitro experiment suggests that bergamot prevents neural cell death where cells are exposed to toxins.*

CAUTIONS Can provoke a phototoxic reaction. May cause a reaction in sensitive skin. Do not use undiluted; patch-test before application. Buy rectified or furocoumarin-free (the ingredient responsible for phototoxicity) bergamot oil through specialty suppliers.

Black pepper

Piper nigrum

Black pepper is a climbing vine with heart-shaped bright green leaves and tiny white flowers, which give way to red berries that turn black as they ripen. Native to India, it is now cultivated throughout South-east Asia and China; the oil is produced in the tropics, Europe and the United States.

KEY PROPERTIES ● Analgesic ● antibacterial ● aphrodisiac ● detoxifying ● digestive ● laxative ● tonic

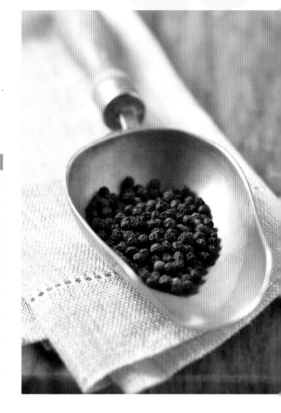

PROFILE

Black pepper essential oil is prepared by steam distillation of the dried, crushed ripe black peppercorns. Ranging from colourless to light yellow-olive green, it has a dry, hot, spicy, pungent aroma with lingering woody overtones. Its overall aroma effect is warming, exciting and stimulating. It blends well with other spicy aromas, such as frankincense, sandalwood and clove; with citrus essential oils such as lemon and bergamot; and with floral fragrances, especially rose, ylang ylang, geranium and jasmine.

APPLICATIONS & EFFECTS

Black pepper essential oil is very helpful in a massage blend for treating digestive upsets, such as colic, constipation, indigestion or a sluggish digestion, loss of appetite, nausea, diarrhoea and heartburn. Black pepper can also be used in inhalations for colds, flu, chills and catarrh, and for fighting viral and bacterial infections.

Black pepper's warming effect also makes it very valuable for easing stiff, tired or sore muscles; improving muscle tone; treating sprains and strains; and possibly improving sporting performance and preventing injuries; as well as for other musculo-skeletal problems, such as neuralgia, arthritis and poor circulation.

AN ANCIENT SPICE

In ancient times, along with myrrh and frankincense, black pepper was used as a preservative agent in the mummification of the Egyptian pharaohs. By 408 CE, when king of the Visigoths, Alaric I, besieged Rome for the first time, the spice was so valuable that he demanded 3000 pounds of it as part of the ransom. In the Middle Ages, black pepper was given to monks on pilgrimage to fortify their bodies and ease aches and pains.

Black pepper has been used in Ayurveda, India's traditional medical system, for more than 4000 years.

It has long been regarded as an aphrodisiac, so use it in massage blends to add a touch of fiery passion. You can also use it to add interest, exotic intrigue and depth to home-made fragrance, room freshener and aftershave recipes.

MIND & MOOD

The oil's piquant aroma is considered comforting, stimulating, elevating and strengthening to the spirit; burn or inhale it to help overcome mental fatigue, nervousness, indifference, vagueness and self-doubt, and to create an atmosphere conducive to confronting fears or emotional blocks, making decisions and taking action.

CAUTIONS Generally regarded as non-sensitising, although its rubefacient and circulation-enhancing properties may mean it can irritate sensitive skin; use in low dilution and patch-test first. Will counteract homoeopathic treatment.

Cedarwood

Cedrus atlantica

Also known as Atlas cedarwood, cedarwood was a key ingredient in embalming resins used to preserve Egyptian mummies, whose tissues have survived to the present day. One of the most ancient of the essential oils, it was also used as a temple incense, cosmetic and medicine.

KEY PROPERTIES ● Antifungal ● anti-infection ● diuretic ● expectorant ● insecticidal ● sedative

PROFILE

Cedarwood essential oil is extracted via steam distillation from the tree's wood chips and shavings, sawdust and leaves. It has a complex, balsamic, spicy aroma and is strongly antiseptic, antifungal and astringent, blending well with strongly camphoraceous scents, such as rosemary, cypress, pine and hyssop, as well as with sweeter floral types, including ylang ylang, rose, jasmine and clary sage.

APPLICATIONS & EFFECTS

Cedarwood is an excellent addition to any massage oil, and is especially recommended for treating respiratory conditions such as bronchitis, coughs, asthma and catarrh. Include it in a gargle for a sore throat, or combine it with pine or eucalyptus essential oil in a steam inhalation to reduce nasal and lung congestion. Its astringent ability means it plays a valuable role in any recipes for shampoos, skin toners or facial washes for over-oily and blemished skin.

Include cedarwood essential oil in a circulation-enhancing application or bath for arthritis and rheumatism and possibly cellulite; as an antiseptic wash for urinary tract infections and

pruritis; as an antifungal household treatment; and as an insect repellent and air freshener.

MIND & MOOD

Cedarwood is a popular and effective tool for meditation, relaxation and visualisation, guided imagery and self-empowerment, self-esteem building and emotional release techniques.

Nervous tension, negativity, fear, anxiety, stress, anger, depression, insomnia, premenstrual syndrome (PMS), lack of trust, aggression, hypersensitivity, indecision, mental exhaustion and conflicted loyalties could all benefit from the use of cedarwood essential oil.

Use it as a vaporiser blend for the bedroom in cases where resentment, insecurity and feelings of being overwhelmed are interfering with libido and sexual expression.

CAUTIONS Avoid during pregnancy. Never use internally. Always dilute before using, as it may irritate sensitive skin. Do not confuse with other cedar oils such as cedarleaf or thuja (*Thuja occidentalis*).

Atlas cedarwood is believed to have originated from the mighty 'Lebanon cedar', famed in the Bible as a building wood because it repelled insects.

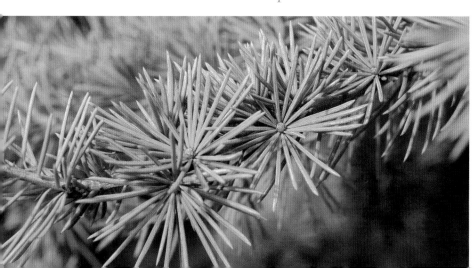

Chamomile

Matricaria recutita (German), *Anthemis nobilis* (Roman)

There are two main types of chamomile that have been used medicinally for more than 2000 years. Roman chamomile was one of the ancient Saxons' Nine Sacred Herbs, while German chamomile is nicknamed *alles zutruat*, meaning 'capable of anything'.

KEY PROPERTIES • Analgesic • anti-allergenic • antispasmodic • balancing • digestive • pain-relieving • sedative

Early Druid priests called chamomile 'the plant's physician', as it improved the health of plants growing near it.

PROFILE

Although the two varieties have different chemical compositions, they have similar medicinal properties. Chamomile essential oil is extracted via steam distillation from the flower heads of both species. The oil has a delightful, refreshing apple-like scent and exceptional soothing and calming properties, due primarily to its active ingredient, an anti-inflammatory compound called azulene. It blends well with the citrus aromas, such as neroli, and with other sweet floral or spicy scents, such as clary sage.

APPLICATIONS & EFFECTS

Chamomile is excellent for infections and all conditions involving inflammation, ranging from chronic conditions such as arthritis to temporary ones such as colitis and diarrhoea.

Other physical conditions that may benefit from a compress, inhalation blend or massage oil containing chamomile essential oil, include asthma; headache and migraine; acne; boils, abscesses and infected cuts; earache; dermatitis; eczema; psoriasis; arthritis, bursitis and joint inflammation; sprains, strains and tendonitis; burns, blisters and ulcers; period pain; muscle cramps and aches; wind; stomach ulcers; broken capillaries; cold sores; and symptoms of menopause and premenstrual syndrome (PMS).

CALMING CHAMOMILE

- *Chamomile tea may prevent complications of diabetes, including vision loss and nerve damage, according to an animal study.*
- *Germany's Commission E, an expert committee established to review the efficacy of more than 300 herbal treatments as medicines, has ratified the use of chamomile and its extracts in topical treatments for skin problems.*

While chamomile tea may be taken internally for these and other conditions, such as toothache, the essential oil may not; however, topical applications using the essential oil may be combined with internal doses of the tea to maximise its efficacy.

Anti-inflammatory, anti-allergenic, healing and calming, it is a soothing inclusion in both hair- and skincare preparations, including treatments for acne, burns, cuts, dermatitis, eczema, urticaria, all other dry and itchy skin conditions, bites and rashes.

MIND & MOOD

Chamomile is excellent for stress-related complaints, including nervous tension, insomnia, anxiety, fear and anger; it is especially helpful for those sensitive people who are susceptible to panic, over-excitement or negativity.

Use it as an inhalation or massage oil, or in a bath. Or try it in a vaporiser to ease depression, calm a stressed household, release past emotional blocks, encourage communication and have a spiritually grounding effect.

CAUTIONS Avoid during the first trimester of pregnancy. Do not take internally. May cause dermatitis, sneezing or wheezing in individuals who are allergic to the ragweed family of plants; always use diluted in low concentrations and patch-test first.

Clary sage

Salvia sclarea

The essential oil from this dramatically tall perennial aromatic herb, which is native to southern Europe, is widely regarded as 'the female helper', because it has a particular affinity with ailments associated with women's major life-stages – puberty, motherhood and menopause.

KEY PROPERTIES ● Antibacterial ● antidepressant ● aphrodisiac ● astringent ● deodorant ● hypotensive ● sedative

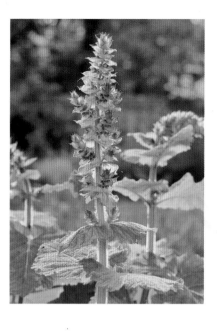

PROFILE

Clary sage essential oil is derived via steam distillation from the flowering tops of the plant. It has a warm, sweet aroma, with strong musky, nutty overtones, and is much used in perfume manufacturing. Clary sage blends well with other herbal aromas, such as rosemary and lavender, as well as the spicy scents, such as frankincense, juniper, neroli, vetiver and petitgrain.

Medieval herbalists called this herb 'clear eye', a reference to its use in assisting eye disorders.

APPLICATIONS & EFFECTS

Clary sage is also a valuable ingredient in skincare, both for its anti-ageing benefits – it has the ability to regenerate skin cells and help reduce the appearance of wrinkles – and because it regulates and normalises the production of oil in the skin, which makes it useful for treating conditions such as acne, skin infections and dandruff.

Clary sage is particularly helpful for a wide range of women's health problems, including irregular or absent periods, the symptoms of premenstrual syndrome (PMS), lowered libido and the hot flushes of menopause, along with other disorders of the genito-urinary system, such as leucorrhoea.

While it is not recommended during pregnancy, it is a powerful uterine tonic and hormone balancer, and may be used – under the supervision of a qualified health professional – to encourage labour, counter pain and help the labouring mother feel calmer and more in control.

Clary sage's warming, muscle-relaxant and antispasmodic effects make it a very helpful essential oil in massage blends or hot compresses that ease digestive disorders, such as constipation and flatulence. The same properties make it an appropriate choice for treating respiratory conditions, such as asthma and chest and throat infections, and circulatory problems, such as varicose veins, high blood pressure and migraine.

MIND & MOOD

This essential oil also has potent emotional and spiritual benefits. Inhale its 'grounding' aroma to reduce tension, anxiety, depression, fear, panic and stress and nervous system-related disorders, such as impotence, and possibly to help heal emotional and sexual trauma.

Of all the essential oils, it has the most pronounced euphoric and relaxant effects, as well as an ability to enhance mood and sexual energy, and to create a sense of profound wellbeing and contentment.

FUTURE POTENTIAL

It seems that clary sage essential oil may have both anti-inflammatory and pain-relieving applications. A recent chemical analysis that has been published in Planta Medica suggests that it may have future applications as an antimicrobial treatment, with some of its key ingredients being shown to have some beneficial effects against the bacteria that commonly cause disease, including Staphylococcus aureus and Escherichia coli, as well as the yeast Candida albicans.

CAUTIONS Avoid clary sage during pregnancy, although it is considered safe during labour. Do not use while drinking alcohol, as it may increase narcotic effect. May cause headache in some individuals.

Cypress

Cupressus sempervirens

This evergreen belongs to one of the most ancient botanical families, and has long been used in many different cultures as a symbol of life after death, often being planted in cemeteries; similarly, the essential oil has a long traditional use in sacred and funeral rites.

A cypress tree can live for centuries, hence its Latin name sempervirens, which means 'ever-living'.

KEY PROPERTIES ● Antirheumatic ● antiseptic ● decongestant ● deodorant ● diuretic ● sedative ● vaso-constrictive

PROFILE

Cypress essential oil is extracted via steam distillation from the tree's leaves, cones and twigs. Pale yellow to light green in colour, it has a fresh, sharp, spicy aroma, with earthy, woody and balsamic overtones. It is such a powerful astringent that the medieval herbalist Nicolas Culpeper described cypress cones as 'drying and binding, good to stop fluxes of all kinds'.

APPLICATIONS & EFFECTS

This essential oil is thought to be most appropriate for use where either an

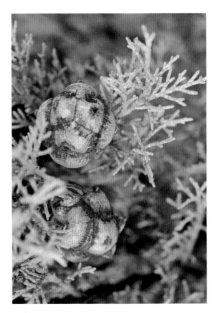

ANCIENT MEDICINE

Cypress has been highly valued as a medicine and aromatic incense for thousands of years. Ancient texts show that Assyrian physicians used the oil to treat snakebites and battle wounds, while the Egyptians used it as a mummification ingredient and also burned its branches in their temples as a tribute to Anubis and Sokar, the gods of death who guarded the gate to the underworld.

excess of fluid or swelling exists, such as in the case of water retention, or where there is an excessive loss of fluid, such as with heavy perspiration and sweaty palms or feet.

Other relevant conditions could include haemorrhoids, heavy periods, nosebleeds, puffy skin, hot flushes, arthritis, cramps, cellulite, oedema, poor circulation and varicose veins.

Cypress essential oil's strong antispasmodic effects make it an effective inclusion in aromatherapy remedies for respiratory complaints, including asthma, bronchitis and spasmodic coughing. Use it in a vaporiser or massage blend, or inhale a few drops from a tissue or handkerchief.

It is also a valuable ingredient in skincare, especially toning and astringent remedies for conditions caused by the over-production of oil; bath vinegars and salts; men's colognes and aftershaves; and, thanks to its ability to reduce perspiration and counter the growth of bacteria that cause odour, for deodorants for underarms and feet. When laundering your pets' bedding, try adding 5–10 drops to the washing water – it will get rid of odours and, as a bonus, help repel fleas.

MIND & MOOD

From an emotional perspective, the scent of cypress essential oil is said to strengthen the mind and fortify the spirit, and it is recommended for easing transitions, including the grief experienced at the passing of someone close or the end of a job or relationship; fear of change; feelings of hopelessness, indecision and discomfort with being alone with one's thoughts; and sadness.

Other psychological applications include irritability, nervous tension, restlessness, impatience, distrust, anger and stress-related conditions such as premenstrual syndrome (PMS).

CAUTIONS Avoid in pregnancy and in cases of hypertension. Although generally regarded as non-irritant, its astringency may not be tolerated by some sensitive individuals; only use in dilution and always patch-test first.

Eucalyptus

Eucalyptus globulus

There are more than 700 varieties of eucalyptus, including lemon-scented eucalyptus (*Eucalyptus citriodora*) and the most common species, the blue gum (*E. globulus*). Several of these varieties yield an essential oil, but it is the oil from the blue gum that is most commonly used in aromatherapy.

Botanist Ferdinand von Mueller called eucalyptus 'the fever tree' because of its use in treating malaria.

KEY PROPERTIES ● Antiseptic ● antispasmodic ● circulatory ● decongestant ● deodorant ● disinfectant ● expectorant

PROFILE

Eucalyptus essential oil is extracted via steam distillation from the tree's fresh or partially dried leaves. Pale yellow in colour, with a clean, sharp, pungent aroma, it blends well with other head-clearing aromas, such as pine, rosemary and lavender, and also with spicy scents, such as cedarwood, thyme and marjoram.

APPLICATIONS & EFFECTS

Rich in eucalyptol, which provides the penetrating scent, eucalyptus essential oil is well known as a trusty natural remedy for a wide variety of respiratory ailments; it also has a variety of household uses, thanks to its potent aroma and infection-fighting abilities.

As well as being an exceptionally effective decongestant, it has powerful medicinal, anti-infective and fever-reducing effects, specifically against cold and flu viruses and common disease-causing bacteria such as *Staphylococcus*: according to the French aromatherapist Dr Jean Valnet, a room spray containing eucalyptus essential oil will kill up to 75% of airborne pathogens.

In addition to being an old favourite for inhalations and chest rubs for coughs, colds, flu, bronchitis, sinusitis, hay fever, asthma, throat infections, catarrh and croup, and for use as a fumigant in sick rooms,

POWERFUL GERM FIGHTER

● *The Australian Aboriginals have long used the healing prowess of eucalyptus. When Captain Arthur Phillip arrived on the continent with the First Fleet, he noted that they used poultices of the crushed leaves to help heal wounds.*
● *According to an Italian study, eucalyptus essential oil in a test tube situation showed some activity against a variety of influenza viruses.*

this essential oil may also be used in topical remedies for skin disorders, including minor burns, cuts, blisters and scratches; viral infections such as cold sores; bacterial infections, including acne, boils, abscesses and ingrown hairs; and also stings and insect bites.

In addition, it is an effective ingredient in massage blends and compresses for all manner of muscular and circulatory conditions, such as aches and pains, bruises, arthritis, poor circulation, sprains, strains and fibrositis, and nervous system disorders, including exhaustion, neuralgia, headache and migraine.

Eucalyptus essential oil's cooling effect makes it a helpful addition to a bath or compress for a child with chickenpox, or any patient with a fever, itching, swollen glands or inflammatory skin condition, including the blisters that appear with shingles.

It is also an effective insect repellent. Try combining it with lavender essential oil in a room spray to purify the air, keep your home smelling clean and fresh, and to deter insect pests such as flies and mosquitoes.

MIND & MOOD

Its head-clearing scent is also thought to have psychic benefits. Use it in an aromatherapy burner when you feel discouraged, dull, confused, insecure or are unable to concentrate or feel enthused about life.

CAUTIONS Never take it internally, as it is highly toxic. Exercise caution when storing or using it near small children. Avoid if taking homoeopathic medicines, or if you have a history of epilepsy. Generally regarded as non-sensitising, but may cause skin irritation in sensitive individuals.

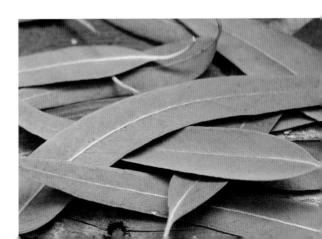

Frankincense

Boswellia carterii

One of the most ancient of scents, thought to repel evil spirits and encourage communion with the heavens, frankincense was burned in the religious rituals of early Egypt, Rome, China and India. It was also widely used in perfumery, skincare, cremation, embalming and mummification.

KEY PROPERTIES ● Antidepressant ● anti-inflammatory ● diuretic ● expectorant ● immune-stimulating ● sedative ● tonic (uterine)

PROFILE

Frankincense essential oil is obtained via steam distillation from the resin or 'tears' collected from the papery bark of the frankincense shrub. Clear to pale gold in colour, this oil has a strong, balsamic, warm, rich aroma with spicy and sweet overtones. It blends particularly well with citrus scents, such as orange and lemon, and with other spicy aromas, including cedarwood, cypress, juniper and patchouli.

APPLICATIONS & EFFECTS

Powerfully astringent, tonic and antiseptic, it has been much used in soaps, cosmetics and perfumes as well as in pharmaceutical products such as muscle-relaxant liniments.

Frankincense boasts exceptional rejuvenating, healing and anti-ageing properties. In addition to treating specific afflictions – such as boils, scars, wrinkles, dermatitis, ulcers, acne and pimples – it may be used in different recipes for masks, bath and massage blends, and compresses to help heal cuts, rashes and grazes, and counter infection.

It is particularly helpful for mature skin, as it has a pronounced tonic effect, tightening sagging skin, boosting micro-circulation of blood and lymph to the skin's surface, giving skin a natural glow, and minimising the appearance of fine lines as well as possibly slowing down the formation of new ones.

When breathed in, it has a marked relaxant and calming effect, making it an excellent choice in inhalations, baths and massage for treating colds, bronchitis, catarrh, laryngitis, flu, coughs and asthma, as it helps to slow and deepen the breathing and deconstrict tight muscles in the chest. It also acts as a pulmonary antiseptic to treat infection and reduce congestion and mucus production.

A uterine tonic, frankincense has a long traditional use in remedies for a wide range of ailments of the genito-urinary tract. It may be helpful in massage or bath blends and also compresses for treating heavy periods, period pain, cystitis; during labour; and for post-partum depression.

MIND & MOOD

This calming and balancing effect also makes frankincense one of the best essential oils for anxiety, nervous tension and stress-related conditions, such as obsessive thinking, and also for creating an atmosphere suitable for meditation, as it encourages introspection and focus.

From a spiritual perspective, it is thought to help deepen understanding and bring peace, and it is recommended for anyone who feels unable to move forward in life, due to insecurity, fear, low self-esteem, apathy, trauma, sorrow or physical or emotional weakness.

The resin that oozes out of the bark of the frankincense shrub is collected as small, pebble-like granules, which are sold as incense, or 'tears'.

CAUTIONS Avoid in pregnancy. Although frankincense is widely regarded as being non-irritating, always patch-test massage blends containing any essential oils.

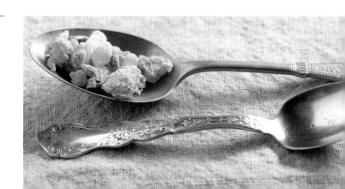

Geranium

Pelargonium graveolens

Many of the more than 500 varieties of geranium are wonderfully scented – for example, with lemon and apple. However, the essential oil is derived from this species, also known as the rose pelargonium, or Bourbon-style geranium, which hails from the Madagascar region in the Indian Ocean.

KEY PROPERTIES ● Antibacterial ● antidepressant ● anti-inflammatory ● antiseptic ● astringent ● deodorant ● tonic

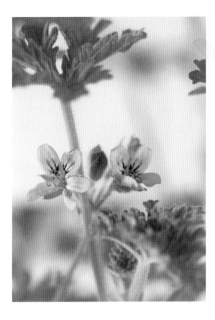

PROFILE

Pale green in colour with a fresh, clean, sweet scent that has flowery overtones of rose, mint and lemon, geranium essential oil is extracted via steam distillation from the leaves, stalks and small pink flowers of rose geranium. It blends well with citrus aromas, notably bergamot and neroli, and with sweet or spicy scents, such as rose, jasmine, lavender, clary sage, patchouli, sandalwood, black pepper, clove and coriander.

APPLICATIONS & EFFECTS

Geranium essential oil's actions are so varied that it's often regarded by aromatherapists as a 'good all-rounder' and 'hormone balancer'.

As an ingredient in skincare blends, it may be useful for any condition where regulating, healing and cellular-regenerating effects are required, including nourishing over-dry skin, balancing skin types that feature both dry and oily patches, and adjusting sebum production in over-oily skin. Skin conditions that may benefit from geranium are acne, bruises, broken capillaries, burns, cuts, dermatitis, eczema, haemorrhoids, wrinkles, ulcers, herpes, shingles and minor wounds.

Its sweet, delicate perfume makes geranium essential oil a delightful inclusion in colognes, bath splashes,

HORMONE BALANCER

Geranium has a mildly stimulating effect on the adrenal cortex, which controls the balance of hormones secreted by other organs, so it may be of value for hormone-related problems, such as menopausal symptoms, premenstrual syndrome (PMS) and heavy periods, and for harmonising the emotions at different female life stages, such as adolescence and post-pregnancy.

> Nicolas Culpeper described geranium as being 'under the dominion of Venus', referring to its use in treating women's health problems.

footbaths and massage blends for the face and body, as well as in an aromatherapy burner to freshen a room, while its insect-repellent properties make it very useful in personal repellents and in topical treatments for ringworm or other viral or fungal infections.

Its diuretic action, combined with its ability to improve the flow of blood, lymph and fluid through the body and its general tonic effect on the liver, makes it of potential benefit for treating conditions where excess fluid retention and poor circulation are involved, such as oedema and puffiness in the lower legs and ankles.

MIND & MOOD

Along with many of the other floral essential oils, geranium's aroma is uplifting, antidepressant and stimulating, making it helpful for relaxing the mind and easing the spirit. When combined with sedative essential oils, such as lavender, it may be used in inhalations and vaporiser blends to nurture the 'inner child'; open the mind to positive energy; calm agitation; and to treat nervous- and stress-related conditions, including insomnia.

It's especially recommended for psycho-emotional states where some degree of 'feeling stuck' is evident, such as rigid thinking or bitterness.

CAUTIONS Avoid during pregnancy. Although generally regarded as non-irritant, it may cause contact dermatitis in sensitive individuals; patch-test before use. May cause agitation or restlessness if used in excess.

Grapefruit

Citrus x *paradisi*

Native to tropical Asia and the West Indies but cultivated mainly in Israel and the United States, the grapefruit, which sports elegant, glossy dark green leaves, bright yellow fruit and delectably scented white flowers, is a cross between the orange (*C. sinensis*) and the pomelo (*C. maximus*).

KEY PROPERTIES ● Antibacterial ● antidepressant ● antiseptic ● astringent ● detoxifying ● digestive ● diuretic ● tonic

Grapefruit is a potent antiseptic that can kill common bacteria, making it useful in household cleaners and air fresheners.

PROFILE

Grapefruit peel is covered with tiny pits that contain essential oil, giving the fruit its distinctive fresh smell. The essential oil is pressed from the outer rind of fresh grapefruit via cold expression. Pale yellow in colour, with a zesty, sweet aroma, it is similar to but stronger and sharper than lemon, with green and fruity overtones. It blends well with other citrus aromas; spicy fragrances, especially cardamom, coriander and petitgrain; and herbal scents such as rosemary.

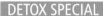
DETOX SPECIAL

This essential oil may be used in a massage blend on the lymph node areas, which may help to remove the toxic metabolic by-products that build up as a result of poor diet, sluggish metabolism, not drinking enough water, shallow breathing, inadequate bowel function and a sedentary lifestyle. It can also be used in a detox body wrap, or an invigorating after-bath body splash to boost circulation and increase metabolic rate, which may help to reduce cellulite and fluid retention.

APPLICATIONS & EFFECTS

Grapefruit essential oil is stimulating to the liver, gall bladder, kidneys and central nervous, immune and lymphatic systems, thereby helping the body to be more active in the elimination of waste.

Grapefruit essential oil is also a valuable inclusion in aromatherapy blends for treating muscular, digestive and circulatory problems, such as cellulite, premenstrual syndrome (PMS), fluid retention, indigestion, nausea, varicose veins and stiffness, as well as remedies to tone and balance oily or combination skin and to clear conditions associated with congestion and infection, such as acne, dandruff, hair loss and greasiness of skin or scalp. Its antiseptic properties also make it helpful for cuts and minor wounds as well as colds and flu.

MIND & MOOD

When it is inhaled, grapefruit has a revitalising, refreshing, uplifting and euphoric effect, and is thought to improve appetite, both the physical appetite for food and the psycho-emotional 'appetite' for life. As with other essential oils, grapefruit may have psycho-neurological benefits for stabilising emotions, strengthening the immune system and countering feelings of depression, anxiety or other mood changes through its effect on the brain's limbic system.

It may be used in a vaporiser blend to treat hangover, moodiness, headache, nervous exhaustion, drug and alcohol withdrawal, overindulgence and jet lag.

From a spiritual perspective, grapefruit is thought to open the mind and the heart to love, happiness and hope, and to bring inspiration and clarity to thought processes.

CAUTIONS This oil can sometimes be phototoxic, so do not use it in bath or massage blends if you are going out in the sunshine. Can cause skin irritation. Compared with other oils, it degrades quickly on exposure to oxygen.

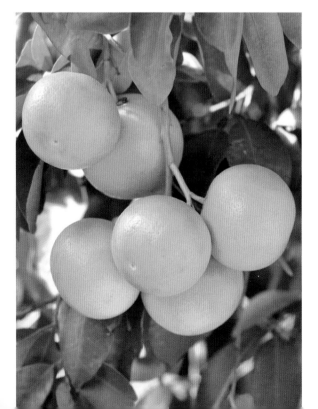

Jasmine

Jasminum officinale, Jasminum grandiflorum

Nicknamed 'the king of the flowers', this dusky-scented, powerfully relaxing essential oil can be derived from two varieties of jasmine – *Jasminum officinale*, an evergreen with highly aromatic, star-shaped white flowers, and *Jasminum grandiflorum*.

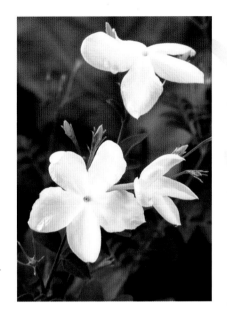

KEY PROPERTIES ● Analgesic ● antidepressant ● anti-inflammatory ● antispasmodic ● aphrodisiac ● sedative ● tonic (uterine)

PROFILE

Jasmine essential oil is extracted from the flowers by a combination of solvent extraction and steam distillation. In its absolute state, the oil is a thick, dark orange-brown and has a rich, heady, exotic, warm and very sweet aroma with floral and musky overtones.

This complex fragrance contains more than 100 chemical constituents, which partly explains why, along with rose, it has never been successfully synthesised. It blends well with other floral aromas, such as ylang ylang, and with citrus, spicy and herbal scents, especially clary sage, neroli, sandalwood and chamomile.

EXOTIC HEALER

● *If hot nights are keeping you awake, take a jasmine-scented bath before bedtime. The very relaxing, calming and soothing aroma may improve sleep and reduce anxiety.*

● *To improve your concentration and mood at work, put 2–3 drops of jasmine essential oil in a burner on your desk. It is thought to have an uplifting effect, creating a positive shift in brain waves and improving reaction times and alertness without making you feel anxious.*

One of Cleopatra's favourite fragrances was jasmine, known for its powerful aphrodisiac qualities.

APPLICATIONS & EFFECTS

Jasmine essential oil has an affinity with sexuality and the expression of intimate feelings, and it may be used in inhalations, baths, massage blends and compresses to treat a variety of women's health problems, including menstrual pain, irregular periods, symptoms of premenstrual syndrome (PMS), chronic emotional stress and loss of libido, impotence and frigidity.

It has been traditionally used in labour and childbirth to relieve pain, strengthen contractions, regulate uterine spasms, expel the placenta post-delivery and promote production of breast milk. It may help promote sexual health and tone both male and female sex organs, balancing the hormones progesterone and oestrogen, and for treating post-natal depression.

Jasmine essential oil is marvellous in skincare recipes, especially those for dry, sensitive or ageing skin, as it has exceptional softening and smoothing effects, and helps to improve the skin's elasticity. It also may be included in remedies for coughs, hoarseness and chest infections.

MIND & MOOD

Jasmine essential oil is particularly valuable in disorders of the nervous system, such as depression, tension, listlessness, emotional imbalance or trauma and pessimism. Noted aromatherapist Robert Tisserand wrote that jasmine 'produces a feeling of optimism, confidence, and euphoria'.

Its profoundly sensual aroma has a unique warming, fortifying and strengthening effect on the emotions, and on a spiritual and psycho-emotional level, it is thought to help overcome bitterness, fear, envy and emotional rigidity, and to open the heart and mind to inner wisdom, calm, romance, love, inspiration and the power of possibility.

CAUTIONS Avoid during pregnancy, although it is considered safe during labour. Generally regarded as non-sensitising, jasmine has been known to cause allergic reactions and headaches in some individuals; patch-test first. Narcotic-like properties; do not over-use.

Juniper

Juniperus communis

This essential oil is derived from an evergreen shrub with blue-green needle-like leaves and berries that are blue-black when ripe. It has been used for centuries as a urinary antiseptic, for respiratory problems, and in treatments for muscular pain, rheumatism and arthritis.

KEY PROPERTIES ● Analgesic ● antirheumatic ● antispasmodic ● astringent ● diuretic ● sedative ● stimulant (circulatory)

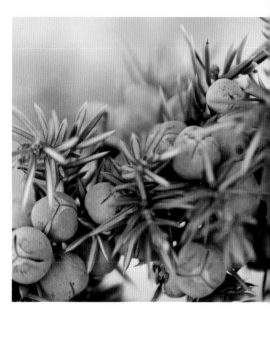

PROFILE

Juniper essential oil is extracted via steam distallation from the unfermented berries of the plant; an inferior oil is made from the needles and wood, but this is not considered suitable for use in aromatherapy. White to pale yellow in colour, it has an invigorating, pungent, woody, balsamic, spicy aroma, with overtones of pine and pepper.

APPLICATIONS & EFFECTS

Of all the essential oils, juniper is one of the most potent diuretic, tonic, purifying, cleansing and detoxifying, and it is very useful in treating any condition where the body needs to speed up its elimination of waste and release fluids. Such conditions include bloating, overindulgence, obesity, premenstrual syndrome (PMS),

> *Juniper branches were once burned in hospital wards to invigorate convalescing patients and protect against infection.*

ANCIENT MEDICINE

Juniper has been used for centuries as both a fragrance and a medicine: it was recorded as an ingredient in the celebrated 'oil of Balanos', a favourite perfume of early Rome. It has also had a long history of use in food products, notably as a flavouring agent for gin – juniper is what gives gin its unique flavour, aroma and even its name, as the word 'gin' comes from genevrier, the French for juniper – and in pharmaceutical preparations, including laxatives, personal care and aftershave products.

cellulite, arthritis, rheumatism or gout, coughs, colds, flu and chest infections, muscular aches and pain, puffy ankles and calves, and sprains or strains.

It is also helpful for skin problems that are slow to heal, and may be linked to toxic residues in the body and possibly constipation, such as allergies, acne and boils. Its traditional use as an appetite stimulant – as in the classic aperitif, gin and tonic – means the essential oil may also be valuable in helping to boost appetite and improve sluggish digestion.

Juniper essential oil has a special affinity with the genito-urinary system, making it a valuable inclusion in inhalations, baths, massage blends and compresses for cystitis, kidney and urinary tract infections; scanty, irregular, painful or absent periods; poor urinary flow; genital warts; jock itch; vaginal discharge; and urinary retention caused by an enlarged prostate.

Its powerful astringent effects make it a particularly good choice in skin toners for oily skin and remedies for the external treatment of haemorrhoids, either in a sitz bath or as a compress or wash.

MIND & MOOD

Juniper is said to clarify, stimulate and focus thoughts, especially in challenging situations. On a psycho-emotional plane, it is considered deeply purifying and healing to the mind as well as the spirit; use it to strengthen resolve, encourage vitality and a positive attitude, and improve courage in cases of general exhaustion, anxiety, jet lag, poor memory and stress-related conditions such as pre-exam jitters, insecurity and fear, and during convalescence.

CAUTIONS Avoid during pregnancy, as it stimulates the uterine muscle. Should not be used by anyone with kidney disease as it may have a nephrotoxic effect. May cause skin irritation in some sensitive individuals; always patch-test first.

Lavender

Lavandula angustifolia, Lavandula officinalis

Of all the essential oils, this time-honoured favourite, with its delightful scent, probably best deserves the description of versatile all-purpose remedy, having been used since ancient times for a wide variety of medicinal, therapeutic, home and beauty care purposes.

Lavender's name derives from the Latin lavare – to wash – probably because it was once widely used for personal bathing and laundry.

KEY PROPERTIES ● Analgesic ● anti-inflammatory ● antispasmodic ● decongestant ● deodorant ● insect repellent ● sedative

PROFILE

Lavender essential oil is extracted via steam distillation from the flowers of two varieties – *Lavandula angustifolia and L. officinalis.* The oil is clear to pale yellow in colour, with a floral, refreshing, slightly herbal, sweet and camphoraceous scent, with balsamic, woody overtones. It blends well with almost all the other essential oils, including citrus, herbal, spicy and floral types. When used at both a physical and emotional level, it is balancing, calming and soothing.

APPLICATIONS & EFFECTS

Although this herb has long been used in healing, it was not until the early twentieth century, when chemist René-Maurice Gattefossé burnt his hand and noted that lavender essential oil resulted in faster healing, that research into the properties of essential oils began.

Lavender essential oil is ideal for treating burns, scalds, cuts, bites, stings, grazes and other minor skin injuries, and is a helpful ingredient in any homemade lotions, toners, creams and massage blends. It promotes healing and minimises scarring by stimulating the cells in a wound to regenerate more quickly.

Its natural antibacterial, antiseptic and oil-regulating effects make it useful and safe for acne and other

STRESS-LESS SCENTS

● *According to a Japanese study, linalool, a substance found in lavender, lowers elevated levels of neutrophils and 'switches off' stress-induced activity in more than 100 genes.*

● *Another study has described how an aromatherapy massage with lavender essential oil given to patients with brain tumours significantly reduced their blood pressure, pulse and breathing rate, inducing both physical and emotional relaxation.*

inflammatory skin conditions, such as pimples and eczema, while its decongestant and antimicrobial properties make it effective in treating colds, coughs, bronchitis, catarrh, laryngitis, whooping cough, asthma, flu and sinusitis. It is also an effective insect repellent for both personal and household use.

Using lavender essential oil, a natural sedative, in inhalations or oil burners, or just sprinkling a few drops on your pillow will also improve the length and depth of your sleep. Massaging a few drops neat into the temples will relieve a headache, as will inhaling the aroma.

Lavender can also be used in baths and massage blends to relieve musculoskeletal aches and pains,

especially arthritis, sciatica, sprains, strains, muscle spasms, labour pain and period pain. Not only does it reduce the actual pain but it also eases the anxiety about the pain, which can be a trigger in itself.

MIND & MOOD

The oil's aroma is particularly valuable for nervous and emotional disorders, such as stress, irritability, panic, anger, hysteria, frustration or exhaustion. Spiritually, it is thought to resonate with the crown chakra, or 'third eye', to provide insight, compassion and deep relaxation.

CAUTIONS Avoid in first trimester of pregnancy. Avoid if blood pressure is very low.

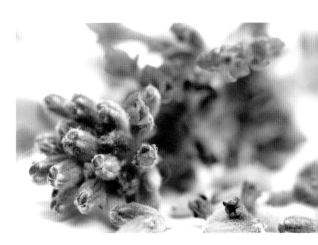

Lemon

Citrus limonum

Thought to have originated in India, the lemon tree was well known to the ancient Greeks and Romans, not only as a food and seasoning but also as a beauty aid and healthcare cure-all, particularly for fighting fever and treating infectious illnesses, such as malaria.

KEY PROPERTIES ● Antibacterial ● antifungal ● antiseptic ● astringent ● detoxifying ● diuretic ● immune-stimulating

PROFILE

Pale yellow-green, lemon essential oil is obtained via expression, or pressing from the peel of the fruit, which is covered with hundreds of tiny sacs, each containing the oil. Limonene, the oil's principal constituent, is primarily responsible for its scent. The aroma is intensely fruity, fresh, citrusy and bright, with sweet overtones.

APPLICATIONS & EFFECTS

Lemon is one of the most useful of the essential oils, and a must-have for any home aromatherapy kit, as it has so many applications.

One of its most important actions is to stimulate the production of white blood cells and act as a tonic to the lymphatic system, thus helping to boost the body's immunity and protect it from infection.

This makes it of great value in fighting fever, colds, flu and other viral infections, such as herpes, upper respiratory ailments, asthma and post-viral fatigue, as well as treating bacterial infections such as gingivitis and boils, and preventing infection in cuts and minor wounds.

Lemon essential oil acts as an anti-hypertensive and an invigorating tonic to the heart and circulatory system, thus helping to reduce high blood pressure, improve poor circulation and help treat varicose veins and arteriosclerosis; as an antirheumatic, so it benefits arthritis, gout and inflamed and painful joints; and as a detoxifier, to help keep cellulite at bay and possibly prevent obesity.

It is an excellent and versatile natural beauty treatment, acting as a mild bleach, which makes it useful for skin pigmentation, while its antiseptic, astringent, cleansing and antibacterial properties make it useful in remedies for oily skin, enlarged pores, acne and body odour. It is refreshing and cooling when you're feeling hot, lethargic, physically and mentally tired, low in energy and in need of a boost.

MIND & MOOD

From a psycho-emotional perspective, lemon essential oil is thought to act as a brain stimulant, increasing joy, renewing zest for life and overcoming black moods. Use this essential oil in a vaporiser or inhalation to counter confusion, brain fog, forgetfulness, lack of focus, depression, difficulty in problem solving, fear, negativity and feelings of being disconnected or overwhelmed.

CAUTIONS In some individuals, may cause irritation or sensitisation. Use with caution on sensitive or damaged skin. Phototoxic, so avoid using on skin that is to be exposed to direct sunlight.

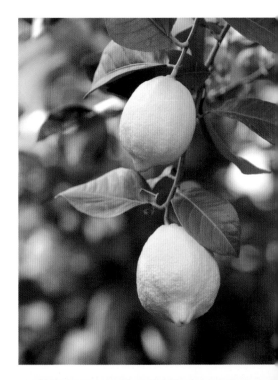

It was the Crusaders who brought lemon trees to Europe from Palestine, where they had discovered lemon's ability to fight infection and also purify water.

Lemongrass

Cymbopogon citratus

Lemongrass is a quick-growing, sweet-smelling grass that is native to Asia; both the whole herb and the essential oil have been used in Indian culture and medicine for centuries to help reduce fever, repel insects and fight disease, and also as a culinary spice and flavouring.

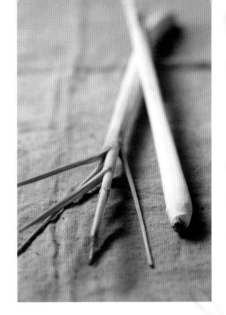

KEY PROPERTIES ● Antibacterial ● antidepressant ● antifungal ● antimicrobial ● astringent ● deodorant ● insecticidal

PROFILE
Lemongrass essential oil is obtained via steam distillation from the young shoots of the lemongrass plant. The main constituent of the oil, which is yellow to light amber brown in colour, is citral, which has a sweet, zesty, fresh and invigorating scent, with strong overtones of citrus and grass. It combines well with spicy scents, such as patchouli, as well as other clean fragrances, such as lavender.

APPLICATIONS & EFFECTS
Lemongrass essential oil is a potent tonic and stimulant. Its traditional use in Indian and Chinese medicine as a treatment for musculo-skeletal conditions causing aches, pain and fever is supported by modern experts, and it may be used in inhalations, massage blends and compresses to reduce the symptoms of arthritis, muscle soreness and spasms, physical tension, headache, bruises and sprains. It is also recommended in massage blends or compresses to ease stomach ache, colitis, constipation and indigestion.

This essential oil is thought to have some immune-stimulating prowess and this, in conjunction with its antibacterial effects, makes it of great value in speeding recuperation from illness, especially post-viral recovery, as well as easing dizziness, palpitations and nervous exhaustion.

Lemongrass has long been used in Ayurveda, India's traditional medical system, to fight infection and fever.

THE MIND BOOSTER
● *In a study published in* Critical Reviews in Food Science and Nutrition, *researchers found that inhaling the scent of lemongrass essential oil increased brain-wave activity, suggesting it may improve speed in performing mental tasks.*
● *According to research published in the* Indian Journal of Experimental Biology, *lemongrass essential oil may help regulate, sedate and slow the central nervous system, and possibly play a role in avoiding brain fatigue and mood swings.*

Lemongrass's pronounced toning and astringent effect makes it an excellent ingredient in topical treatments for sagging skin, cellulite, excessive perspiration, body odour, acne, athlete's foot, enlarged pores, dull skin tone and poor circulation, while its lemony, refreshing scent makes it a good oil to use in bath and body care preparations, albeit with care because of its strength.

As with other citrus-scented oils, lemongrass is a very effective insect repellent, so it may be included in room freshener and potpourri mixes for the home, as well as in blends to launder pet bedding and keep fleas and ticks at bay. Include it in a vaporiser mix and place the burner on a windowsill to discourage flies and mosquitoes.

MIND & MOOD
The zesty aroma of lemongrass is thought to refresh the mind and spirit as well as the body. It is excellent for improving concentration, vitality and overcoming mental fatigue, and for focusing an over-active mind. If you suffer from bad dreams due to stress, try inhaling 2–3 drops of lemongrass essential oil on a tissue to put the dark images and sluggish feeling behind you so you can clear your mind and embrace the new day.

CAUTIONS Avoid during pregnancy. May cause irritation in some individuals. Do not use on sensitive, allergy-prone or damaged skin. Always use this oil in very low dilutions.

Lime

Citrus aurantifolia

The lime is a small evergreen tree with stiff, sharp spines; smooth, oval dark green leaves; and exquisitely scented tiny white flowers, which give way to a sour, pungent fruit about half the size of a lemon.

KEY PROPERTIES ● Antibacterial ● antiseptic ● antiviral ● astringent ● detoxifying ● digestive ● tonic

PROFILE

The lime is grown widely throughout the Mediterranean region and the southern United States, where the essential oil is produced via expression, or the cold pressing of the ripe peel of the fruit, which is covered with multiple tiny sacs, each containing a miniscule amount of the precious oil. Pale yellow to light olive-green in colour, lime essential oil has a sharp, refreshing aroma with citrusy bitter-sweet overtones, and mixes well with other citrus essential oils, as well as lavender, rosemary, clary sage, neroli and ylang ylang. Its overall effect is cooling and revitalising.

APPLICATIONS & EFFECTS

An inferior oil is also produced via the steam distillation of the crushed whole fruit (a by-product of the juice industry), and this is widely used in fragrancing cosmetics, household cleaners and some food products; however, this oil is not considered appropriate for therapeutic use.

The properties of lime essential oil (see above) are similar to those of the other citrus-type oils. A powerful tonic and energiser, it is valuable in physical and emotional health conditions.

To support the body in dealing with a cold or bout of flu, asthma, bronchitis or catarrh, use lime essential oil in a blend in a bath, vaporiser, inhalation or massage oil. It will help clear the head, ease a sore throat, relieve tiredness and fever, and invigorate the spirit.

Lime essential oil is very useful in shampoos, rinses and tonics for oily hair; topical treatments for acne, boils, herpes, insect bites, pimples and warts; baths for oily skin and sluggish digestion; in massage for cellulite, excess fluid, congestion, constipation and lymphatic drainage; and, when mixed with essential oils such as pine and rosemary, which stimulate the circulation of blood, it can be helpful for various aches and pains, arthritis and rheumatism.

MIND & MOOD

Use lime essential oil in a blend for a burner when you are mentally fatigued, restless or exhausted and you need clarity, inspiration, positive energy and a new direction on a perplexing problem.

Just as lime's mouth-watering aroma is thought to have an aperitif effect, sparking the production of digestive juices and giving you an appetite, so is lime essential oil considered to have a positive effect on the mind, emotions and spirit, creating an 'appetite for life'.

It is particularly recommended for countering emotions characterised by gloom and confusion, such as grief, heartache, obsession, self-doubt and sorrow as well as more general stress-related conditions such as anxiety, exhaustion and fatigue.

CAUTIONS May cause irritation, a skin rash or sensitisation in some individuals; patch-test first. May be phototoxic; do not use on skin exposed to direct sunlight. May irritate mucous membranes in some people, so only use in very low dilutions.

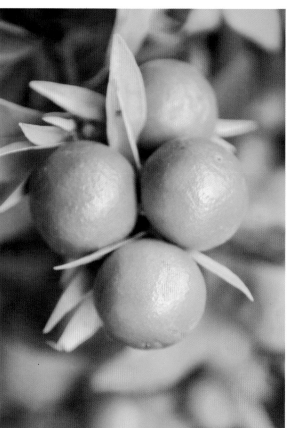

Mandarin

Citrus reticulata

The mandarin is a small evergreen citrus tree native to southern China, with glossy green leaves and sweet-scented white flowers, which are followed by bright orange, loose-skinned fruit. The fragrance of mandarin essential oil is very delicate and sweet, true to the aroma of the fruit.

KEY PROPERTIES ● Antiseptic ● antispasmodic ● digestive ● diuretic (mild) ● laxative ● sedative ● tonic

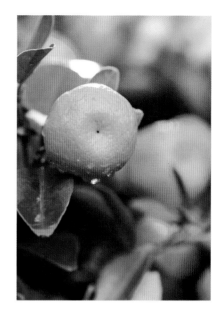

PROFILE

Mandarin essential oil is produced via the cold expression (pressing) of the peel of the fruit. It is a light golden yellow in colour, and has an intensely sweet and refreshing citrus scent with light and delicate floral overtones. Its overall effect is calming, softening and soothing. In addition to aromatherapy, the oil is used extensively in the commercial production of cosmetics, perfumes and soaps, and also as a flavouring agent, notably in liqueurs.

It blends well with other citrus oils, such as neroli and orange, both to enhance the aromatic impact and to increase a blend's therapeutic efficacy. It also combines well with spicy aromas, such as clove, nutmeg and cinnamon, and with herbal ones, notably coriander and lemongrass.

APPLICATIONS & EFFECTS

Use this oil in a massage blend or inhalation to treat stress-related problems, such as insomnia and nervous tension; to stimulate liver function; to improve circulatory system disorders, such as muscle spasms, fluid retention and cellulite; and to ease digestive problems, including abdominal cramping, burping, indigestion, intestinal spasms, hiccups and poor appetite.

One of the few essential oils considered safe for use during

This fruit was so named because it was once a traditional offering to the mandarins, government bureaucrats in Imperial China.

THE CHILDREN'S FAVOURITE

In France, mandarin essential oil is nicknamed 'the children's remedy', as it is considered to be so beneficial for digestive problems in children. To ease colic and indigestion, include the oil in a massage blend and smooth it gently into the abdomen of a baby or toddler, always in a clockwise direction. It is especially appropriate if the stomach upset is of nervous origin, such as anxiety due to the arrival of a new sibling.

pregnancy, mandarin is particularly recommended as a component of a massage blend that can be used daily, from the fifth month onwards, to help prevent stretch marks.

Its tonic effect also makes it an outstanding addition to inhalations and compresses designed to boost the immune system during recovery from illness and in topical home treatments for acne, oily and congested skin, and pimples.

MIND & MOOD

From a psycho-emotional perspective, the scent of mandarin essential oil is considered cheering, uplifting, revitalising and encouraging.

It is recommended for anyone who is feeling physically, emotionally or spiritually fragile, weak, apathetic, disconnected or isolated from others, or discouraged, including the very young and the elderly.

Use mandarin essential oil to stimulate mental energy, creativity and inspiration; create a sense of flow and movement in life; help overcome frustration, trauma and sadness; and counter mental fatigue due to overactivity, restlessness, panic, irritability or depression.

CAUTIONS Generally regarded as non-irritant and non-sensitising but may cause reactions in people who are allergic to citrus. It may also be mildly phototoxic in some people, so don't apply to skin before exposure to sunlight. Use within six months of opening.

Marjoram, sweet

Origanum marjorana

Marjoram is a low-growing, bushy annual herb with dark green oval leaves and clusters of small white or mauve flowers. Native to the southern Mediterranean, it has long been used to flavour food and beverages, as a folk remedy, and in fragrances and cosmetics.

KEY PROPERTIES ● Analgesic ● antibacterial ● antifungal ● antiviral ● digestive ● expectorant ● sedative

Marjoram is also known as wild marjoram and joy of the mountains, as it once grew wild around the Mediterranean.

PROFILE

Marjoram essential oil is made via steam distillation of the dried leaves and flowers. Pale to medium golden yellow, it darkens to amber brown with age. It has a penetrating spicy, woody, herbal aroma with peppery and camphoraceous overtones and an overall warming and relaxing effect. This versatile essential oil blends well with floral oils such as rose and lavender, as well as herbal ones, such as bergamot, and other strongly camphoraceous aromas, such as eucalyptus.

APPLICATIONS & EFFECTS

The fresh or dried herb was used by early European herbalists as a tea or in a bath or compress to ease stomach ache and respiratory complaints, with Nicolas Culpeper writing that it 'is comforting in cold diseases of the head, stomach, sinews, and other parts, taken inwardly or outwardly applied'. His advice holds true nearly 500 years later, as marjoram is also a very effective essential oil to use in a steam inhalation or hot bath to clear the chest and soothe bronchitis, flu, asthma, sinusitis or a cold or cough.

Marjoram essential oil's warming effects make it an excellent choice for massage blends for treatment of musculo-circulatory problems, such as chilblains, arthritis, bruises, aches,

ON THE HORIZON

Marjoram essential oil may have a role to play in ensuring food safety, even extending the shelf life of food. Researchers from the US Department of Agriculture have shown that edible protective food coatings, made from tomatoes and then impregnated with marjoram essential oil, were able to effectively prevent the growth of the three most common bacteria to affect food – Salmonella, Escherichia coli and Listeria.

pain and stiffness, hypertension, palpitations, muscular spasms, rheumatism, sprains and strains, as well as for digestive upsets, such as colic, constipation, wind, indigestion and flatulence.

Marjoram essential oil is especially useful for easing menstrual cramps and the teary distress that often accompanies them. Try adding it to either a warm compress or a massage blend, then enhance the therapeutic effects by placing a hot water bottle on the abdomen immediately after the treatment.

MIND & MOOD

Warming and calming to the spirit as well as the body, marjoram essential oil is often helpful in treating headache, migraine or insomnia, especially if it has been triggered by stress or anxiety. Use it in an inhalation, bath or massage blend to help deal with mood swings and unstable emotions, such as obsession, heartache or panic. Marjoram is particularly recommended for providing support for people who are lonely or grieving, as it conveys a sense of nurturing, confidence and all-embracing protection.

CAUTIONS Avoid during pregnancy. Avoid if there is a history of very low blood pressure, due to its sedative effects. May cause skin irritation in some sensitive individuals; always use in low dilutions and patch-test first.

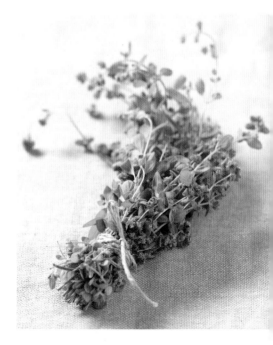

Neroli

Citrus aurantium

Neroli essential oil comes from the sweet-scented flowers of the bitter orange or Seville tree, an evergreen that is native to Asia but is now widely cultivated throughout the world. Most of the oil is currently produced in Italy, Morocco, Egypt and France.

KEY PROPERTIES ● Antidepressant ● antiseptic ● antispasmodic ● aphrodisiac ● deodorant ● digestive ● tonic (circulatory)

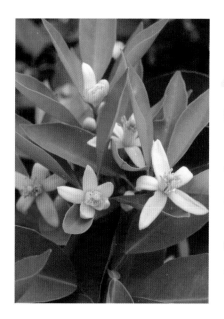

PROFILE

Neroli essential oil is made via solvent extraction and steam distillation from the freshly picked flowers of the bitter orange tree; the distillation process also yields orange flower water.

Pale yellow in colour, with a rich, bittersweet, citrusy aroma and slightly floral overtones, its overall effect is gentle, uplifting and soothing, so it is calming to nervous reflex actions and also has a tonic effect on the entire nervous system.

Neroli essential oil blends well with other floral oils, such as rose, geranium, jasmine, lavender and

Neroli takes its name from that of a princess from Nerola in Italy who was said to have regarded it as her favourite perfume.

ylang ylang as well as citrusy and spicy scents, such as bergamot, lemon and coriander.

APPLICATIONS & EFFECTS

Both the essential oil and the flower water have a long history of use in cosmetics, skincare, perfumery and household applications, while the water has also been a popular culinary ingredient, especially in desserts and beverages. Pure neroli oil is one of the most expensive essential oils, and it is often sold diluted in a base oil, such as jojoba. While the fragrance is still very strong, the therapeutic benefits will not be as pronounced.

Neroli essential oil has several significant benefits for the physical body: it is excellent for nourishing, toning and rejuvenating dry, mature and sensitive skin; it may also help to prevent scarring, wrinkles and stretch marks as well as soothe skin that has been sunburned or exposed to radiation treatment.

It may also be beneficial in some disorders of both the digestive and circulatory systems, including poor

circulation, palpitations, varicose veins, indigestion, colic, intestinal spasms, flatulence and diarrhoea (especially if it is triggered by anxiety).

MIND & MOOD

It is particularly valuable in treating nervous system disorders, especially anxiety, depression, stress, insomnia, premenstrual syndrome (PMS), shock and neuralgia. With its comforting and nurturing effects, neroli is a useful oil to include in an inhalation, bath, compress or vaporiser blend to ease agitation, sadness and irritability, especially during adolescence and menopause, and in a burner blend to create an atmosphere of positive energy, peace and relaxation.

CAUTIONS Generally regarded as non-irritant, non-sensitising and non-phototoxic. However, contact dermatitis, phototoxicity and irritation can occur in sensitive people, so patch-test first.

THE BRIDE'S CHOICE

Neroli is regarded as an aphrodisiac, but unlike other essential oils that boast the same effect, it is not due to any stimulating or tonic effect on male or female hormones. Rather, it is neroli's ability to soothe the nervous apprehension that may be present before a sexual encounter, and also to create a sense of peace and safety, encouraging trust, self-confidence, sensuality and empathy, and removing inhibitions that combine to create its effect. This explains why orange blossom is traditionally included in bridal bouquets and headdresses.

Orange, sweet

Citrus sinensis

Smaller than bitter orange, with fewer or no spines, sweet orange has glossy dark green leaves, fragrant creamy white flowers, and a highly nutritious, juicy, bright orange fruit. A wonderful room freshener, orange essential oil refreshes stale indoor air and dispels unpleasant odours.

KEY PROPERTIES ● Antidepressant ● anti-inflammatory ● carminative ● hypotensive ● sedative ● stimulant (digestive and lymphatic) ● tonic

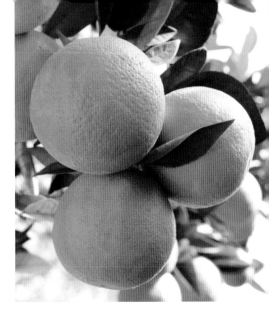

PROFILE

Orange essential oil is extracted by steam distillation or cold expression of the fresh, ripe outer peel of the fruit. A third type of oil, distilled from the pulp and essences – by-products of orange-juice manufacture – is not recommended for aromatherapy.

The expressed oil is a deep yellow-orange in colour, while the distilled oil is pale yellow, or clear. Both essential oils have a light, fresh, fruity aroma with sweet overtones. The overall effect of these essential oils is warming, cheering, uplifting and invigorating, but it is the cold-expressed type – with its stronger, longer-lasting scent and its additional important ingredients – that is considered best for aromatherapy.

Orange blends nicely with other citrus essential oils, such as neroli, as well as with spicy oils such as nutmeg, ginger and clove, and it also adds warmth and depth to exotic scent blends, such as myrrh and patchouli. It adds a rich, expansive note to skin-care and after-shave balms for men.

APPLICATIONS & EFFECTS

As they belong to the same plant family, many of the properties and uses of orange overlap those of neroli. For example, orange – the fruit, dried peel and essential oil – has traditionally been used to treat disorders of the

In Greek mythology, Hera's orchard, a garden of golden apple trees (thought to be oranges) was tended by nymphs called the Hesperides.

ANTIDEPRESSANT ALTERNATIVE?

A research study has shown that citrus essential oils – orange, lemon and bergamot, in particular – have antidepressant effects. In the study, depressed patients who inhaled one of these citrus essential oils each morning needed markedly fewer antidepressant drugs than those who did not. The results suggest that these citrus essential oils may help to improve homoeostatic balance in humans, and are therefore of psychological and physical benefit to both emotional health and the immune system.

respiratory system, such as bronchitis, colds and flu. Use it in an inhalation, compress or massage blend for chest and neck to clear congestion and counter a ticklish cough.

Its mildly tonic and stimulating effect makes it a helpful oil in skincare blends for oily or combination skins, as well as for soothing tiredness and insomnia, either in a bath oil or a massage blend.

Orange also appears to have a nourishing, balancing and harmonising effect on the stomach and intestines, and is recommended in a massage blend for the stomach to treat indigestion, constipation, muscular spasms or cramps, colic in children and nervous diarrhoea.

MIND & MOOD

Like neroli, orange essential oil has a warming, nurturing, comforting effect on your mood and psyche. Try it in an inhalation for nervous tension and stress-related disorders, and as an antidote to exhaustion, apathy and hopelessness.

During the dark winter months, use it in a vaporiser – it will help to alleviate sadness and boredom, and create enthusiasm, energy and a bright, uplifting mood.

CAUTIONS Generally regarded as non-irritant and non-sensitising, but may cause dermatitis in some people who are sensitive to citrus. May be phototoxic, so avoid exposure to sunlight after application. Use within six months of opening.

Patchouli

Pogostemon cablin

This perennial herb has hairy stems bearing large, furry, rounded leaves and pale white and mauve flowers. In its native habitats of Malaysia, China and India, where it has a long history of use as a medicine and perfume, it is known for scenting linen and clothing.

KEY PROPERTIES • Analgesic • antidepressant • anti-infective • aphrodisiac • decongestant • deodorant • insecticidal

PROFILE

It is the leaves of the patchouli herb that provide the essential oil with its distinctive, familiar and earthy scent: every leaf is covered with tiny hairs, each of which is covered with minute droplets of dark amber-brown oil. The leaves are dried and fermented before the oil is extracted by steam distillation. Patchouli has a pungent, deep, penetrating, sweet and rich aroma, with musky, spicy, smoky overtones. Compared with most other essential oils, it is quite thick and viscous.

Patchouli blends well with citrus essences, particularly bergamot and lemon, as well as clean, sharp scents, such as lavender and petitgrain, and spicy types, such as cedarwood and clary sage.

APPLICATIONS & EFFECTS

Patchouli's overall effect is warming, grounding, stimulating, strengthening and enriching. It is also particularly

Indian cashmere shawls were fashionable in Victorian England and, because they were shipped in patchouli leaves to protect them from moths, the scent also became popular.

long-lasting and is thought to improve with age, unlike most other essential oils, explaining its use as a fixative and masking agent in the soap and perfume industry.

One of patchouli's constituents, eugenol – also found in clove – has strong analgesic and anti-infective properties, while another consituent, patchoulene, is said to be similar in structure and effect to azulene, a key anti-inflammatory complement of chamomile essential oil.

Patchouli has been used in traditional Asian medicine for treating a wide variety of ailments, from colds, headaches and nausea to diarrhoea, indigestion and halitosis, even snakebites and scorpion stings. It has also been traditionally used as a household insect repellent and antiseptic, and as a perfume.

Patchouli essential oil is appropriate for inclusion in skin- and haircare remedies, especially those for over-oily scalp and skin conditions, such as pimples and open pores, and for hydrating, renewing and nourishing mature, dry,

wrinkled or fragile skin. Its anti-inflammatory, cell regenerative and antiseptic properties make it valuable in preparations for treating acne, athlete's foot, cracked or chapped skin, dermatitis, some allergies, and minor sores and infections.

MIND & MOOD

Patchouli essential oil has a reputation as an aphrodisiac, so it may be helpful in a vaporiser blend for both soothing nervous conditions and boosting sexual energy, by countering sexual fears, emotional coldness, listlessness, over-sensitivity or conflict, and also by strengthening the connection between the mind, body and spirit.

CAUTIONS Generally regarded as non-irritant and non-sensitising. Use patchouli essential oil in moderation, as its penetrating aroma may cause headache in some sensitive individuals.

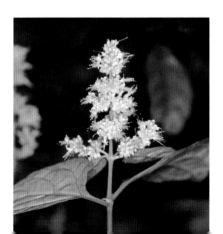

Peppermint

Mentha x piperita

A perennial herb with dark green leaves and small purple flowers, peppermint has been cultivated for centuries – the ancient Egyptians and Romans wrote of peppermint's healing prowess and its use as a culinary flavouring and household insect repellent.

KEY PROPERTIES ● Analgesic ● anti-inflammatory ● antispasmodic ● decongestant ● digestive ● expectorant ● vasoconstrictor

MULTICULTURAL MINT

Peppermint is arguably one of the best travelled culinary herbs. Its refreshing flavour complements a wide variety of ingredients, and it is used in many famous dishes – from Greece's yogurt and cucumber salad and Turkey's lamb and mint koftas to India's sweet teas, pilafs and raitas and Thailand's mint-laced stir-fries.

PROFILE

Peppermint essential oil is obtained via steam distillation from the flowering tops of the plant. Pale yellow to yellow-green with a very fresh, penetrating and minty aroma, with sweet and camphoraceous overtones, the overall effect of peppermint essential oil is stimulating, cooling and revitalising.

This refreshing essential oil has a long history of use in pharmaceutical products, particularly as an ingredient in cough and cold mixtures, as a flavouring for beverages and tobacco, confectionery such as chewing gum, and as a perfume for soap, toothpaste and detergent.

Peppermint was once used in smelling salts, as its stimulating scent helped to relieve nausea and counter the effects of shock.

The main active ingredient of peppermint essential oil, menthol, blends well with other sharp-scented essential oils, such as eucalyptus and lemon, as well as floral spicy types, such as rose, clary sage and marjoram.

APPLICATIONS & EFFECTS

Peppermint essential oil has many useful applications. First, it is a remedy for the digestive system – include it in massage blends for colic, cramps, indigestion, irritable bowel syndrome, flatulence and nausea – and also for respiratory ailments, making it a valuable addition to compresses, steam inhalations and chest or throat rubs for asthma, bronchitis, sinusitis, coughs (especially of a spasmodic nature) and colds.

Compresses and baths containing a few drops of peppermint oil have a pronounced cooling effect on feverish and inflamed conditions; at the same time, peppermint induces sweating, which helps to reduce fever. Other therapeutic uses for a massage blend containing peppermint essential oil include bruises, muscular aches, period pain, migraine and neuralgia.

Adding a few drops to a gargle recipe (do not swallow) makes an effective treatment for bad breath and may help to speed healing of mouth ulcers and oral thrush. A facial steam containing 1–2 drops of peppermint essential oil benefits oily or congested skin, especially acne, due to its anti-bacterial and antiseptic properties.

MIND & MOOD

This essential oil is thought to create clarity, vitality and focus – burn it to boost self-confidence, release toxic emotions or other people's negative attitudes or comments, and increase physical and mental energy. Inhalations can help treat lethargy, mental fatigue, nervous stress and depression: just place a few drops on a tissue and breathe in for a head-clearing effect.

CAUTIONS This oil promotes menstruation, so avoid during pregnancy and lactation. It causes alertness, so avoid using it at night. Use in low concentration, as it may irritate skin, especially sensitive types. Do not use it with homoeopathic remedies, as it will cancel their effect, or store it near them.

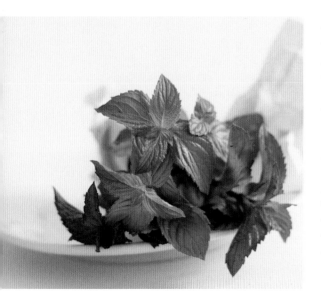

Pine

Pinus sylvestris

Also known as the Scotch, Scots, Norway or Norwegian pine, this tall evergreen conifer has red-brown, deeply grooved bark, long needles and oval brown cones. The only pine tree native to Northern Europe, it is also a popular choice in the United States for Christmas trees.

KEY PROPERTIES ● Antiseptic ● antispasmodic ● astringent ● decongestant ● expectorant ● stimulant ● vasoconstrictor

The famed Arabian physician and philosopher Avicenna prescribed inhalations and compresses of pine for patients with chest infections.

PROFILE

Pine essential oil is produced via steam distillation of the needles; an inferior grade of oil is also made from the twigs, cones, bark and wood, but this is not considered suitable for aromatherapy.

The essential oil is clear to very pale yellow in colour, and has a strong, balsamic, resinous aroma, with camphoraceous, turpentine-like overtones. Its overall aroma effect is cooling, invigorating and refreshing.

Pine essential oil blends well with rich, spicy aromas, such as cedarwood and frankincense, as well as other clean, stimulating scents, such as tea tree, lavender, rosemary, eucalyptus and lemon.

APPLICATIONS & EFFECTS

Much used commercially in warming creams and liniments for treating and preventing sporting injuries, poor circulation, neuralgia, sciatica, muscular stiffness and soreness, as well as the aches and pains of arthritis, gout and rheumatism, it is recommended in home aromatherapy recipes for the same purposes.

Pine's head-clearing aroma and powerful expectorant, fever-reducing and antiseptic effects make it valuable in inhalations or chest rub remedies for coughs, colds, flu, asthma, bronchitis, catarrh, laryngitis, sinusitis and

A VERSATILE SCENT

Native Americans once burned pine needles in 'sweat lodges', as they were thought to clear the mind and strengthen the spirit before battle. In Japan, the aroma of pine is synonymous with bathing and relaxation, because the tubs that are used for communal bathing are usually made from pine wood. These days, in the United States, Europe and Australia, pine is widely used as a fragrance in household cleaners, soaps, air fresheners and detergents.

a sore throat. Its brisk fragrance and ability to counter excessive perspiration and odour makes it a natural fit for aftershave or men's cologne recipes, bath blends, room fresheners, deodorant powders or sprays.

It can also be used for its insect-repellent and antifungal effects in treatments for lice and athlete's foot.

MIND & MOOD

Pine essential oil may have an antidepressant effect. Try using it in an inhalation to stimulate the brain, aid clear thinking, and ease fatigue and nervous exhaustion.

Pine is also considered to remove negative energy and promote focus and perseverance. Add it to a burner

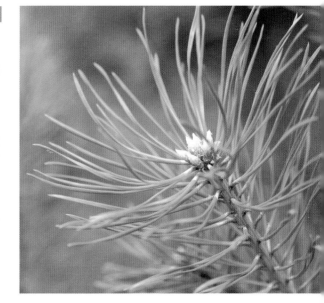

to create a bracing atmosphere when you feel listless or lethargic and want to overcome apathy or depression due to stale memories, envy or bitterness, or when you need to get started on a new project.

CAUTIONS Generally regarded as non-irritant, but may cause sensitisation in some people. Use in low concentrations; do not use on damaged, allergy-prone or fragile skin. Patch-test first. Do not confuse with other pine oils, such as dwarf pine (*Pinus pumilio*), which are classified as hazardous.

Rose

Rosa centifolia, Rosa damascena

Records indicate that the famed Arab doctor and alchemist Avicenna created rose essential oil, possibly by accident, in tenth-century Persia. Since then, the rose has enjoyed great significance as an ingredient in health, household, cosmetic, religious and culinary preparations.

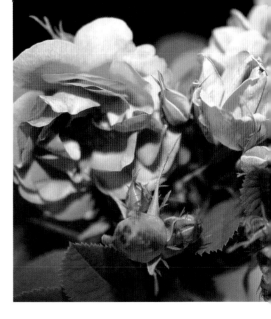

KEY PROPERTIES ● Antidepressant ● anti-inflammatory ● antispasmodic ● astringent ● sedative ● tonic (heart, liver, stomach, uterus)

PROFILE

Two main varieties of cultivated rose are used for the extraction of essential oil – the cabbage or maroc rose (*Rosa centifolia*), which grows to 2.5 m, with numerous pale pink or pink-purple musky-scented flowers, and the smaller damask rose (*Rosa damascena*), with its deep pink, honey-scented flowers, which grows to between 1 and 2 m.

There are two main types of rose essential oil – rose otto, which is made via steam distillation of the fresh petals, most often from the damask rose, and rose absolute, made by solvent extraction of the fresh petals, usually from the cabbage rose.

Both oils are suitable for use in aromatherapy, although the otto is considered superior. However, producing it is highly labour-intensive: it takes hundreds of blossoms to make a tiny amount of this expensive oil.

Rose otto is pale yellow in colour with a beautiful rich, sweet, mellow aroma, with overtones of vanilla and spice. Rose absolute is usually a darker yellow-orange in colour with a similar deep, sweet aroma.

The overall effect of both oils is sensual and nurturing; reputed to be aphrodisiacs, both contain more than 300 constituents. Rose essential oil blends well with other floral essential oils, as well as citrus and spice types.

The rose has traditionally been called the 'queen of the flowers', and is associated with Venus, the goddess of love and beauty.

SOOTHING SCENT

According to Japanese research, rose essential oil demonstrates a powerful 'anti-conflict' effect, comparable to that achieved with the use of benzo-diazepine drugs, but without the side effects. Although this experiment was conducted on animals, the researchers concluded that it was reasonable to expect the same effects – of easing mental and emotional conflict and stress – in humans.

APPLICATIONS & EFFECTS

Much loved for its feminine fragrance, rose essential oil may be included in all manner of facial, body and bath treatments; it is particularly recommended for thread veins, eczema, acne, dandruff, scarring, wrinkles and dryness, and for mature, sensitive or fragile skin in need of rejuvenation.

Its hormone-balancing qualities make it very effective in treating disorders of the female reproductive system, such as period pain, heavy periods, irregular menstruation, pre-menstrual syndrome (PMS), lowered libido and post-natal depression, as well as genito-urinary, digestive, musculo-skeletal and circulatory problems, such as palpitations.

MIND & MOOD

The oil's physical effects may be less important than its ability to support the spirit and heal the emotions. As well as easing nervous tension, headaches, depression, insomnia and other stress-related disorders, it is thought to heal the 'inner child' and encourage the expression of love and enjoyment of sensuality. Use it in a massage blend to counter grief, sadness, apathy, envy, vulnerability, sexual fears, self-image problems and shyness.

CAUTIONS Generally regarded as being non-irritant and non-sensitising; however, the absolute form may irritate sensitive skin, so patch-test first. Avoid during the first two trimesters of pregnancy.

Rosemary

Rosmarinus officinalis

In the Middle Ages, the 'herb of remembrance' was burned to counter the plague – it would at least have repelled disease-carrying fleas. For many centuries it continued to be burnt in sickrooms as a fumigant – until the twentieth century it was burnt in French hospital wards.

KEY PROPERTIES ● Analgesic ● antiseptic ● antispasmodic ● astringent ● decongestant ● stimulant (circulation, adrenal cortex) ● tonic (liver, skin, nervine, digestion)

PROFILE

Rosemary essential oil is obtained via steam distillation of the flowering tops and stems of the herb; oil may also be made by distilling the entire plant, but this is regarded as being of inferior quality for aromatherapy.

Rosemary essential oil is colourless to pale yellow with a strong, fresh, herbal, camphoraceous aroma with woody, balsamic overtones. Its overall effect is invigorating, refreshing and strengthening, and it blends well with other herbal and spicy scents, including basil, pine, citronella, cedarwood, oregano, thyme and coriander as well as citrus oils, especially orange.

APPLICATIONS & EFFECTS

Rosemary essential oil has a long history of use as a medicine, especially for respiratory and muscular complaints, and, being strongly antiseptic, as a fumigant and pest repellent. In the days before refrigeration, it was used to wrap meat to prevent it from rotting, and was also burned in hospitals to counter infection and deter fleas and flies, and in religious rituals, such as exorcisms.

Its stimulating and warming properties make it a useful ingredient in body and bath treatments for ailments of the musculoskeletal and circulatory systems, including varicose veins, arteriosclerosis, muscular aches,

> *Rosemary is said to have once had white flowers; they turned blue when the Virgin Mary hung her cloak on a rosemary bush as she rested.*

pains or weakness, sprains and strains, rheumatism, arthritis, period pain, headache, cramps, fluid retention, swelling, gout, backache and poor circulation. Use it in a massage blend before exercise to stimulate your circulation and so prevent injury.

Traditionally, rosemary essential oil has been used for its effect on the central nervous system and the brain. The whole herb is an excellent tonic for the digestion, liver and gall bladder; similarly, a massage blend containing rosemary essential oil may benefit indigestion, constipation, poor appetite and flatulence.

Rosemary's head-clearing quality makes it helpful for many respiratory problems, including asthma, colds, flu, bronchitis, tonsillitis and sinusitis; it also has beauty tonic benefits, especially for oily skin, acne or pimples, oily hair, dandruff and hair loss, and in various toiletry recipes.

MIND & MOOD

On a psycho-emotional level, rosemary essential oil is thought to awaken the spirit, clarify problems and strengthen conviction – burn or inhale it to find purpose and enthusiasm.

Inhalations are valuable for apathy, debility, fatigue, amnesia, lethargy, depression, exhaustion, nervous tension, mental sluggishness and problems with both concentration and memory.

CAUTIONS Avoid during pregnancy, or if you have a history of high blood pressure or epilepsy. Do not use on damaged or sensitive skin. May irritate sensitive skin.

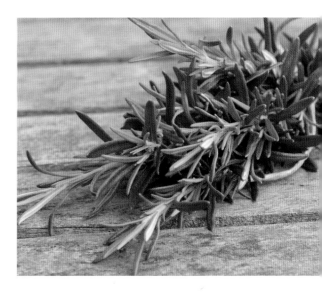

Sandalwood

Santalum album, Santalum spicatum

Traditionally, sandalwood comes from a small evergreen, semi-parasitic tree native to India, but this variety has been over-forested, jeopardising its supply of essential oil. Australian sandalwood, the *spicatum* species, has a similar perfume, effects and chemical composition.

....

KEY PROPERTIES ● Antibacterial ● antidepressant ● anti-inflammatory ● antiseptic (urinary and pulmonary) ● astringent ● diuretic ● sedative

Sandalwood incense is traditionally used in meditation to open the 'third eye' and encourage spiritual connection.

PROFILE

Sandalwood essential oil is extracted via steam distillation from the dried roots and heartwood of the tree. Pale yellow to green-brown in colour, it has an exotic, strong, soft, deep aroma, with woody, sweet and balsamic overtones. Its overall aroma effect is warming, comforting, nurturing and enticing. Sandalwood's aroma develops on the skin, and the scent clings to fabric for a long time.

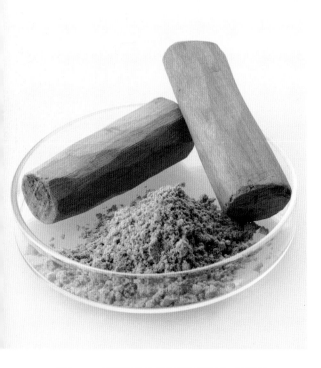

POWERFUL PROTECTION

● *This oil has been shown to have a potent antimicrobial effect against antibiotic-resistant infections such as* Staphylococcus aureus, *which may be acquired in hospitals.*
● *Another study found sandalwood has significant anti-larval activity, suggesting it may have potential in ensuring water safety in areas where mosquito infestation is a problem.*

APPLICATIONS & EFFECTS

One of the oldest known fragrances, sandalwood has been used in Asia and India for centuries as an incense, cosmetic, perfume and embalming material. Its ability to repel insects and pests once made it a popular material in buildings and furniture. It has also been a key ingredient in Ayurveda, India's traditional medical system, where it has been prescribed for stomach ache, urinary tract infections, skin problems and sexual conditions.

More recently, it has been used as a fixative in commercial skincare manufacture and perfumery, especially in oriental-style fragrances and men's products. It blends well with floral essential oils, such as rose and jasmine; with other spicy scents, such as black pepper; and with sharper fragrances, such as juniper and pine.

Use sandalwood essential oil in inhalations, compresses or chest rubs to ease respiratory problems, such as bronchitis, asthma, catarrh, coughs, laryngitis and a sore throat.

Sandalwood's soothing antibacterial properties make it useful in treatments for oily skin, rashes, acne, itching, eczema, dry, cracked or chapped skin, and as an aftershave, as well as in a sitz bath to relieve the sting of cystitis.

It is particularly recommended for regenerating and nourishing dry, mature or fragile skin, and in massage blends to ease backache or relieve the bloating and teariness of premenstrual syndrome (PMS).

MIND & MOOD

This essential oil is said to help ground emotions and create an atmosphere of comfort and tranquillity, making it suitable for vaporiser, inhalation or massage blends to be used in times of irritability and apprehension, as well as for helping with insomnia, mood swings, depression, nausea and other stress-related disorders.

CAUTIONS Generally regarded as being non-irritant and non-sensitising; however, may cause contact dermatitis in some sensitive individuals. Always use diluted, and patch-test first.

Tea tree

Melaleuca alternifolia

This small, shrubby tree with needle-like leaves and tiny yellow or mauve flowers is native to Australia. Like eucalyptus and clove, which belong to the same plant family, it is a powerful infection fighter and immune-system booster.

KEY PROPERTIES • Antibiotic • antifungal • antiparasitic • antiseptic • antiviral • expectorant • immunostimulant

Tea tree was so named because Captain Cook observed Australian Aboriginals brewing the leaves with water to make a medicinal tea.

PROFILE

Tea tree essential oil is obtained via steam distillation from the plant's leaves and twigs. Pale yellow, sometimes with a slight green tinge, it has a sharp, medicinal, camphoraceous aroma, with spicy, piney, woody and lemony overtones. Its overall aroma effect is invigorating, cooling and cleansing. A very useful essential oil for the home first-aid kit, tea tree blends well with other head-clearing essential oils, such as eucalyptus, pine and rosemary; citrus scents, such as lemon; floral fragrances, notably lavender, clary sage and geranium; and spicy scents, such as clove.

APPLICATIONS & EFFECTS

Tea tree essential oil has a very wide range of uses. It may be used in compresses, baths or skin treatment blends for all manner of minor skin disorders and infections, including abscesses, boils, warts, acne, cold sores, athlete's foot, sunburn, smelly feet, dandruff, abrasions, insect bites, cuts, fungal nail infections, jock itch, oily skin, pimples and rashes.

Tea tree essential oil is also an effective treatment for viral and bacterial infections of the respiratory system, such as colds, flu, asthma, bronchitis, catarrh, coughs and sinusitis, as well as other infectious diseases, such as chickenpox.

THE BUG BUSTER

Clinical research studies demonstrate that tea tree essential oil dramatically reduces both the count and effect of airborne bacteria. One study showed that tea tree essential oil was effective against methicillin-resistant Staphylococcus aureus *both on the skin and in the atmosphere. In another study, tea tree-based body wash and nasal ointment were found to perform better than conventional triclosan-based products.*

Add tea tree essential oil to a bath or massage blend to stimulate sweating and reduce fever, which helps the body to fight the infection, or use it in an inhalation or vaporiser. Diluted and used in a sitz bath, it is helpful for minor bacterial and fungal genito-urinary infections, such as cystitis, thrush, pruritis and vaginitis.

Tea tree makes an excellent household antiseptic – to counter dust mites, add a few drops to the final rinse water when laundering bed linen, and also use it in a room spray to kill airborne bacteria and repel mosquitoes.

MIND & MOOD

With a bracing effect on both the emotions and the body, this oil is a good choice for vaporiser or massage blends to stimulate thought, improve self-confidence and enhance mental clarity. Use it to restore focus and boost energy following a shock or debilitating experience.

CAUTIONS Generally regarded as non-irritating; however, may cause skin reactions in sensitive or allergy-prone individuals, so always use diluted, and patch-test first.

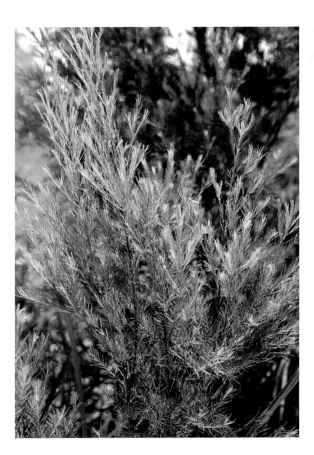

Thyme, sweet

Thymus vulgaris

Sweet thyme, also known as garden thyme, is a small, perennial herb with strongly aromatic grey-green leaves and tiny pink or white flowers. Originally native to the Mediterranean, it has been recognised and used as a medicinal plant for many centuries.

KEY PROPERTIES ● Antioxidant ● antiseptic ● antispasmodic ● antitussive ● aperitif ● disinfectant (pulmonary) ● stimulant (digestion, circulation, immune system, nervous system)

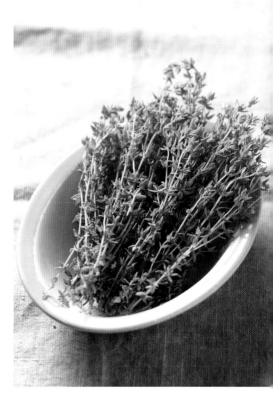

PROFILE

Thyme essential oil is derived via steam distillation from the leaves and flowering tops of the plant. Usually pale yellow in colour, it has a strong, sweet, herbaceous aroma with fresh green overtones; its overall aroma effect is warming, stimulating and gentle. It blends well with light, fresh aromas, such as lavender, lemon and bergamot, as well as sharper scents such as pine and eucalyptus, and herbal ones such as rosemary and marjoram.

APPLICATIONS & EFFECTS

Thyme has a long history of use in cooking and, like many essential oils made from culinary herbs that were once used to preserve food as well as flavour it, it has significant antibacterial effects, as well as particular applications in digestive disorders, such as in a warming massage blend for indigestion or diarrhoea.

This strongly germicidal essential oil is a good immune stimulant, making it an excellent choice for home aromatherapy treatments for asthma, bronchitis, catarrh, bad breath, sore throat, coughs, colds, laryngitis, flu, sinusitis and mouth and gum infections. Try it in a chest rub or inhalation to ease congestion, support the body during illness and relieve fatigue during recovery.

TAKE YOUR THYME

Research indicates that resveratrol, a key component of red wine, interferes with the action of the COX-2 enzyme, which is linked to cancer and heart disease. But those who don't like red wine may one day be able to achieve a similar effect with treatment based on thyme essential oil. Japanese scientists have found that thyme essential oil has the ability to reduce COX-2 activity in cells by nearly 75%.

A Greek study suggests that thyme essential oil may destroy Staphylococcus *bacteria, which is super-resistant to antibiotics.*

Thyme essential oil also boosts circulation and has a mild hypertensive effect, so it elevates blood pressure slightly and also stimulates appetite – two qualities that make it particularly beneficial in cases of post-viral fatigue, lethargy, nervous exhaustion, general debility and depression.

Use thyme essential oil in topical remedies for cystitis and urethritis, and for skin disorders, including acne, abscesses, burns, bites and stings. Its insecticidal properties make it a helpful ingredient in hair-care preparations for repelling lice as well as household sprays and potpourris to keep pests such as moths and mosquitoes at bay.

MIND & MOOD

From a psycho-emotional perspective, thyme essential oil is considered soothing to the mind and spirit; use it in inhalations or a vaporiser blend to help build vitality, support healing, create a feeling or atmosphere of freedom and movement, and to restore balance and focus.

CAUTIONS Avoid during pregnancy, or if you have high blood pressure. Generally non-irritant. Red thyme or wild thyme essential oils are not recommended for aromatherapeutic use. Always purchase thyme oil made from the linalol chemotype.

Ylang ylang

Cananga odorata

The ylang ylang tree grows widely in the Philippines, Indonesia and Madagascar, where much of the oil is produced. Its graceful arching branches bear beautiful, highly scented flowers in pink, mauve and yellow, so it's not surprising that it's widely regarded as an aphrodisiac.

KEY PROPERTIES ● Antidepressant ● antiseptic ● aphrodisiac ● euphoric ● hypotensive ● sedative ● stimulant (circulation)

Ylang ylang's exotic name — pronounced ee-lang ee-lang — means 'flower of flowers'.

PROFILE

Ylang ylang essential oil is made via steam distillation from the flowers. There are several different grades, with 'ylang ylang extra' (which is collected first) considered the superior grade for perfumery and aromatherapy.

The pale yellow oil has an intensely sweet, rich, floral, heady aroma and slightly spicy, musky overtones. It has a long history of use in cosmetics, especially in high-quality fragrances, and its overall aroma effect is sensual, soothing, warming, exotic and intoxicating.

Ylang ylang's aroma blends well with floral fragrances, such as rose, geranium and jasmine; with citrusy oils, such as neroli, bergamot and orange; and with spicy, piquant scents, especially black pepper, rosewood and frankincense.

A VICTORIAN FAVOURITE

A popular perfume in the Victorian era, ylang ylang was a key ingredient in Macassar oil, a men's hair tonic that helped achieve smooth hairstyles but also left stains on chair- and sofa-backs. So it became fashionable to protect the fabric with lace-trimmed cloths, hence these doily-like mats became known as 'antimacassars'. Today you'll find the non-perfumed disposable version on aircraft seats.

APPLICATIONS & EFFECTS

Ylang ylang essential oil has a pronounced effect on the respiratory and circulatory systems, and it has also been shown to lower blood pressure as well as slow down the breathing rate and reduce a too-rapid heartbeat.

The essential oil is also excellent for both dry and oily skin types, as it has a regulatory, balancing and toning effect on the secretion of sebum; it also eases skin irritation and redness, so it is useful in treatments for acne, bites and fever.

MIND & MOOD

Use ylang ylang in aromatherapy treatments for palpitations, shock, fear, anger and insomnia. It also lifts the spirit, helping to create an atmosphere of creativity, sensuality and warmth. Use it in an inhalation or burner to counter feeling withdrawn, guilty, rigid or emotionally cold.

It is also recommended for premenstrual syndrome (PMS) and stress-related disorders, including anxiety, depression and nervous tension. Ylang ylang's calming, antidepressant and aphrodisiac qualities can help to overcome frigidity and impotence, especially when they are caused by poor self-image, jangled nerves or fears of sexual inadequacy.

CAUTIONS Avoid if you have a history of low blood pressure or sleep apnoea, as it has sedative and hypotensive effects. May cause headache and nausea in some people. Generally safe, but may irritate some sensitive people; use in dilution and patch-test first.

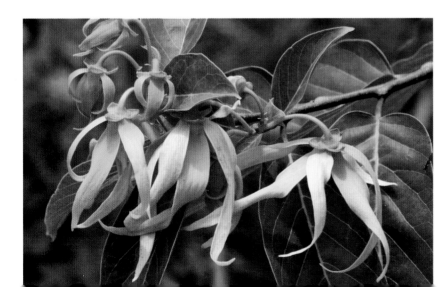

Carrier oils

Natural base oils are used to 'carry' and apply essential oils to the body and, being rich in nourishing essential fatty acids, vitamin E, proteins, antioxidants to slow ageing, and other valuable nutrients, they offer considerable benefit to your skin and hair.

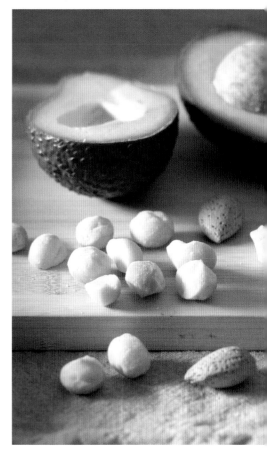

TYPES OF CARRIER OILS

Carrier oils usually have little or no aroma, and should, in most cases, be cold-pressed and unrefined. A refined oil, in contrast, may have been extracted via extreme heat and possibly chemical solvents, and may contain artificial colouring and deodorising agents, while mineral ('baby') oil is derived from petroleum.

Here is a list of the most important carrier oils and their characteristics, but you could also use safflower, borage, coconut, sesame and sunflower oils.

Almond oil (*Prunus amygdalus*)
This light-textured, pale yellow carrier oil has a mild nutty aroma and a slightly sticky, slippery feel, which makes it a great choice in massage blends for face and body. Also known as sweet almond oil, it is very soothing and nourishing and contains linoleic acid (LA) and vitamin E, which are helpful for itchy, dry or cracked skin.

Apricot kernel oil (*Prunus armeniaca*)
Fine-textured apricot kernel oil is rich in the free radical-fighting antioxidants, vitamin E and A, as well as a rejuvenating fatty acid called oleic acid. Healing as well as calming and soothing, it is helpful for delicate, dry, sensitive and irritated skin.

Avocado oil (*Persea americana*)
This lushly textured green oil is not only rich in essential fatty acids but also contains generous amounts of vitamins E and D, beta-carotene and linoleic acid (LA), which supports the health of cell membranes. With its excellent penetration and deeply moisturising effects, avocado oil is good for all skin types, but especially for dry, damaged, under-nourished and ageing skin.

Evening primrose oil (*Oenothera biennis*)
This light golden oil is excellent in nourishing aromatherapy blends to restore suppleness, speed cellular renewal, hydrate skin and help heal psoriasis and eczema.

Grapeseed oil (*Vitis vinifera*)
Pale green grapeseed oil is very light-textured and easily absorbed by the skin. Almost completely odourless, it is suitable for all skin types.

Jojoba (*Simmondsia chinensis*)
Traditionally used as a skin treatment, jojoba is a delicate, non-greasy liquid wax that is good for all skin types, especially where smoothing rough-ness, deep cleansing and moisturising or the regulation of sebum production are required.

Macadamia nut oil (*Macadamia integrifolia*)
A fine-textured, clear golden oil, this contains palmitoleic acid, an essential fatty acid found naturally in sebum, so it not only has a natural affinity with the skin but is also highly moisturising, emollient and softening.

Olive oil (*Olea europaea*)
The yellow-gold 'virgin' olive oil, made from the second pressing of the hard, unripe fruit of the olive tree, is most suitable for home aromatherapy use, but both the 'virgin' and 'extra virgin' forms have a pronounced fruity aroma and also contain the skin-nourishing essential fatty acid, alpha linolenic acid, or ALA.

Rosehip oil (*Rosa rubiginosa*)
This rich orange-red oil contains essential fatty acids, antioxidants and retinoic acid, which all help to maintain the health of cell membranes and also to regenerate and rejuvenate skin tissue, making it useful for reducing scarring, stretch marks, wrinkles and pigmentation; soothing sunburn; and improving skin elasticity.

Sunflower oil (*Helianthus annuus*)
Soothing, with a mild nutty aroma, this light-textured oil ranges from a light yellow to gold in colour and

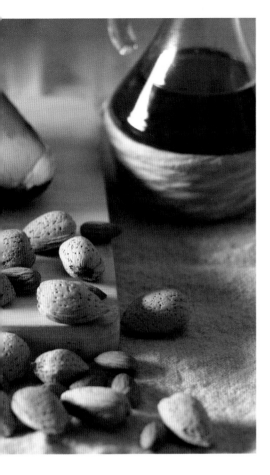

Don't confuse sesame oil with the pungent, dark brown culinary oil, which is made from the toasted seeds.

contains skin-enhancing lecithin, vitamin E and omega-6 fatty acids. Suitable for all skin types, it is an excellent carrier oil.

Wheatgerm oil *(Triticum vulgare)*
This thick yellow-orange oil, with its strong aroma, is not suitable as a sole carrier oil, but you can add a small amount to massage blends to enhance penetration and skin repair and conditioning. Its high content of vitamins A, E and D is thought to extend the shelf life of oil blends. Wheatgerm oil is suitable for all skin types, especially for healing burns, scars and stretch marks.

BLENDING OILS
As essential oils are very potent, you must always dilute them before using them in aromatherapy recipes. In this book, most of the blends for topical application have been made up in a ratio of 10 drops to 20–30 ml (about 2–3 tablespoons) of carrier oil, the amount required for a full body

massage for an average-sized person, or for 3–4 applications on a particular area, such as the shoulders.

For facial blends, or for anyone with sensitive or damaged skin, halve this ratio to about 5 drops per 20 ml (2 tablespoons). Most of our topical recipes blend 3–6 essential oils with 1–2 carrier oils (or with another base, such as salt, cream or aloe vera gel), with the aim of producing a fragrance that smells attractive and provides the maximum therapeutic benefits.

Make up small amounts of blends at a time, as both the essential and carrier oils will start to oxidise on contact with the air. An essential oil blend should last for up to six weeks at room temperature, or three months in the refrigerator.

Try adding a little wheatgerm or vitamin E oil to blends, as they act as mild natural preservatives.

STORING CARRIER OILS
Keep unblended carrier oils in dark glass bottles in a cool, dark place away from heat and moisture. Check the use-by date on the labels as a guide to how long they will last. Unblended carrier oils usually last up to nine months at a very cool temperature (about 10°C). You can also store carrier oils in a refrigerator, although some will solidify.

CAUTIONS Always patch-test a recipe blend before using it. See the cautions for pregnant women on page 14.

MAKING YOUR OWN BLEND

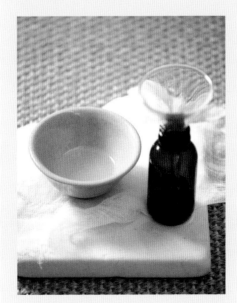

1 Carefully measure 20–30 ml (2–3 tablespoons) of your carrier oil, such as almond oil, and pour it into a small bowl.

2 Add up to 10 drops of your chosen essential oil, one drop at a time. Warm a little in your hands, and test the fragrance.

3 Use a small kitchen funnel to pour it into a small, dark glass bottle, available from essential oil suppliers and pharmacies.

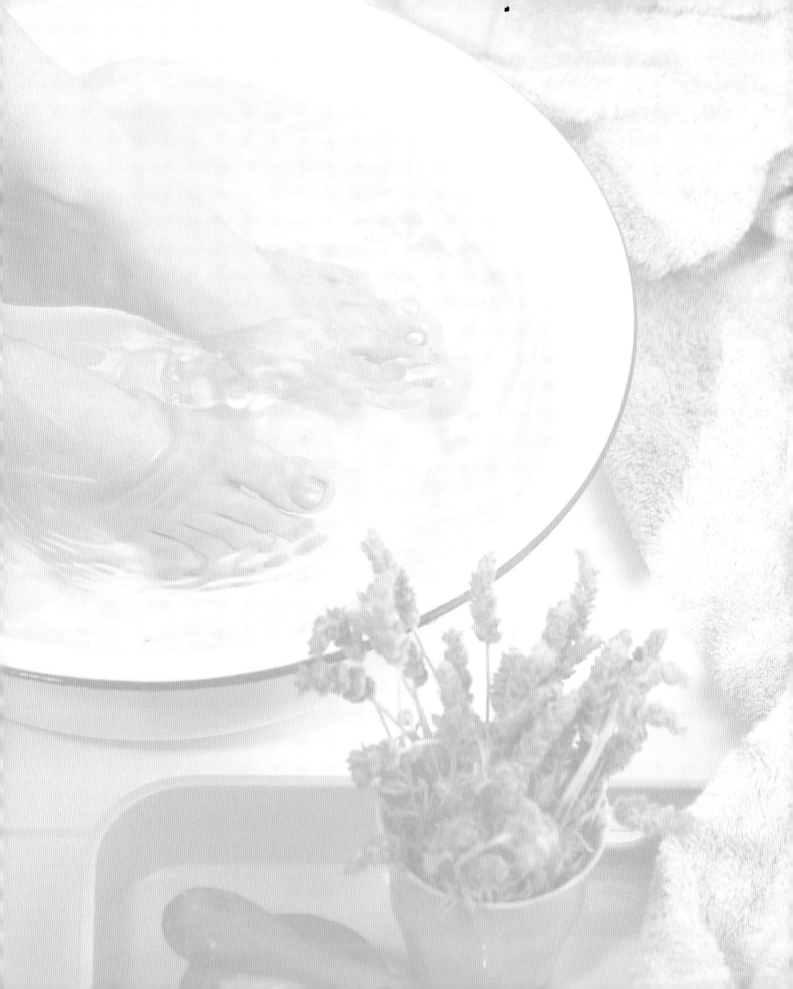

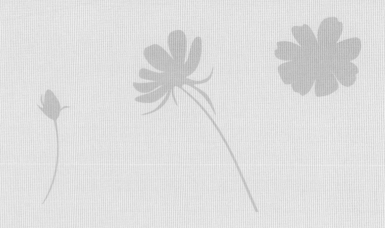

Aromatherapy
BLENDS

Brain and nervous system

Aromatherapy is one of the gentlest yet most effective self-help treatments for problems associated with the brain and nervous system, helping to support, strengthen and relax as well as increase alertness and concentration.

Computer eye strain

If computer eye strain triggers headaches, keep a small jar of this headache balm handy.

3 drops lavender essential oil
3 drops peppermint essential oil
3 drops geranium essential oil
1 drop eucalyptus essential oil
3 tablespoons unscented base cream or sweet almond oil

1 Combine the essential oils with the base cream or sweet almond oil, and store in a small glass jar or pot.
2 To use, massage lightly into the temples and back of the neck.

Headache

The hot water in this footbath dilates blood vessels, increasing blood flow to your feet and drawing it away from your head, while the cold compress constricts blood vessels in your head.

3 drops rosemary essential oil
3 drops lemongrass essential oil
5 drops lavender essential oil

1 Soak your feet for 10 minutes in a basin of hot water mixed with the first two essential oils.
2 At the same time, hold a compress dipped in 125 ml (½ cup) of ice-cold water mixed with 5 drops lavender essential oil to your forehead.

MIGRAINE

Next time you have a migraine, try treating the intense pain with one of these aromatherapy blends.

● Soak a face washer in 125 ml (½ cup) of cool water mixed with 3 drops each of lavender and peppermint essential oils. Wring it out and place it across your forehead and temples. Change it frequently as the face washer warms up.

● Mix 5 drops of lavender essential oil with 1 tablespoon of sweet almond oil, and use the blend to massage your temples, hairline and back of the neck lightly but firmly, as long as touching your head does not intensify the pain.

● A warm, comforting compress on the back of the neck will boost blood flow to the brain: soak a face washer in 125 ml (½ cup) of warm water to which you have added 5 drops of marjoram essential oil. Wring it out and hold on the back of the neck.

Nerve pain

Try this balm for neuralgia.

3 drops peppermint essential oil
3 drops marjoram essential oil
3 drops eucalyptus essential oil
1 drop coriander essential oil
3 tablespoons sweet almond oil

Mix together well, and massage into the affected area.

Jet lag

Essential oils with calming, mood-boosting and balancing effects may help to counter jet lag.

3 drops lavender essential oil
3 drops chamomile essential oil
3 drops neroli essential oil
¼ cup natural sea salt

1 Mix the essential oils with the natural sea salt.
2 Add the mixture to a bath filled with warm – not hot – water, and soak for 10–15 minutes.

Mental fatigue

Try a stimulating footbath to invigorate your mind and body.

3 drops pine essential oil
3 drops rosemary essential oil
3 drops lavender essential oil
1 drop clary sage essential oil
2 tablespoons Epsom salts

1 Add this mixture to a flat-bottomed pan that is large enough to fit your feet, and fill it with cold water, swishing to disperse it evenly.
2 Sit quietly for 10 minutes, soaking your feet and practising some deep breathing.

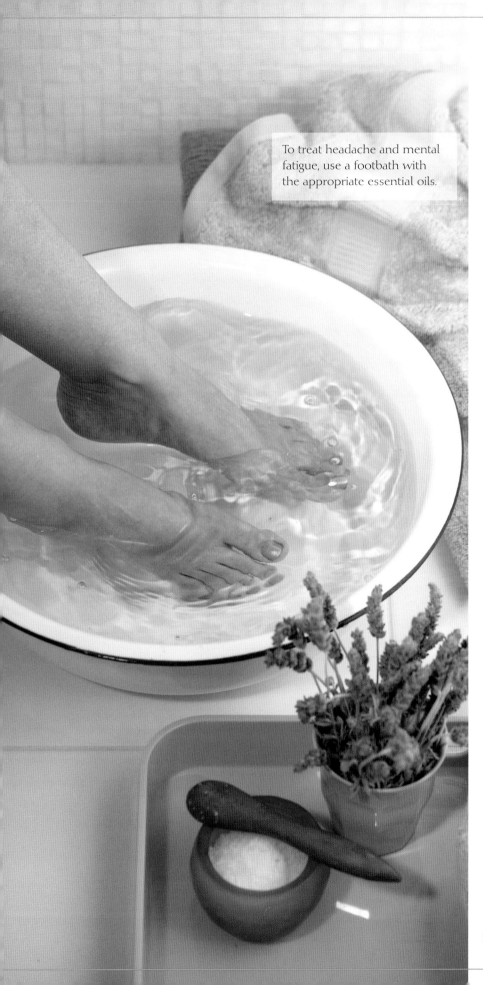

To treat headache and mental fatigue, use a footbath with the appropriate essential oils.

Poor memory

Stimulate your memory with this aromatherapy mix.

2 drops rosemary essential oil
2 drops peppermint essential oil
1 drop lemon essential oil

1 Place the essential oils in the dish of an aromatherapy burner with 3 tablespoons of water.

2 Light a tea-light candle to heat the mixture, and place it near or on your desk.

3 Alternatively, place 1 drop of each of the oils on a handkerchief or tissue, and inhale at intervals throughout the day.

What's the alternative?

Here are a couple of natural memory boosters.

• The nutritional supplement lecithin is a source of the neurotransmitter acetylcholine, vital for communicating nerve impulses to and from the brain.

• The gotu kola herb has been used by Ayurvedic doctors to improve memory, while modern research confirms that ginkgo, long used in Traditional Chinese Medicine as a brain tonic, does in fact boost the circulation of blood and oxygen to the brain.

Digestive and urinary systems

The digestive system involves not only the stomach, kidneys and colon but also the liver, gall bladder and nervous system, and your nutritional status, emotional state and immunity can all affect it.

Colitis (Crohn's disease)

This inflammatory condition is exacerbated by stress, so it may be improved by abdominal massage with a soothing aromatherapy blend.

3 drops lavender essential oil
3 drops lemon balm essential oil
3 drops chamomile essential oil
1 drop ylang ylang essential oil
3 tablespoons sweet almond oil

Mix well, and apply daily to the lower abdomen, using the palm of the hand in a clockwise motion.

Constipation

Rather than depend on laxatives, which have an irritating 'scouring' effect and, over time, can make the bowel lazy, try a warming massage oil blend to get things moving.

3 drops marjoram essential oil
3 drops rosemary essential oil
3 drops fennel essential oil
1 drop black pepper essential oil
3 tablespoons sweet almond oil

Mix well, and massage into the lower abdomen, in a clockwise direction, and also into the lower back, over the spine.

Cystitis

Sandalwood is used as a urinary antiseptic in Ayurveda, India's traditional medical system.

1 cup Epsom salts
1 cup bicarbonate of soda
5 drops sandalwood essential oil
5 drops tea tree essential oil

Fill a bathtub with comfortably warm water, then add the mix. Soak for 15–20 minutes.

What's the alternative?

Naturopaths suggest the following remedies for treating cystitis.

- Unsweetened cranberry juice helps to prevent *Escherichia coli* bacteria, which cause cystitis, from adhering to the walls of the bladder.

- Bearberry tea, a natural antiseptic and diuretic, flushes bacteria out of the body faster.

- Extra vitamin C helps fight infection by stimulating the body's immune function.

Diarrhoea

If the diarrhoea is due to anxiety or stress, try this massage blend.

3 drops lavender essential oil
3 drops chamomile essential oil
3 drops ginger essential oil
1 drop neroli essential oil
3 tablespoons sweet almond oil

Mix well, and massage gently over lower abdomen and back.

Gastric ulcer

Although this condition is caused by a bacterium, *Helicobacter pylori*, it is also associated with extreme emotional stress, poor eating habits and acid-provoking foods. An aromatherapy massage blend containing healing and relaxing essential oils may help.

3 drops chamomile essential oil
3 drops lavender essential oil
3 drops rose essential oil
1 drop marjoram essential oil
3 tablespoons sweet almond oil

Combine the oils and massage into the abdomen, paying particular attention to the upper region over the stomach.

Taking a teaspoon of herbal bitters in water before meals will improve digestion and stimulate the liver to produce bile, the body's natural laxative.

Haemorrhoid cream

This cream will help to shrink the swollen vein.

- 3 drops cypress essential oil
- 3 drops geranium essential oil
- 3 drops juniper essential oil
- 1 drop myrrh essential oil
- 3 tablespoons unscented moisturising cream or aloe vera gel

Mix well, and apply as required.

Indigestion

Try this calming compress.

- 3 drops clary sage essential oil
- 3 drops coriander essential oil
- 3 drops ginger essential oil
- 1 drop black pepper essential oil

1 Combine, and add to 125 ml (½ cup) of hot water.
2 Soak a face washer in the mixture, wring it out, and fold it over the stomach, then cover with plastic film and a heat pack.

Vomiting

If vomiting is due to a gastrointestinal infection, try this blend.

- 3 drops lavender essential oil
- 2 drops tea tree essential oil

In a burner, burn the essential oils with 2 tablespoons of water to cleanse the air.

Irritable bowel syndrome

Relieve symptoms of cramping, flatulence, bloating and alternating bouts of diarrhoea and constipation with this calming massage blend.

- 3 drops chamomile essential oil
- 3 drops lavender essential oil
- 3 drops peppermint essential oil
- 1 drop marjoram essential oil
- 3 tablespoons sweet almond oil

Mix well, and massage gently into the lower abdomen.

GINGIVITIS

If your gums are inflamed, rinse with one of these antibacterial blends after cleaning your teeth; do not swallow.

- *Combine 3 drops each of thyme, mandarin and myrrh essential oils and 1 drop of lemon essential oil with 3 tablespoons of vodka and 100 ml of warm water. Mix well.*
- *Brew 100 ml of strong, strained, red raspberry leaf tea. While it is still warm, add 1 drop of sage essential oil and 3 drops each of fennel, rosemary and thyme essential oil. Mix well.*

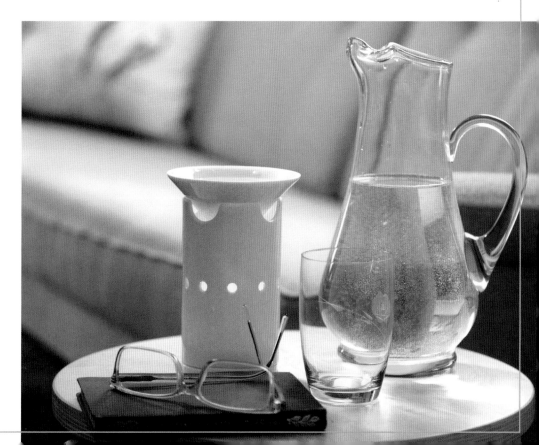

Musculoskeletal and circulatory systems

The human body is a complex engineering system that some of us rarely appreciate. The combination of massage and aromatherapy is an effective way to alleviate pain and keep muscles, bones and joints in good working order.

Arthritis

This bath blend will help shift the build-up of toxins, such as uric acid, and also improve circulation.

3 drops black pepper essential oil
3 drops marjoram essential oil
3 drops lemon essential oil
1 drop cypress essential oil

Combine, and add to a warm bath.

What's the alternative?

Naturopaths suggest these remedies for reducing the chronic pain of osteoarthritis.

- Together, glucosamine and chondroitin curb inflammation and provide the building blocks of cartilage, thus increasing the padding in joints and slowing damage over time.

- Used topically, cayenne cream is an effective pain reliever. The capsaicin in cayenne inhibits the production of substance P, a chemical involved in sending pain messages to the brain.

- Take 1 teaspoon each of apple cider vinegar and honey in a glass of hot water first thing each morning.

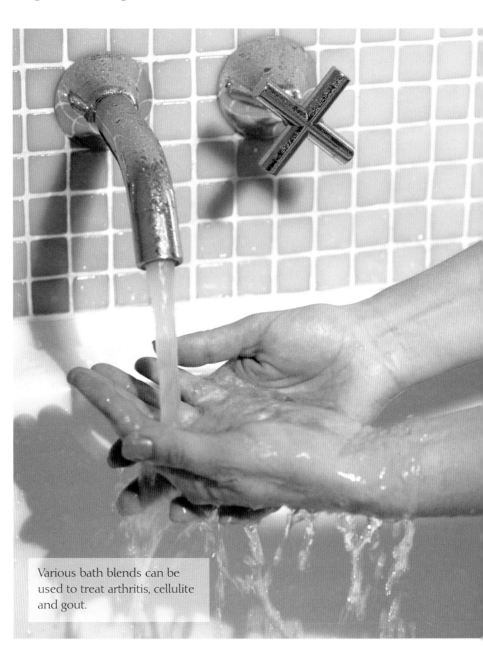

Various bath blends can be used to treat arthritis, cellulite and gout.

*Anti-spasmodic and anti-inflammatory essential oils
applied to a sore muscle or joint will be absorbed
into the surrounding tissues.*

Cellulite

Essential oils with stimulating and detoxifying properties may help to boost metabolism and possibly counter cellulite.

3 drops juniper essential oil
3 drops grapefruit essential oil
3 drops peppermint essential oil
1 drop black pepper essential oil
¼ cup Epsom salts
¼ cup sea salt

Combine, and add to a bath.

Cramp

Antispasmodic and warming essential oils are very helpful for cramps.

3 drops lavender essential oil
3 drops marjoram essential oil
3 drops rosemary essential oil
1 drop sandalwood essential oil
3 tablespoons sweet almond oil

Combine, and massage briskly into the affected muscles.

Gout

The redness, swelling and throbbing of gout tends to target one joint at a time and is usually worse at night. To ease the pain, try an evening bath.

3 drops chamomile essential oil
3 drops lavender essential oil
2 drops ginger essential oil
2 drops bergamot essential oil

Combine, and add to a bath.

Hypertension

Regular massage over the long term with essential oils with antihypertensive properties can help to reduce blood pressure and also regulate breathing and heart rate.

3 drops lavender essential oil
3 drops sandalwood essential oil
3 drops mandarin essential oil
1 drop ylang ylang essential oil
3 tablespoons sweet almond oil

Combine, and massage across chest and upper back, using long, sweeping strokes out to the shoulders and inhaling deeply at the same time.

Muscular aches

Make a soothing massage oil.

3 drops wintergreen essential oil
3 drops juniper essential oil
3 drops eucalyptus essential oil
1 drop bergamot essential oil
3 tablespoons sweet almond oil

1 Combine, and massage into affected area.
2 Cover area with plastic wrap and then a warm wheat bag or heat pack; replace it as it cools.

Sciatica

When the pain is not too bad, try a preventive massage treatment to boost circulation and reduce spasm in the surrounding muscles.

3 drops geranium essential oil
3 drops marjoram essential oil
3 drops rosemary essential oil
1 drop pine essential oil
3 tablespoons sweet almond oil

Combine, and work the mixture thoroughly into buttocks and legs.

Varicose veins

Help improve varicose veins with this massage blend.

5 drops cypress essential oil
5 drops bergamot essential oil
5 drops juniper essential oil
1 drop lemon essential oil
3 tablespoons sweet almond oil

Combine, and massage lightly into the affected area, always moving upwards towards the heart.

Bursitis

Ease the pain of the bursa, fluid-filled sacs that facilitate movement in the knee, shoulder and elbow joints.

5 drops cypress essential oil
5 drops lavender essential oil
5 drops peppermint essential oil
1 drop juniper essential oil

1 Combine the oils with 125 ml (½ cup) of cold water.
2 Dip a face washer in the liquid, wring out lightly and place over the affected area. Cover with a cold pack. Repeat 2–3 times daily.

Respiratory system

The air we need to sustain life can also contain pollutants and disease-causing microbes, bacteria and fungi. Essential oils help to optimise the health of the mucous membranes lining the respiratory organs and also protect them.

Antispasmodic

Try burning these antispasmodic oils in a vaporiser.

2 drops lavender essential oil
2 drops marjoram essential oil
2 drops rose essential oil

Combine with 2 tablespoons of water.

Asthma

Use this massage blend to help open out the chest and shoulders.

3 drops lavender essential oil
3 drops peppermint essential oil
3 drops chamomile essential oil
1 drop eucalyptus essential oil
3 tablespoons sweet almond oil

Mix well, and massage into the thoracic area with long strokes.

To help clear the head and prevent the spread of flu germs, place 1 drop each of eucalyptus, tea tree and lavender essential oils on the pillow.

Bronchitis

A steam inhalation with essential oils that act as pulmonary antiseptics will combat infection, lower fever and ease coughing.

2 drops eucalyptus essential oil
2 drops lemon essential oil
2 drops rosemary essential oil

1 Add the essential oils to a basin filled with very hot water.
2 Tent the head with a towel and inhale the steam for 10 minutes, keeping the face 20 cm away from the water's surface. Repeat 2–3 times daily.

Catarrh

This inhalation will break down congestion and clear the head.

2 drops peppermint essential oil
2 drops eucalyptus essential oil
2 drops thyme essential oil

1 Add the essential oils to a basin filled with boiling water.
2 Tent the head with a towel and inhale the steam for 10 minutes, keeping the face 20 cm away from the water's surface.

Colds

At the first sign of a cold, massage this immune-enhancing blend into the chest and throat.

3 drops geranium essential oil
3 drops rosemary essential oil
3 drops eucalyptus essential oil
1 drop lemon essential oil
3 tablespoons sweet almond oil

Combine, and massage into the chest and throat. Pay particular attention to the lymph glands in the neck, and inhale deeply.

What's the alternative?

Naturopaths suggest these nutritional supplements for a cold.

- Vitamin C shortens the duration and minimises symptoms, and vitamin A maintains the health of your mucous membrane surfaces, including the lungs.

- Zinc lozenges help, possibly by destroying the virus itself, and the herb echinacea is one of the best for stimulating activity of the 'natural killer' cells that engulf incoming bacteria, viruses and fungi.

- Garlic tablets or capsules will help to boost immunity and clear a cold.

Earache

Gentle massage with this blend may help to ease the pain.

> 2 drops lavender essential oil
> 2 drops chamomile essential oil
> 1 drop peppermint essential oil
> 2 tablespoons sweet almond oil

Combine, and massage around the ear. Do not insert essential oils into the ear.

Flu

Burn this blend in a room where a flu patient is resting.

> 2 drops tea tree essential oil
> 2 drops lemon essential oil
> 2 drops pine essential oil

In a vaporiser, burn the blend with 2 tablespoons of water.

Hay fever

Try a head and neck massage with this blend.

> 2 drops peppermint essential oil
> 2 drops lemon essential oil
> 1 drop lavender essential oil
> 2 tablespoons sweet almond oil

Mix well, and gently massage into the scalp, hairline, temples and back of the neck.

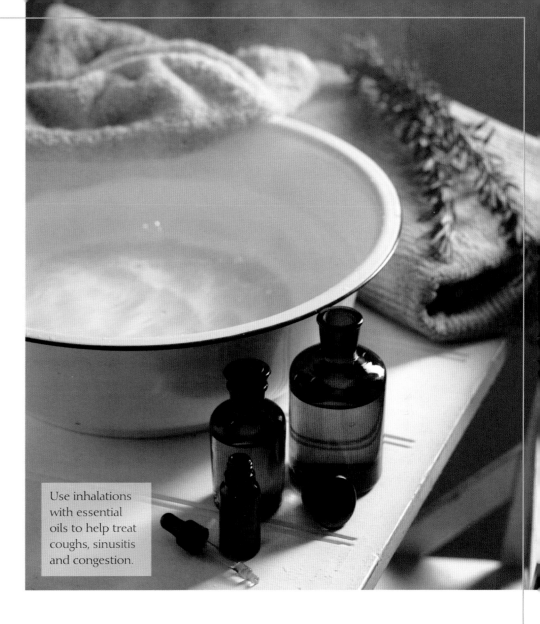

Use inhalations with essential oils to help treat coughs, sinusitis and congestion.

Sinusitis

If the pressure is getting to you, warm, moist steam will enhance the penetration of essential oils into your breathing passages.

> 2 drops eucalyptus essential oil
> 2 drops pine essential oil
> 2 drops peppermint essential oil

Add the essential oils to a basin filled with very hot water. Tent the head with a towel and inhale deeply, keeping the face 20 cm away from the water's surface.

Sore throat

Lemon juice helps to shrink any swelling; tea tree essential oil is an antimicrobial and antifungal; cayenne reduces substance P, a chemical that transmits pain from the throat's nerve endings to the brain; and salt discourages bacteria.

> juice of ½ lemon
> 1 drop tea tree essential oil
> good pinch cayenne
> 2 teaspoons salt

Combine with 125 ml (½ cup) of warm water. Gargle for 1 minute. Do not swallow.

Skin

Your skin protects against the invasion of micro-organisms, supports a vast network of nerve endings and excretes toxins. Skin problems often signal organ dysfunction, and aromatherapy-based treatments can help hasten healing.

Acne

Make an antiseptic toner that will help balance over-active sebaceous glands and counter bacterial infection.

2 drops lavender essential oil
2 drops tea tree essential oil
2 drops chamomile essential oil
1 tablespoon witch hazel
1 tablespoon apple cider vinegar
3 tablespoons distilled water

1 Combine the ingredients, and store in a dark glass bottle.
2 Shake well and apply to skin with a cottonwool ball. Avoid eye area.

Athlete's foot

After bathing, dust your feet with this powder, paying particular attention to between the toes.

3 drops lavender essential oil
3 drops tea tree essential oil
3 drops patchouli essential oil
1 drop pine essential oil
¼ cup cornflour

Combine the ingredients, and sift to disperse the oils.

Boils

Repeat this treatment three times daily to ease inflammation, draw out pus and prevent further infection.

3 drops tea tree essential oil
3 drops thyme essential oil
3 drops myrrh essential oil
1 drop lavender essential oil
1 tablespoon Epsom salts

1 Add ingredients to ¼ cup of very hot water, and mix well.
2 Soak a face washer or cottonwool ball in the mixture, wring out, and place over affected area. Replace with a fresh hot application as it cools and dries.

Cold sores

These essential oils help speed the healing of cold sore blisters and also prevent further infection.

2 drops lemon balm essential oil
2 drops eucalyptus essential oil
2 drops tea tree essential oil
1 tablespoon vodka

Mix well, and store in a small dark glass bottle. Apply with a cottonbud.

BITES AND STINGS

Essential oils that have antiseptic properties can be used in these first aid treatments.
- *To clean and prevent infection, apply 1 drop of neat tea tree or lavender essential oil.*
- *To relieve itching, combine 1 drop of calendula essential oil and 3 drops each of peppermint, lavender and tea tree essential oils with 2 tablespoons of witch hazel. Store in a dark glass bottle, shake before use, and apply with a cottonwool ball.*

Eczema

Ease itching, inflammation and redness with a cooling compress. If itching is severe, add crushed ice to the mixture, ensuring that no chips of ice are caught in the cloth or towel, as they may scratch the skin.

2 drops chamomile essential oil
2 drops lavender essential oil
2 drops calendula essential oil
1 drop geranium essential oil

1 Combine with 125 ml (½ cup) of cool water.
2 Soak a clean, soft towel in the liquid, wring it out and place over the affected area.

*Sponge sunburnt skin with a blend
of ½ cup tepid water, 3 drops each of lavender,
chamomile and geranium essential oils
and 1 tablespoon of bicarbonate of soda.*

Hives

Lemon balm, chamomile and jasmine essential oils are all helpful for itchy or inflamed skin.

3 drops lemon balm essential oil
3 drops chamomile essential oil
3 drops jasmine essential oil
2 tablespoons witch hazel

Mix well, and dab on hives to reduce the swelling.

Minor burns

Use this blend to hasten healing and help prevent scarring.

2 drops calendula essential oil
2 drops hypericum essential oil
2 drops lavender essential oil
2 tablespoons rosehip oil

Combine the ingredients, and massage in a few drops daily.

Psoriasis

Stress both triggers and worsens this condition. These essential oils have antidepressant properties.

2 drops rose essential oil
2 drops chamomile essential oil
1 drop clary sage essential oil
3 tablespoons water

Combine, and burn in a vaporiser to release the fragrance.

What's the alternative?

Naturopaths believe psoriasis is triggered by poor digestion and the build-up of toxins in the body. The following remedies may help.

• Sarsaparilla tea, which has a long history of use for treating skin problems.

• Milk thistle, as it improves liver function.

• Flaxseed oil, which is rich in the essential fatty acids that help reduce inflammation.

Scars

To help heal scarring, massage this blend into the affected area daily.

3 drops lavender essential oil
3 drops neroli essential oil
3 drops calendula essential oil
1 drop tea tree essential oil
2 tablespoons rosehip oil
3 x 1000 IU vitamin E capsules

Combine the ingredients, and mix together thoroughly.

Shingles

Ease the pain of blisters with this soothing blend.

3 drops lavender essential oil
3 drops bergamot essential oil
3 drops patchouli essential oil
1 drop eucalyptus essential oil
3 tablespoons aloe vera gel
1 x 1000 IU vitamin E capsule

Mix the oils with the contents of the capsule, and use a cottonbud to apply the mixture to blisters.

Mind and emotions

The health of the mind and the body are inextricably linked. In addition to reducing stress and enhancing relaxation, aromatherapy may help specific emotional and mental health problems.

Anger
Ease feelings of rage and restore a sense of control.

3 drops lavender essential oil
3 drops bergamot essential oil
3 drops peppermint essential oil
1 drop ginger essential oil
3 tablespoons sweet almond oil

Mix well, and massage the blend into the neck and chest, inhaling deeply.

Anxiety
Ylang ylang essential oil has a harmonising and balancing effect, but if you experience severe anxiety, see your doctor.

2–3 drops ylang ylang
essential oil

1 Sprinkle the oil on a cottonwool ball and inhale deeply.
2 Tuck the ball inside your shirt or bra, where your body warmth will help release the aroma through the day.

Change
Heighten alertness and also open your mind to the positive aspects of future possibilities.

2 drops juniper essential oil
2 drops lemongrass essential oil
2 drops clary sage essential oil

In a vaporiser, burn the essential oils with 3 tablespoons of water.

The blues
Listen to soothing music while soaking in this bath blend.

3 drops lavender essential oil
3 drops ylang ylang essential oil
3 drops geranium essential oil
1 drop grapefruit essential oil
3 tablespoons honey

Combine, and add to a warm bath. Soak for 15 minutes.

Insomnia
Lying awake night after night is slow torture, but a soothing pillow spray can help.

3 drops lavender essential oil
3 drops rose essential oil
3 drops ylang ylang essential oil
1 drop marjoram essential oil
2 tablespoons rosewater

1 Combine the ingredients with enough water to make up 50 ml.
2 Shake well before use, and lightly mist the pillows and bedding before going to bed.

Grief
The spicy, warming scents of this blend are gentle and supportive.

3 drops patchouli essential oil
3 drops ginger essential oil
3 drops rose essential oil
1 drop frankincense essential oil
3 tablespoons sweet almond oil

FEAR
Essential oils with a strong, clear scent can have a stabilising effect, helping to dispel nervousness, enable clarity of thought, and make you feel more grounded and 'here now'.
* *In a vaporiser, burn 2 drops each of rosemary and cedarwood essential oils to create an energising and positive atmosphere.*
* *Place 2 drops each of orange and lemongrass essential oils on a handkerchief and inhale deeply.*
* *Place 1 drop each of frankincense, myrrh and sandalwood essential oils on a cottonwool ball and inhale deeply. Tuck it into your bra or shirt pocket so the scents stay with you all day. When combined, these oils have a profoundly peaceful effect.*

Mix well, and use as a soothing rub for tense shoulders, or for relaxing the chest and neck and regulating breathing after bouts of crying.

Mild fatigue
Fatigue is often a symptom of another problem – for example, stress, anxiety, lowered immunity or infection.

3 drops clary sage essential oil
3 drops geranium essential oil
3 drops rose essential oil
1 drop basil essential oil
3 tablespoons cream or honey

Combine, and add to a warm bath. Soak for 15–20 minutes.

Stress

Use this blend for self-massage or, better still, ask someone else to do it for you.

- 3 drops lavender essential oil
- 3 drops sandalwood essential oil
- 3 drops rose geranium essential oil
- 1 drop basil essential oil
- 3 tablespoons sweet almond oil

Combine the ingredients, and massage into your neck.

What's the alternative?

These natural remedies can help ease you into dreamland.

- **Herbal helpers** Valerian, an effective sleep aid, works best when taken with other sedating herbs such as passionflower in tablets, tea or as a tincture.

- **Warm milk and honey** Milk contains calcium, which relaxes muscles, and tryptophan, which converts to serotonin, the soothing neurotransmitter. Honey helps tryptophan cross the blood–brain barrier to be converted to serotonin.

- **Bach flower remedies** Try mimulus (for specific fears and post-traumatic recovery – great for worry-warts); aspen, for generalised anxiety; and white chestnut, for fretting, agitation and obsessive thoughts.

CAUTIONS ● Depression should be treated by a doctor. ● Avoid taking natural sleep aids with conventional sedatives or drugs that make you sleepy, as excessive drowsiness may result.

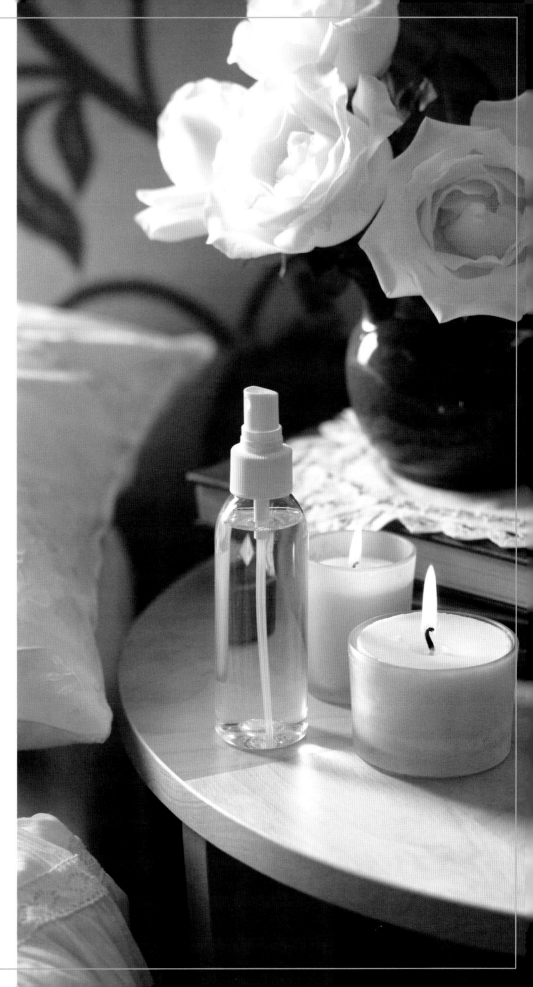

Women's health

Aromatherapy and massage help in treating many common hormonal conditions, such as premenstrual syndrome (PMS) and menopausal symptoms, and they can also help to ease emotional and physical discomforts.

Heavy periods

A compress containing essential oils that have a uterine tonic effect may help regulate menstrual flow.

> 3 drops cypress essential oil
> 3 drops geranium essential oil
> 3 drops rose essential oil
> 1 drop marjoram essential oil

1 Combine the essential oils with 125 ml (½ cup) of cool water.
2 Dip a face washer in the liquid, wring it out lightly and place across the abdomen. Repeat 2–3 times daily.

Labour

Jasmine essential oil stimulates the uterus to contract during labour while lavender essential oil soothes the nerves and eases anxiety. Do not use this blend during pregnancy.

> 3 drops jasmine essential oil
> 3 drops lavender essential oil
> 3 tablespoons sweet almond oil

Mix well, and use as a massage blend for the lower back during labour.

Loss of periods

Several essential oils can stimulate menstruation, but you must avoid them if there is any chance at all of falling pregnant.

> 3 drops fennel essential oil
> 3 drops marjoram essential oil
> 3 drops basil essential oil
> 1 drop myrrh essential oil
> 3 tablespoons sweet almond oil

Combine the oils, and use to massage the lower back and abdomen.

Menstrual cramps

An aromatic bath can help to ease period pain.

> 3 drops lavender essential oil
> 3 drops chamomile essential oil
> 3 drops marjoram essential oil
> 1 drop cypress essential oil
> 3 tablespoons honey

Combine, and add to a warm bath. Soak for 15–20 minutes.

Morning sickness

This can be quite debilitating.

> 2 drops lavender essential oil
> 2 drops chamomile essential oil
> 1 drop peppermint oil

1 Combine the oils with 125 ml (½ cup) of cool water.
2 Dip two face washers in the liquid, wring out lightly, and place one across the stomach and the other across the forehead.

Perineal healing

Help speed healing of the perineum if it has been torn during childbirth.

> 5 drops lavender essential oil
> 5 drops tea tree essential oil
> ¼ cup sea salt

Add the ingredients to a shallow bath filled with lukewarm water, and use daily.

Baby blues

Post-natal depression should always be monitored by a doctor, but inhaling essential oils that have balancing and uplifting effects may help to restore balance and counter the feeling of negativity in the first few weeks.

> 3 drops jasmine essential oil
> 3 drops clary sage essential oil
> 3 drops ylang ylang essential oil
> 1 drop mandarin essential oil

Combine the oils, and add to a bath.

Essential oils have hormone-like and stress-relieving properties that help to ease transition into different life stages.

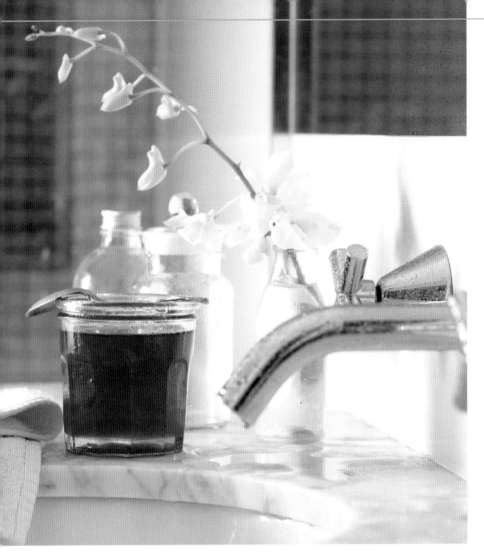

- *If night sweats are a problem, try this soothing bath before bedtime. Add 3 drops each of chamomile, cypress and clary sage essential oils with 1 drop of lime essential oil and 1 cup of strong, strained sage tea to a warm – not hot – bath.*
- *To ease irritability and mood swings, burn 2 drops each of rose geranium and bergamot essential oils with 3 tablespoons of water.*
- *Combine 3 drops each of rose, ylang ylang and neroli essential oils with 1 drop of jasmine essential oil and 3 tablespoons of sweet almond oil. Use this blend of oils, with their antidepressant, feminine qualities, to gently massage the breasts, belly and thighs.*

Stretch marks

From the seventh month of pregnancy, massage with this blend.

2 drops lavender essential oil
2 drops geranium essential oil
3 tablespoons sweet almond oil

Combine, and massage a small amount daily into the belly, hips, buttocks and thighs.

Vaginal thrush

A shallow bath containing this blend can ease pain and, being anti-fungal, help to prevent further infection.

3 drops lavender essential oil
3 drops tea tree essential oil
3 drops myrrh essential oil
1 drop sandalwood essential oil

Combine, and add to a shallow bath.

Premenstrual syndrome (PMS)

Nervous tension, anxiety and tearfulness can be helped with this massage blend.

3 drops clary sage essential oil
3 drops rose essential oil
3 drops sandalwood essential oil
1 drop mandarin essential oil
3 tablespoons sweet almond oil
2 x 250 mg evening primrose oil capsules

Combine the oils with the contents of the capsules, and apply daily to the lower abdomen and back, always working towards the heart, and inhaling deeply, for 5–10 days prior to your period, or whenever the symptoms are prevalent.

What's the alternative?

Naturopaths recommend the following remedies for treating PMS/PMT.

- The herb chaste tree (*Vitex agnus-castus*) has sedative, regulatory and antispasmodic properties, and also helps balance hormone levels. You'll find the tablets and capsules at health food stores.

- A healthy liver helps keep your hormones under control, so drink 3 cups of dandelion tea a day in the week leading up to your period. Add 1 teaspoon of fresh chopped ginger, and sweeten with honey if you like.

Aromatherapy blends for full body massage

Essential oils have many properties that affect the brain and body, and may be combined to enhance physical, emotional and nervous health and general wellbeing. Try creating your own blends for full body massage.

Beating burnout

If left unchecked, a build-up of mental, nervous and physical stress can spiral into burnout and exhaustion. This blend will help the body cope better with stress and also prepare it for quality relaxation and sleep.

> 3 drops lavender essential oil
> 3 drops sandalwood essential oil
> 3 drops chamomile essential oil
> 1 drop marjoram essential oil
> 3 tablespoons sweet almond oil

Confidence booster

Essential oils help to ease symptoms of anxiety and also encourage feelings of mental acuity, concentration and creative vigour. Use this blend before starting a new job or making a major presentation at work.

> 3 drops peppermint essential oil
> 3 drops clary sage essential oil
> 3 drops geranium essential oil
> 1 drop bergamot essential oil
> 3 tablespoons sweet almond oil

To promote confidence, burn 2 drops each of lime and ginger essential oils in a vaporiser with 3 tablespoons of water.

Cool down

A full body massage with this combination is both stimulating and calming for someone who is ill.

> 3 drops lavender essential oil
> 3 drops bergamot essential oil
> 3 drops basil essential oil
> 1 drop eucalyptus essential oil
> 3 tablespoons sweet almond oil

Detox special

Detoxifying the body can have long-lasting benefits for overall health, not only helping to tone and restore the lymphatic system and kidneys but also softening and nourishing the skin, encouraging the elimination of dangerous waste and easing the mind.

> 3 drops lemon essential oil
> 3 drops grapefruit essential oil
> 3 drops frankincense essential oil
> 1 drop peppermint essential oil
> 3 tablespoons sweet almond oil

Energy breakthrough

A full body massage using stimulating and rejuvenating essential oils will help to release a feeling of being emotionally 'stuck', and also stimulate fresh thinking and clarity of vision.

> 3 drops eucalyptus essential oil
> 3 drops basil essential oil
> 3 drops lemon essential oil
> 1 drop pine essential oil
> 3 tablespoons sweet almond oil

Healing the heart

When a person is feeling very low and dispirited following the end of a relationship, a regular full body massage with the following blend will help to calm the heart, and encourage feelings of acceptance, safety and peace.

> 3 drops rose essential oil
> 3 drops mandarin essential oil
> 3 drops marjoram essential oil
> 1 drop rosemary essential oil
> 3 tablespoons sweet almond oil

Immune support

The refreshing essential oils in this blend will help the body to stimulate the production of white blood cells, which destroy pathogenic bacteria and viruses.

  3 drops tea tree essential oil
  3 drops thyme essential oil
  3 drops eucalyptus essential oil
  1 drop orange essential oil
  3 tablespoons sweet almond oil

Love and light

When a negative mind set makes everything seem depressing or unsafe, restore feelings of openness and hope with a blend that encourages a positive attitude.

  3 drops orange essential oil
  3 drops sandalwood essential oil
  3 drops coriander essential oil
  1 drop black pepper essential oil
  3 tablespoons sweet almond oil

COMFORT AND KINDNESS

When a loved one is suffering or grieving, a practical way to comfort them is to offer a full body massage, using a blend that has warming and nurturing qualities that help to ease painful transitions.

  3 drops patchouli essential oil
  3 drops orange essential oil
  3 drops sandalwood essential oil
  1 drop lemon essential oil
  3 tablespoons sweet almond oil

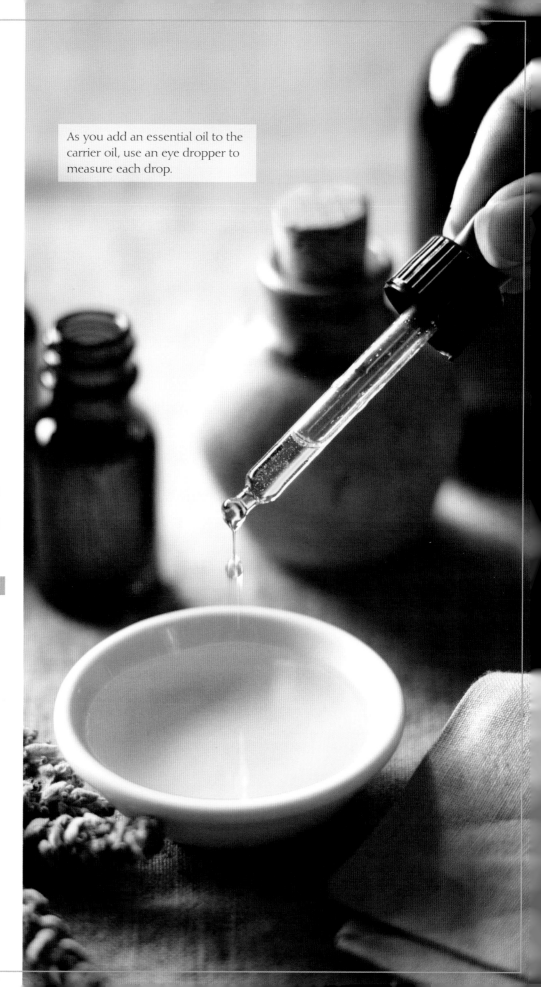

As you add an essential oil to the carrier oil, use an eye dropper to measure each drop.

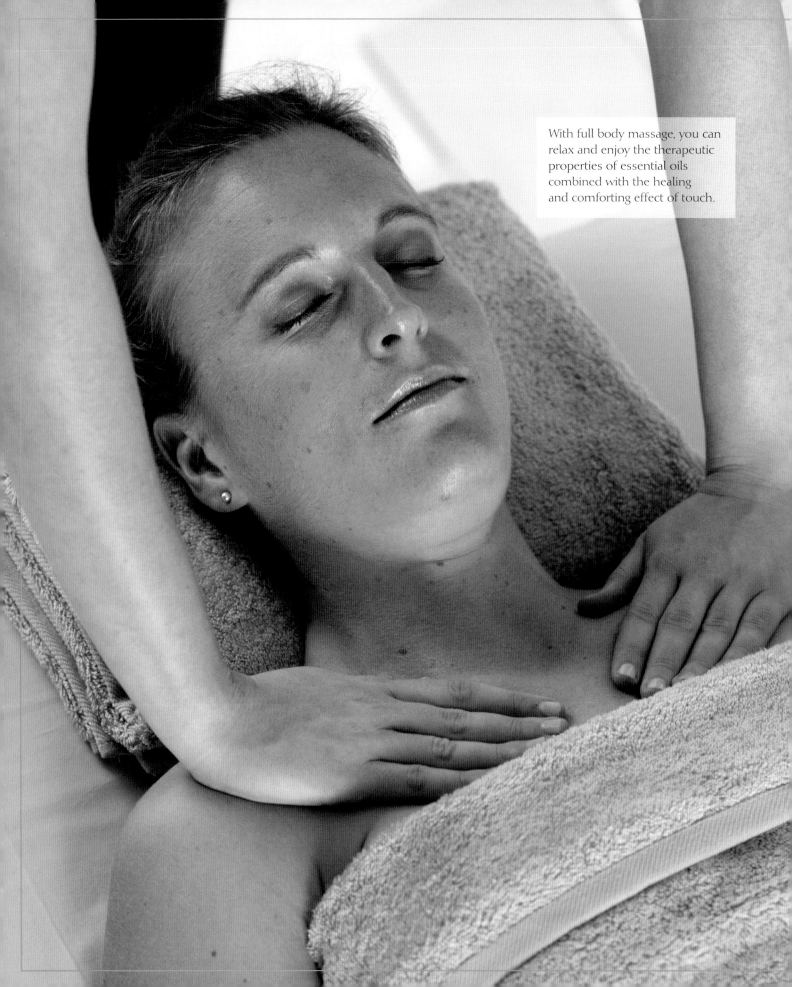

With full body massage, you can relax and enjoy the therapeutic properties of essential oils combined with the healing and comforting effect of touch.

Overcoming obstacles

This blend will generate a sense of empowerment, acceptance and strength, and also help ground a person's emotions, encourage self-belief and rally their ability to overcome difficulties.

3 drops basil essential oil
3 drops lemon balm essential oil
3 drops geranium essential oil
1 drop vanilla essential oil
3 tablespoons sweet almond oil

Restoring balance

Being unsettled and agitated can spiral out of control into full-blown anxiety or a panic attack. This blend is an effective 'circuit-breaker', ideal for creating feelings of stability and strength and enabling a more balanced view of a situation.

3 drops peppermint essential oil
3 drops lavender essential oil
3 drops marjoram essential oils
1 drop lemon essential oil
3 tablespoons sweet almond oil

Romance rehab

Encourage relaxation, affection, intimacy and sensual sensations in a partner by treating them to a full body massage with a blend of revitalising essential oils.

3 drops neroli essential oil
3 drops ylang ylang essential oil
3 drops jasmine essential oil
1 drop ginger essential oil
3 tablespoons sweet almond oil

Soul soother

The gentle, sweet floral aromas of jasmine, lavender and rose work well together to relieve physical and mental exhaustion, while the addition of a stimulating note of pine helps to expand the mind, move past emotions of frustration and anger, and create a fresh outlook.

3 drops jasmine essential oil
3 drops lavender essential oil
3 drops rose essential oil
1 drop pine essential oil
3 tablespoons sweet almond oil

STRENGTHENING THE SPIRIT

Low energy levels, mood swings and nervous tension may be the result of trauma and shock. Try a full body massage with essential oils that will help clear negative energy, fortify the emotions and uplift the spirit.

3 drops lavender essential oil
3 drops cypress essential oil
3 drops peppermint essential oil
1 drop lemon balm essential oil
3 tablespoons sweet almond oil

Time out

Use this aromatherapy blend to create a sense of stillness and feeling centred, and to enhance a full body massage for someone who urgently needs some 'time out'.

3 drops ylang ylang essential oil
3 drops orange essential oil
3 drops sandalwood essential oil
1 drop lemongrass essential oil
3 tablespoons sweet almond oil

Weekend warrior

If you throw yourself into competitive exercise on the weekend after a sedentary week, you may suffer aches and pains, even injury, if your muscles are not sufficiently relaxed and warm beforehand. A regular full body massage will help to boost circulation of blood and lymph, relax muscles and also increase energy.

3 drops peppermint essential oil
3 drops cypress essential oil
3 drops lavender essential oil
1 drop pine essential oil
3 tablespoons sweet almond oil

During labour, sponge your face and neck with cool water containing a few drops of calming lavender essential oil.

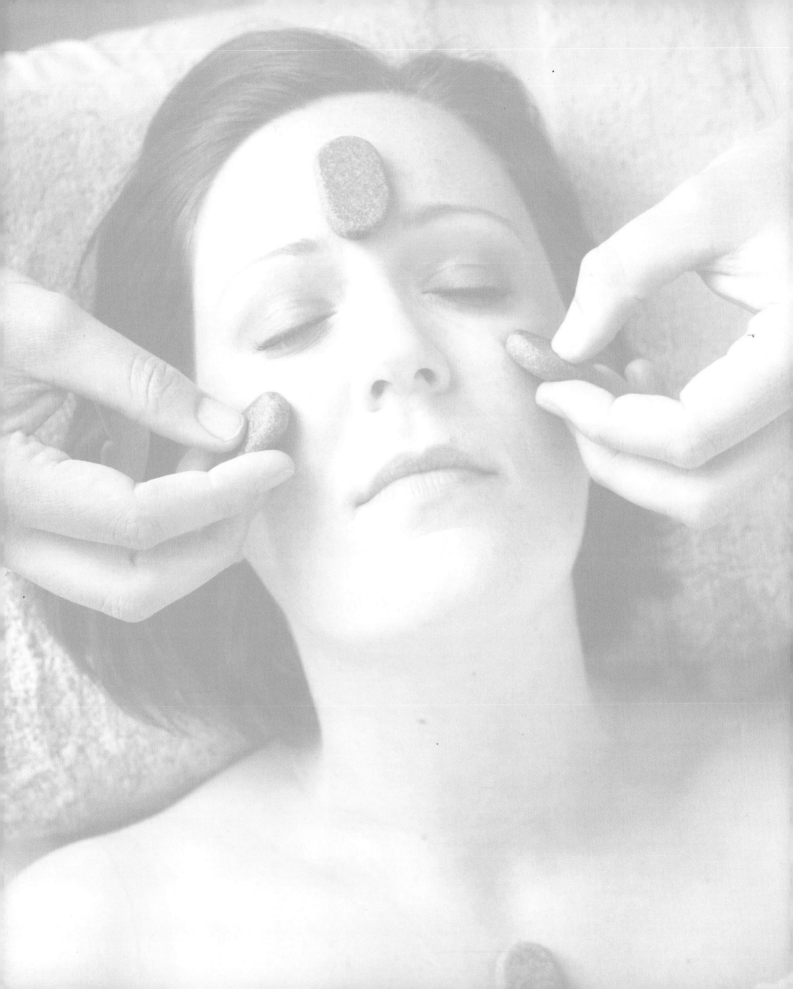

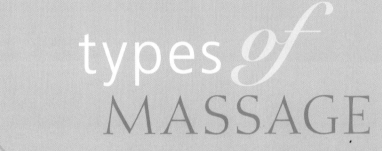

types *of* MASSAGE

Aromatherapy massage

This gentle holistic therapy combines the therapeutic effects of touch with the healing properties of essential oils, helping to both balance the physical and emotional ailments of the body and promote a sense of wellbeing.

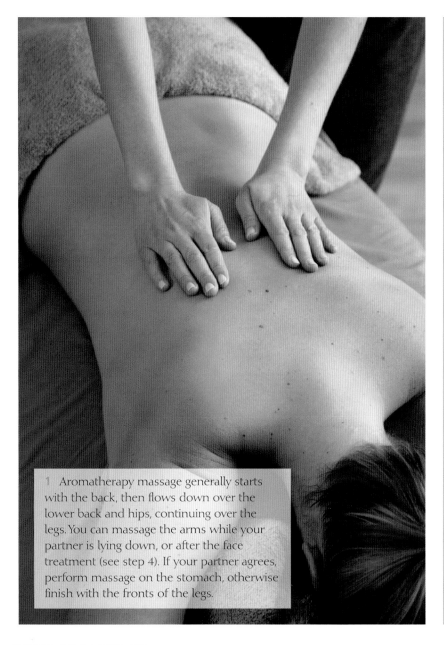

1 Aromatherapy massage generally starts with the back, then flows down over the lower back and hips, continuing over the legs. You can massage the arms while your partner is lying down, or after the face treatment (see step 4). If your partner agrees, perform massage on the stomach, otherwise finish with the fronts of the legs.

KEY PRINCIPLES

● The benefits of aromatherapy massage are obtained by both touch and smell. In addition to the therapeutic benefits of essential oils, aromatherapy treatment provides relief from muscular tension, anxiety and stress, and also improves circulation.

● Soft tissue manipulation, rhythmic slow movements and other gentle techniques promote deep relaxation so the receiver feels nurtured and healed. The effect of this style on the nervous system can have both uplifting and energising results, even when using the gentle techniques.

● To avoid overstimulation, do not let the massage take more than 45–60 minutes. Although this sequential treatment is always performed the same way, the blends are chosen according to specific conditions (see pages 62–81).

● There are various forms of aromatherapy massage, but Micheline Arcier developed this unique technique – which combines Swedish massage techniques, acupressure, lymphatic drainage, polarity therapy and reflexology – in the 1940s.

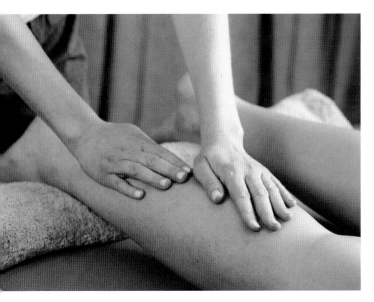

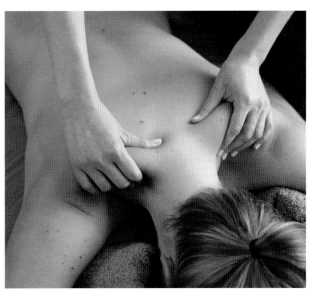

2 Gentle stroking movements, the main techniques used in aromatherapy treatment, can be applied any time to promote the feeling of relaxation. Using flat hands, slide rhythmically over each area to increase the circulation and enhance the absorption of the essential oils.

3 To smooth away any tightness around the shoulder and upper back area, apply some additional kneading techniques, which may also ease a tension headache as well as any aches or stiffness in the neck. Put your hands close together and gently squeeze the muscles in alternating movements.

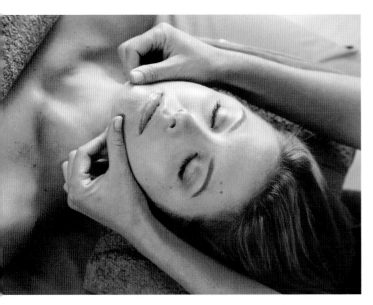

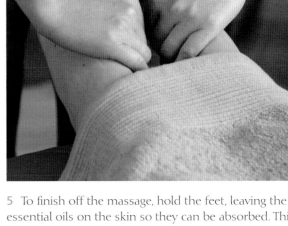

4 The front sequence often starts with a relaxing scalp massage, followed by a facial. The combination of a highly aromatic fragrance and smooth, nurturing strokes results in complete relaxation. A clay mask blended with essential oils is sometimes incorporated in the treatment to promote deep cleansing and healing of the skin.

5 To finish off the massage, hold the feet, leaving the essential oils on the skin so they can be absorbed. This also helps prolong the enjoyable, relaxed mood. It is common for a therapist to give the client a small bottle of the massage blend so she can use it between sessions and recall the blissful feeling of the treatment at home.

CAUTIONS ● See 'Safety and cautions', page 134. ● Always check your partner's medical history for any contraindications, sensitivities and allergies. ● Unless you are qualified, check the properties of each oil you use, and keep the correct ratio of essential oils to base oil.

➲ 'Aromatherapy blends', page 62
● 'Beauty or facial massage', page 102
● 'Before you start', page 126 ● 'Full body sequence for aromatherapy massage', page 154

Swedish massage

Created by Per Henrik Ling, Swedish massage has evolved into the most popular massage style in Western culture. This wonderfully therapeutic technique relies on using oils as well as gentle rhythmic touch and movement to relax and rejuvenate the mind and body.

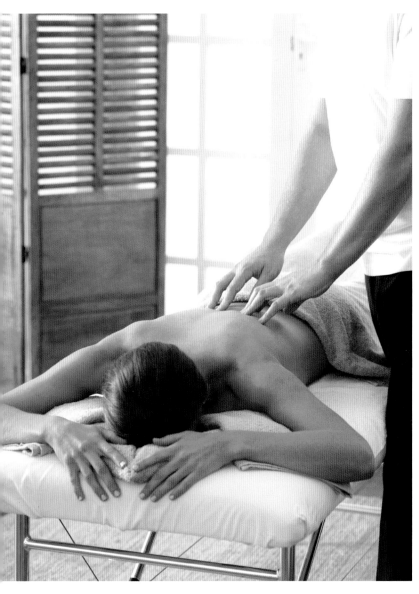

KEY PRINCIPLES

● Swedish massage is usually performed in a calm environment, with candles, soft music and the burning of certain oils all helping to create a relaxed atmosphere. It can be applied to anyone, from the elderly to babies and children.

● This massage technique moves restricted muscles, thus releasing tension and tightness by increasing blood flow and circulation. It has also been known to work on the nervous and lymphatic systems (see page 104).

● The main techniques for Swedish massage are applied at different times for various effects. For the full sequence, which includes the front of the body, see pages 138–53.

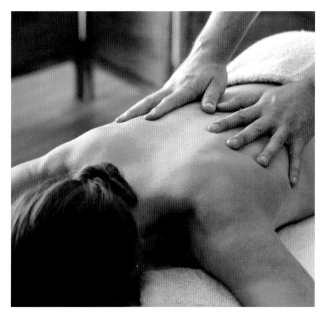

1   Once your partner is on the table and draped with towels, begin by palpating the back to accustom her to your touch. Simply push your fingertips down into the skin and muscles to identify any tightness or particular areas you should avoid.

2   Using both hands, apply essential oil to the back with gentle gliding movements. This technique, called effleurage, relaxes your partner while stimulating blood flow and warming up her muscles. Use it as you begin and end on a particular area.

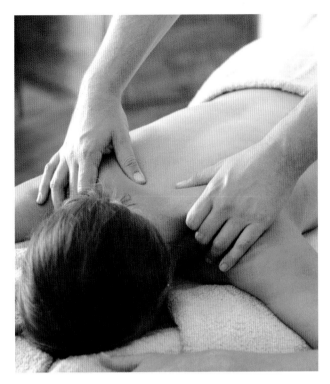

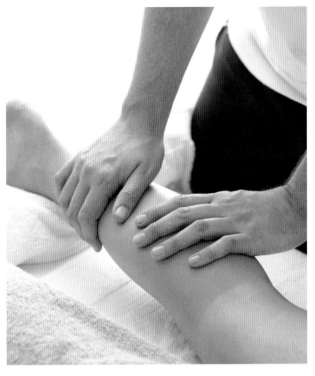

3 Once you have warmed up the back, work your way up the body towards the shoulders, neck and back of the arms. This area is renowned for being tense and tight, so kneading, which causes the muscles to soften and become more pliable, is often used to release tension. Next, cover the back.

4 Begin working on the legs. Apply effleurage first, then petrissage, always working upwards. To shake the muscles free, you may need to use vibration on the front and back of the thighs and calves.

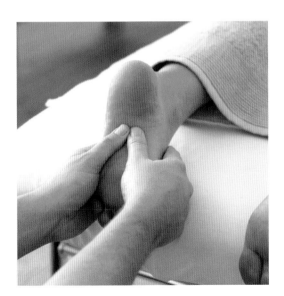

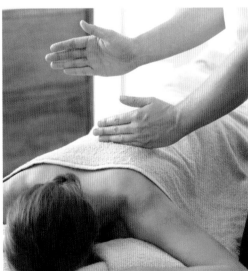

CAUTIONS
● See 'Safety and cautions', page 134.
● Avoid massaging over the spine at all times, and be careful when working close to bony landmarks such as the hips and shoulders.

5 Using soft, rhythmic circular movements with your fingers and thumbs, continue the massage on the feet, emphasising the toes and tendons; your partner should experience a sense of bliss. Apply similar techniques to the ones used in step 4.

6 Cover your partner, then apply various percussion techniques over the towel to the whole body underneath. Use techniques such as cupping around the thoracic area to loosen muscles, and hacking and pummelling over the rest of the body to stimulate nerve endings.

➔ *'Full body sequence for Swedish massage', pages 136–53*

Deep tissue or therapeutic massage

This treatment usually focuses on alleviating certain muscular and skeletal conditions, including tension headaches and poor posture, and it will often take a series of treatments to restore the client's health.

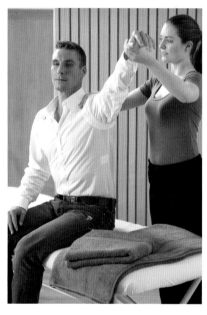

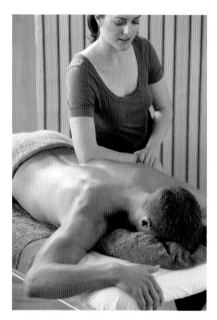

1 The therapist first ascertains the client's problem, then does range of movement and other specific tests to determine what is causing it. After agreeing on a treatment plan, she drapes the client and begins the massage.

2 She starts by palpating the back area. After identifying the tight and restricted areas, she adds oil and applies effleurage and petrissage to warm and loosen up the muscles. A forearm technique works into the deeper layers of the back and helps break up muscular tension.

CAUTIONS ● See 'Safety and cautions', page 134. ● A trained therapist will take care not to use too much pressure, as the client can be sore, or even bruised, for a few days afterwards.

KEY PRINCIPLES

● *As a therapeutic massage works much deeper in the body, a trained therapist will do a thorough consultation before the treatment to establish if there are any general or local contra-indications to the massage.*

● *This more vigorous style is based on Swedish massage (see page 86). In this case techniques such as effleurage and kneading comprise the preliminary moves of warming up the client's muscles and relaxing him.*

● *Once the circulation is flowing, deeper techniques – using the forearms and elbows, soft fists, supported hands or thumbs, and trigger point therapy or myofascial release – can be applied to relieve tension and access the deeper muscles.*

● *A deep tissue massage can be performed in 30, 60 or 90 minutes or longer. Stretching and corrective exercises are often given at the end of the treatment, not only to help correct posture but also to achieve a better muscular balance.*

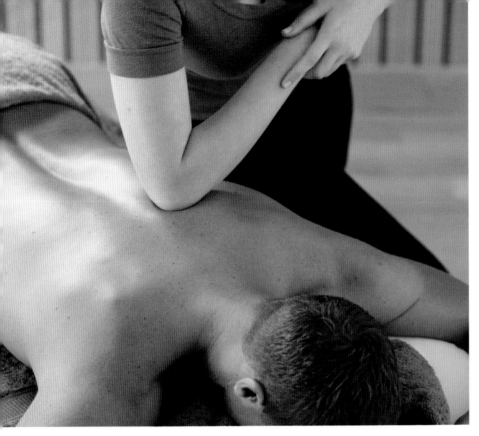

3 Once the superficial and intermediate back muscles have been loosened, the therapist uses an elbow to access the deeper layers. Starting from the lower back, she massages up to the shoulder blade area, taking care not to move over the spine. This technique breaks up adhesions and fascial restrictions lying deep in the muscles.

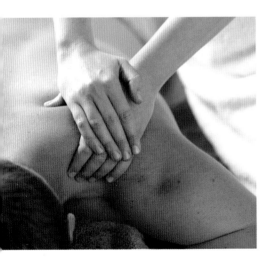

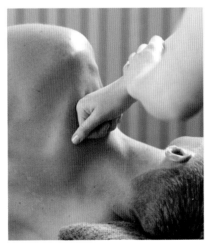

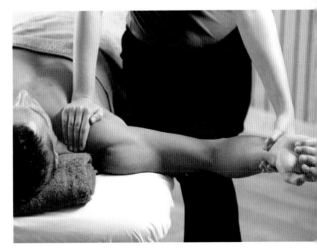

4 With supported hands, she massages over the trapezius and shoulder muscles, perhaps using a trigger point technique. She holds a supported thumb for 20–30 seconds. When the pain decreases, she then releases the pressure and applies the same techniques to the other side.

5 Next, she massages the neck area with a scooping movement to warm up the muscles, before positioning the client on his side and applying a soft fist technique, starting at the shoulders and moving down into the neck. She repeats this technique on the other side.

6 With the client lying face up, and carefully draped, she massages one side of the chest with her hands or palms, pulling the arm out as she does so to stretch the muscles. She repeats this on the other side of the chest before finishing the treatment on the arms or neck.

Shiatsu

Shiatsu is more than just a massage – the nurturing touch of the practitioner brings a sense of calmness and deep wellbeing as she treats the person holistically, looking at physical, mental and emotional imbalances.

CAUTIONS
● See 'Safety and cautions', page 134.
● Avoid strong direct pressure on certain points, especially during pregnancy (see page 232).

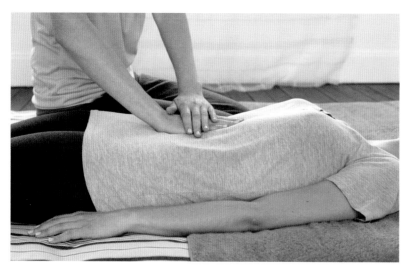

1 Treatment usually begins with diagnosing the *hara* (stomach area), back, pulse or tongue. The general state of the client's health can be read by observing, for example, her body and facial expression. Diagnosis is an important part of the treatment, as it helps to determine which part of the body to work on and which points on the meridians to address.

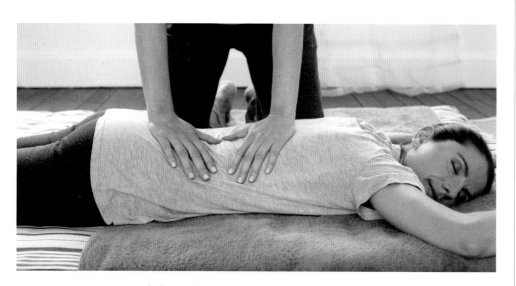

2 To rebalance the flow of *chi*, the therapist applies pressure to different points along the meridians.

KEY PRINCIPLES

● Shiatsu *literally means 'finger pressure', although the thumbs, palms, elbows, forearms, knees and feet are used in the treatment. It is based on the philosophy of the five element theory in Traditional Chinese Medicine (TCM) – the meridians (energy channels),* tsubo *(pressure points), oriental diagnosis, the concept of* yin *and* yang, *and the* chi *(or* ki, *the energy).*

● *Shiatsu works on the* chi *that flows through the body in different channels called meridians. There are twelve main meridians, with both physical and energetic functions, running on both sides of the body, and each is linked to the organs. The massage includes applying pressure, stretching, holding and joint rotations, and may also include corrective exercises and lifestyle changes.*

● *Massaging the points removes the feeling of tension as well as any physical and emotional blockages, restoring the natural balanced flow of* chi. *Both the giver and the receiver will benefit from the Shiatsu treatment, and feel truly relaxed yet energised.*

● *Shiatsu is traditionally performed on a mat or futon on the floor, but it can also be done with the receiver lying fully clothed on a massage table or sitting in a chair.*

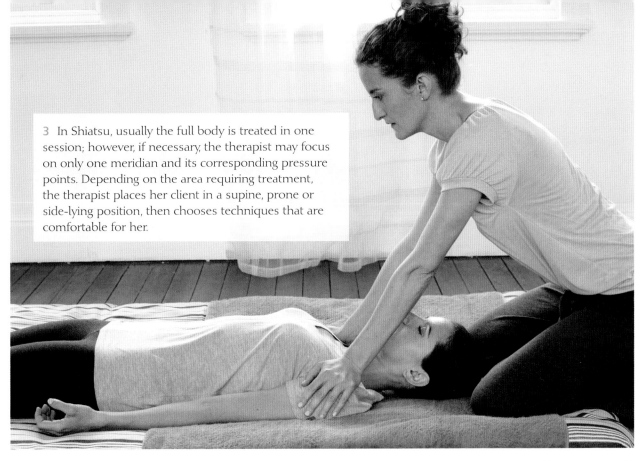

3 In Shiatsu, usually the full body is treated in one session; however, if necessary, the therapist may focus on only one meridian and its corresponding pressure points. Depending on the area requiring treatment, the therapist places her client in a supine, prone or side-lying position, then chooses techniques that are comfortable for her.

MAIN SHIATSU POINTS

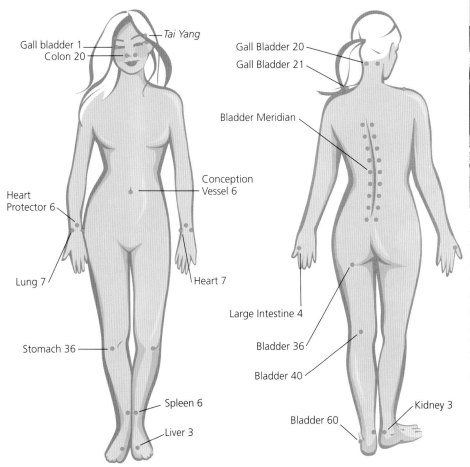

Tai Yang
Gall bladder 1
Colon 20
Heart Protector 6
Lung 7
Heart 7
Stomach 36
Spleen 6
Liver 3
Conception Vessel 6

Gall Bladder 20
Gall Bladder 21
Bladder Meridian
Large Intestine 4
Bladder 36
Bladder 40
Bladder 60
Kidney 3

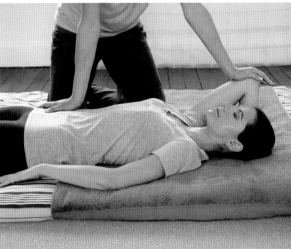

4 Shiatsu generally involves a variety of stretches, which originated in Western osteopathic techniques or oriental massage methods. The aim of these is to activate certain meridians and help bring them to the surface. There are also exercises that help stretch certain meridians, but only professional therapists can apply these.

Eastern or Chinese massage

Chinese massage is one of a range of different treatments – including acupuncture, cupping and Chinese herbs – that trained practitioners use in Traditional Chinese Medicine (TCM). The massage is usually applied through clothing.

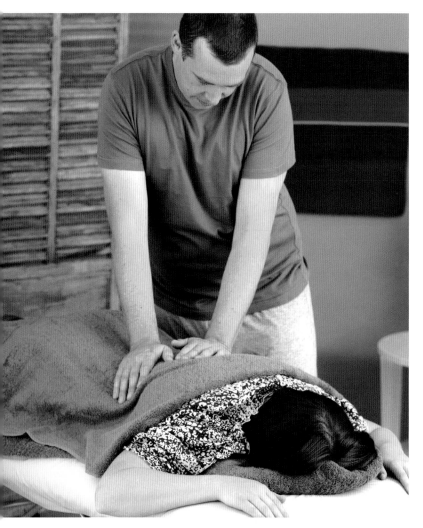

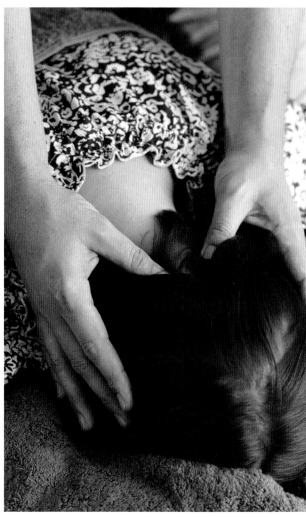

1 After the initial consultation, the practitioner begins the massage on the back area. With his thumbs or elbows, he uses the press method or compression technique to warm up the muscles and stimulate blood flow. As he works along the spine, he applies pressure downwards, holding and then slowly releasing.

2 This technique is fantastic for alleviating pain and restriction in the neck and shoulder area. Using the thumbs to press specific points at the base of the head assists with headaches, tension and eye strain.

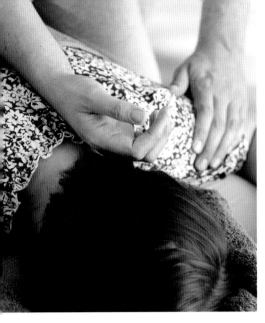

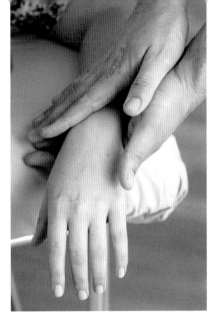

3 The therapist moves onto the shoulders and legs before using the roll method. With a soft and flexible wrist, he rolls his wrist back and forth so the back of his hand makes rhythmical contact, warming the recipient's muscles and massaging away tension.

4 Pressing and rolling the arms and fingers releases any tension within them. The therapist stimulates each limb by holding it with his fingers and thumbs, pulling and plucking so they make a clicking sound.

THE MERIDIANS

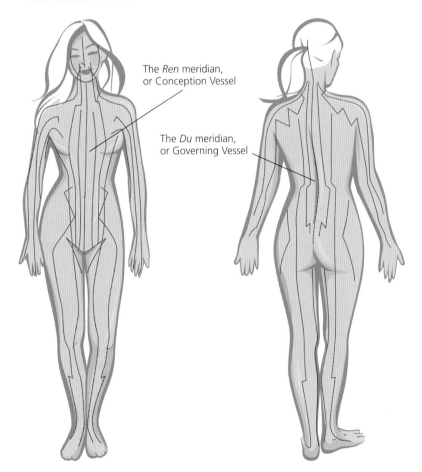

The *Ren* meridian, or Conception Vessel

The *Du* meridian, or Governing Vessel

Thai massage

Thai massage is a wonderful technique that allows you to enjoy a treatment on a futon or table while staying fully clothed. For an hour or more, a Thai massage therapist will press, pull, stretch and manipulate your body to restore it to its natural balance.

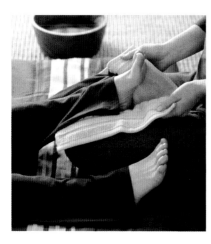

1 It's traditional to start by carefully and thoroughly washing the feet with warm water and a cloth before pressing, massaging and stretching the feet and toes.

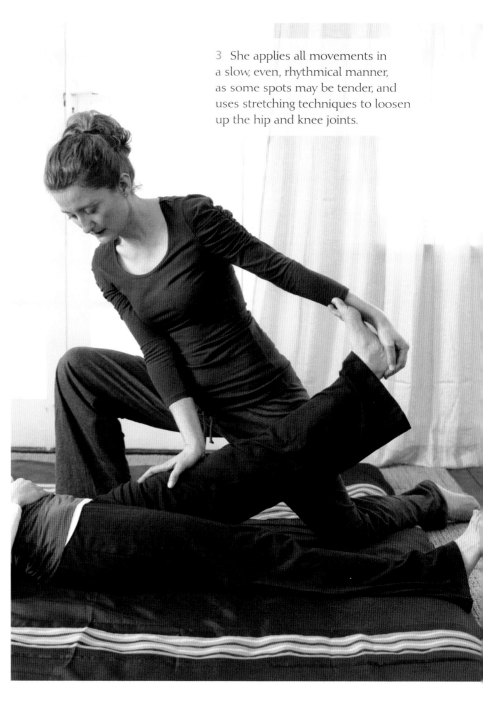

3 She applies all movements in a slow, even, rhythmical manner, as some spots may be tender, and uses stretching techniques to loosen up the hip and knee joints.

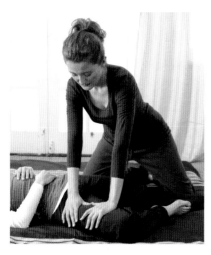

2 The therapist massages one side of the leg, then progresses to the other, positioning the leg so she can access the different meridian or *Sen* points with her palms and thumbs.

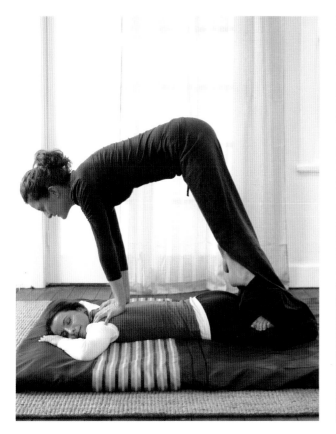

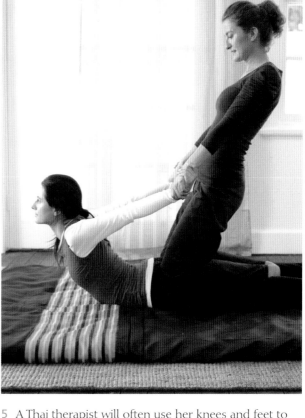

4 She then massages the arms, chest and face before turning the client over and massaging the backs of her legs, buttocks, back and shoulders.

5 A Thai therapist will often use her knees and feet to apply pressure on the stronger areas as well as give a range of stretches, including the cobra stretch.

KEY PRINCIPLES

● *Originally practised by Buddhist monks in temples, traditional Thai massage works on the belief that* Sen *or energy lines run through the body. The trained therapist works on these energy lines to release any blockages and also to allow the muscles and joints to return to their optimal movement. During the treatment, the recipient can experience healing on physical, emotional and mental levels as her body's natural equilibrium is restored to balance.*

● *Treatments start with the feet but focus on the legs, where the energy lines affecting the upper half of the body are located. The therapist treats the rest of the body by using her thumbs, hands, palms, knees and feet to manipulate the muscles and stretch them out.*

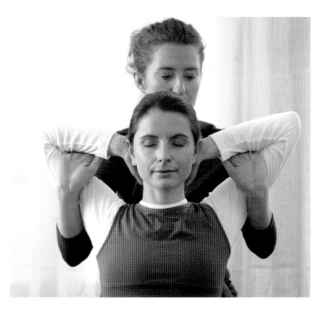

6 The receiver should sit up so the therapist can massage her neck and shoulders efficiently, using her forearms and elbows to push down and loosen the muscles of the shoulders. She then massages the neck with thumb and finger pressure. This revitalising treatment ends with stretches to both the shoulders and the neck.

CAUTIONS ● See 'Safety and cautions', page 134.
● As Thai massage involves a lot of stretching, take care when working with the elderly; anyone with circulatory, heart or disc conditions; and those individuals with knee or hip problems.

Indian massage

Originally developed by Indian women to keep hair thick and healthy and the scalp relaxed and tension-free, this massage style, part of the ancient Ayurvedic healing system, has been practised in India for more than 1000 years.

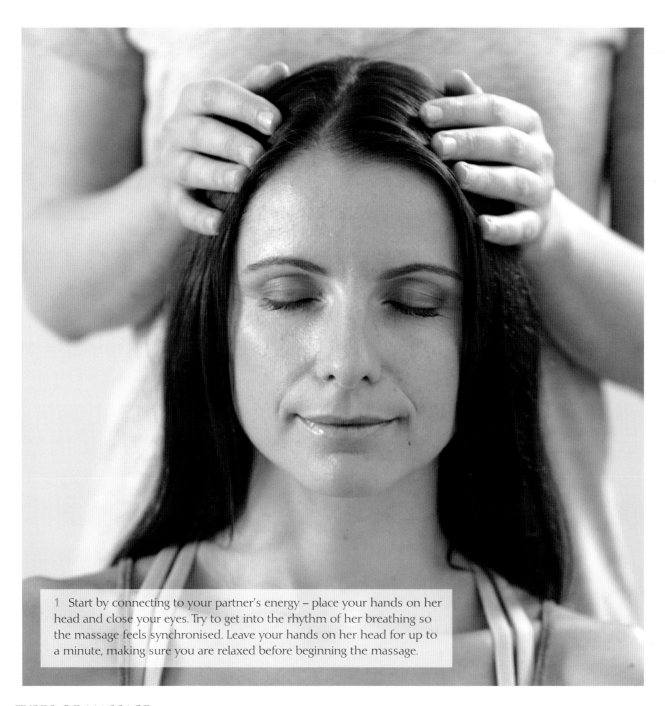

1 Start by connecting to your partner's energy – place your hands on her head and close your eyes. Try to get into the rhythm of her breathing so the massage feels synchronised. Leave your hands on her head for up to a minute, making sure you are relaxed before beginning the massage.

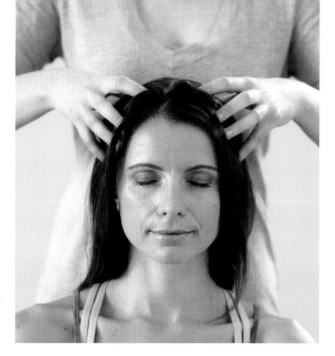

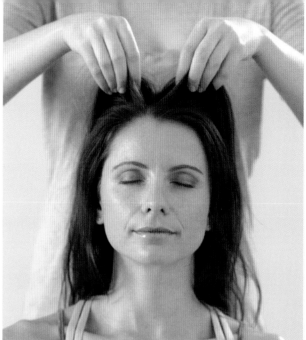

2 Gently begin by moving your fingers and thumbs in circles over your partner's scalp so she relaxes and unwinds. Slowly apply a little firmer pressure, making sure you have covered the entire scalp, then work in more firmly with your fingertips, devoting specific attention to the temples.

3 This technique is called ruffling or plucking. Placing your hands in a C-shape, pluck your partner's hair, ruffling it as you lift it up. Repeat this a few times, then slowly move your hands in a zigzag motion, trying not to pull her hair too hard.

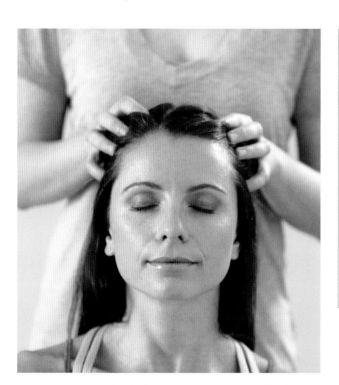

4 A great way to finish the treatment is to stroke the hair away from the face. Starting at the edge of the scalp, use your fingers and move them back through the length of the hair a few times. As you near the end of the move, grab the ends of the hair and lightly pull.

KEY PRINCIPLES

● *Becoming more and more popular in other parts of the world as more people visit the East and experience it, Indian head massage is often used during or at the end of treatments.*

● *Head massage plays an important role in Indian family life, and women often practise it on other family members, using herbs, spices and oils, depending on seasonal availability; hairdressers and barbers also practise it as part of their trade.*

● *This wonderfully relaxing and soothing treatment helps relieve tension, stress and anxiety, quietening the mind and easing headaches. It also stimulates the circulation of the scalp, nourishing the roots and helping promote strong and healthy, lustrous hair. You can apply it with or without oil.*

CAUTIONS ● See 'Safety and cautions', page 134. ● Do not apply the massage if your partner has a migraine, inflammation of the scalp or any recent whiplash or neck injury.

Hawaiian massage

Kahuna ('healer') or Lomi Lomi ('massage') massage is a wonderfully flowing and energetic style that originated in Hawaii. The therapists use their arms and hands over your body while they move freely around the table.

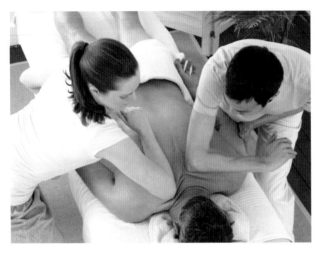

1 Loosely drape your partner with a sarong or towel. Starting at one shoulder, massage with your hands, warming up the area before gently working in with your forearms around and down the arm. Continue the move with your other arm massaging down the back.

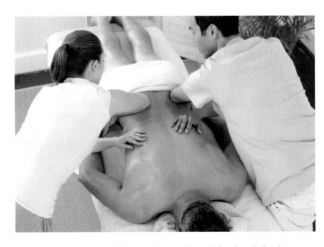

2 Massage up and down that side of the back before treating down one side of the leg, then come back up. Pay specific attention to the hip area, using your forearms around the lower back. Rotate your hands so you massage the side of the hip, then go back down the leg.

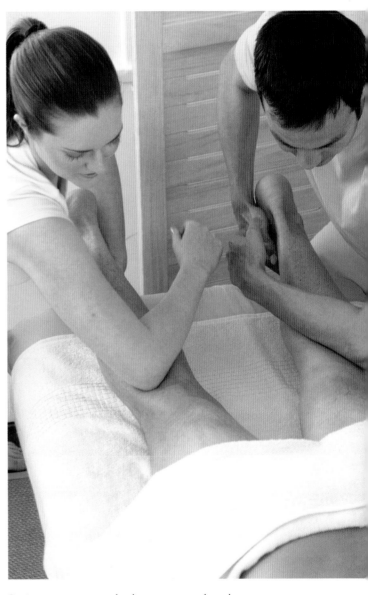

3 As you massage the leg, cup your hands so your fingertips are treating the muscles underneath. Move onto the lower leg, bending it at the knee and massaging one foot with your forearm and hand before moving back up the lower leg. Continue on the back.

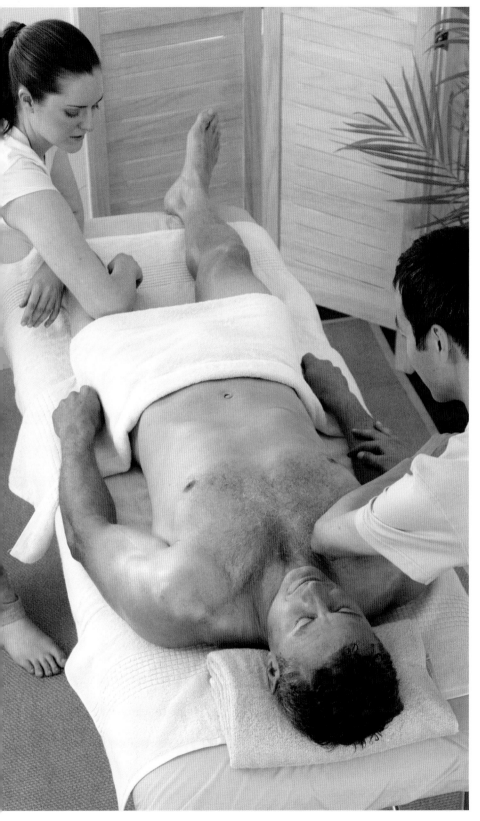

● *Also known as loving hands,
Hawaiian massage is based
on a philosophy of healing
called* Huna, *which advocates
that everything seeks harmony
and love, and that the flow of
energy through the body can
be blocked by ideas or beliefs
as well as tight muscles.*

● *The therapist's goal is to
release blockages in the body
while redirecting energy, so
she uses oil to massage over
the body from the head to
the toes, working in fluid
rhythmical motions with her
hands and forearms, and
perhaps humming and adding
dance movements, working
down one side of the body
at a time. Hawaiian massage
is often applied intuitively, as
the therapist senses what the
body needs. Treatments can be
given by one or more people.*

CAUTIONS ● See
'Safety and cautions',
page 134. ● Some-
times the breasts are
included in the massage,
so before you start,
check whether it's
acceptable for your
partner. You might
feel a little unbalanced
after the treatment
as your energies
realign themselves.

4   Complete these moves on both sides before carefully turning over your
partner. Re-drape him with the sarong or towel before massaging the chest
and arms. Finish with both sides of the legs. Allow your partner time to
become alert after this powerful massage, as it is quite deep and he might
feel rather light-headed afterwards.

Hot stone massage

Fast becoming one of the most popular treatments in the beauty, spa and massage industries, hot stone massage involves placing hot stones on the *chakra* points and massaging them into the body with oil.

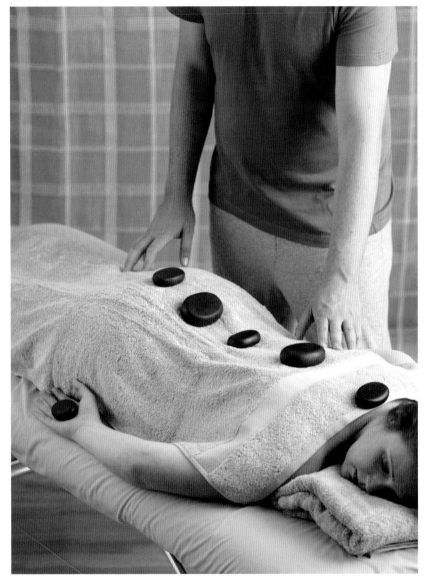

CAUTIONS ● See 'Safety and cautions', page 134.
● This treatment should not be given to anyone who is pregnant or has diabetes or circulatory, heart, respiratory, skin or blood pressure conditions.

KEY PRINCIPLES

● The current hot stone movement originated in the United Kingdom and the United States in the early 1990s, but the Chinese, Japanese, Hawaiians and Native Americans have used stones and rocks for centuries for different forms of healing, including cleansing the body and warming the abdomen to assist digestion.

● Typically, basalt, marble and sometimes jade stones are used. Basalt, a volcanic rock, is used because of its heat-retaining properties. The stones are heated in a water heater and placed over the body to warm the muscles before the massage and also to stimulate the seven major chakra points. They are then massaged into the body to stimulate blood flow as well as release tension and stress.

● Marble stones, which are naturally cool, are placed in a bowl of chilled water and then used to massage certain parts of the body, including the face.

1　The therapist consults his client before asking her to undress and lie face down on the table. First, he drapes the body, then he removes the hot stones from the special water heater and dries them. Without removing the towel, he places the stones on the specific *chakra* points of the back and on the palms of the hands.

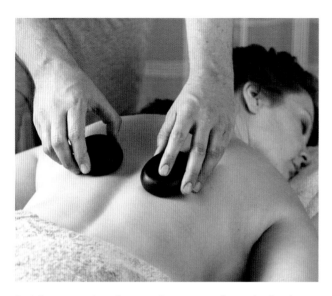

2 After removing the standing stones from the back area and the palms, he uses oil to apply effleurage over the back before using petrissage with the hot stones to work out muscular tension and adhesions. He massages the backs of the legs, then turns her over, redraping her before placing the stones on the *chakras* on the front.

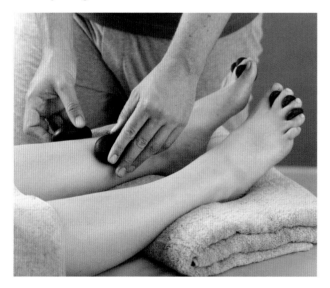

3 With the client's legs undraped, the therapist applies oil and begins massaging the feet. Once the legs are warmed and relaxed, he uses the stones to massage the heels, then positions stones between the toes before continuing the treatment on the legs.

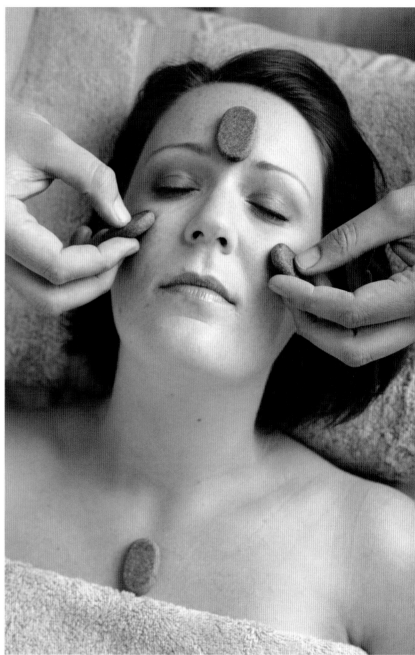

4 The therapist then gently massages the abdomen, always in a clockwise direction. He applies effleurage to the chest area and arms with oil, then kneads with the stones before finishing on the face with marble stones.

Beauty or facial massage

Create a salon or day spa at home with a beauty or facial massage –
a fantastic way to cleanse, moisturise, revitalise and treat your skin.
Take special care to choose products that best suit your skin type.

KEY PRINCIPLES

● *Facial massage, which assists in the body's natural skin-shedding process and the removal of follicle blockages, comprises four stages: basic cleansing; deep cleansing, which focuses on your skin type and its condition; Swedish massage; and, finally, a mask.*

● *After the first round of cleansing, which removes makeup and dirt so the skin is easier to assess, choose products that suit your partner's skin. Deep cleansing involves exfoliation, although brush cleaning and vaporising can also be used.*

● *Using cream or oil, apply Swedish massage to the face. This extremely relaxing technique improves lymph flow and circulation and also soothes nerve endings. Finally, apply a setting, non-setting or specialised mask. Once you have removed the mask, finish this nourishing treatment with toner and moisturiser.*

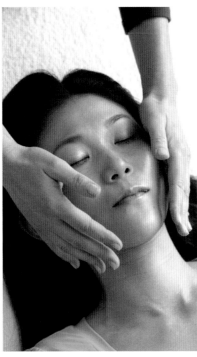

1 After an initial consultation, and with your partner lying face up, remove any makeup or dirt by cleansing her face, neck and décolletage. Taking your time, apply cleanser – use special products such as milks, lotions, creams and antibacterial washes – to all areas, then repeat.

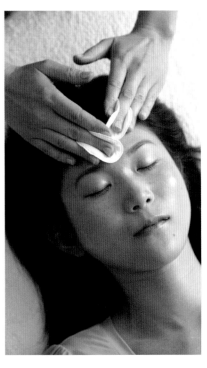

2 Now that the skin is clean and clearer, determine exactly which products to use. Take special note of the condition of the skin and whether it is dehydrated, blemished, sensitive or mature. Then exfoliate the skin, wait for the recommended time, or until it is dry, and remove it slowly and gently.

CAUTIONS ● See 'Safety and cautions', page 134. ● Be careful if your partner has hypersensitive skin or sinus issues.

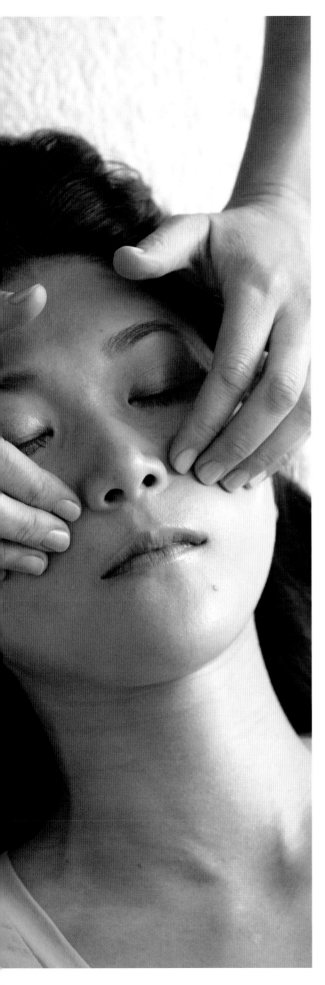

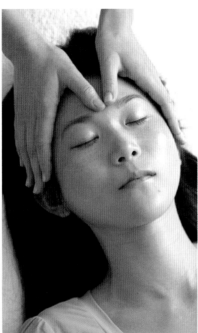

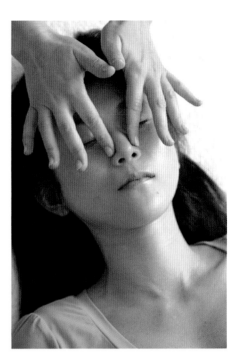

3 The next stage is a Swedish massage to the face and neck. With flexible hands and smooth motions, apply slow rhythmical strokes (left and above left), using mainly effleurage, with some kneading (above right), frictions and light tapping. This helps to strengthen and tone muscles in the face and also soften the skin.

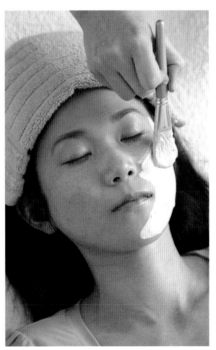

4 Apply a mask, either a powdery substance mixed with liquid or a mix made from natural products such as strawberries, yoghurt or honey. Wait until it dries, then remove it completely. Clean the face with warm towels before applying toner and, finally, moisturiser.

Lymphatic massage

With sessions as brief as 20 minutes for acute conditions, this wonderfully gentle massage style, designed to cleanse the body, is a fantastic way to boost the immune system, treat cellulite and remove excess fluid from the body.

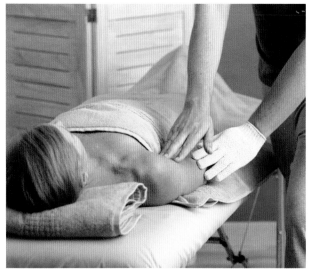

1 Once your partner is settled on the table, you could place a relaxing eye pad, to which you've added 2 drops of lavender essential oil, over her eyes. Then, using either a soft brush or a glove, apply a skin-brushing technique over the areas to be massaged. Apply the techniques in a light rhythmic manner, always towards the heart.

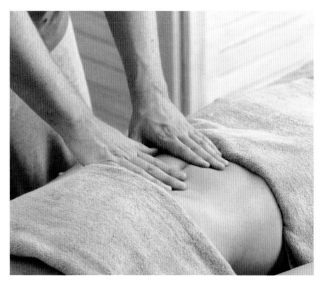

2 The sequence continues with some deep abdominal breathing to assist with relaxation. Use a gentle rocking movement with the palms of your hands, called pulsing, to nurture your partner. Then begin the massage on the neck area, always using soft pressure, and continue on the areas where you have brushed the skin.

KEY PRINCIPLES

● *Lymphatic massage was developed during the 1930s by Dr Emil Vodder and Dr Estrid Vodder, who used it to treat a variety of conditions, including sinus infections, acne and swollen lymph nodes resulting from sickness. It is now used in hospitals and by qualified massage therapists to treat a variety of ailments and conditions, from oedema and arthritis to sports injuries.*

● *This technique is designed to maximise the lymphatic system, which is responsible for the body's immune system, and relies on muscle movement and contraction to* move around the lymph fluid. Skin brushing stimulates the skin and also improves its circulation, texture and function. These techniques help remove any excess fluid from the muscles and joints, making lymphatic massage an effective treatment for swollen ankles resulting from accidents or sprains.

● *Although lymphatic massage is gentle, the techniques of stretch effleurage, palpation and vibration might leave the receiver feeling a little unsettled at first, but after the treatment she should feel as if her body is functioning more efficiently.*

CAUTIONS ● See 'Safety and cautions', page 134.
● Except for basic conditions such as puffy ankles or blocked sinuses, only a trained therapist should administer lymphatic massage. ● As the body eliminates toxins and wastes released from lymph nodes and nodules during the massage, the receiver might feel a little worse before she feels better.

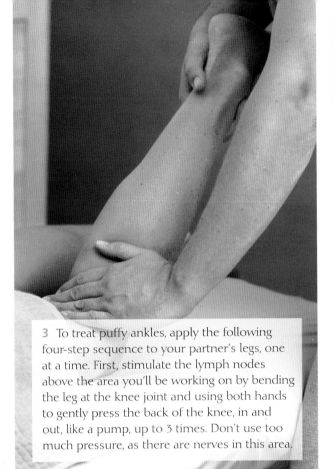

3 To treat puffy ankles, apply the following four-step sequence to your partner's legs, one at a time. First, stimulate the lymph nodes above the area you'll be working on by bending the leg at the knee joint and using both hands to gently press the back of the knee, in and out, like a pump, up to 3 times. Don't use too much pressure, as there are nerves in this area.

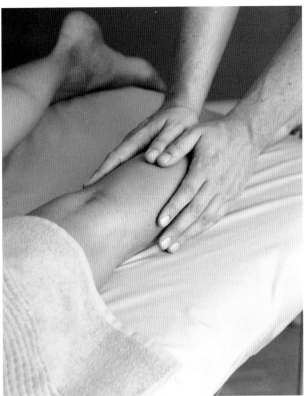

4 Place both palms on the lower leg. Slowly and gently move them up, imagining that you are pushing any fluid up the leg. Repeat up to 5 times. This prepares the leg to receive any extra fluid from the ankles.

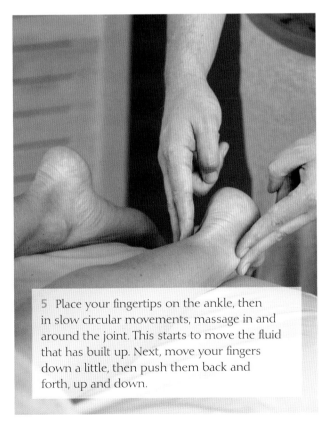

5 Place your fingertips on the ankle, then in slow circular movements, massage in and around the joint. This starts to move the fluid that has built up. Next, move your fingers down a little, then push them back and forth, up and down.

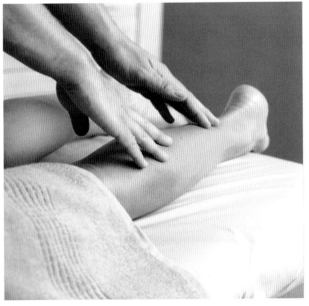

6 To finish, gently stroke back up the leg, making sure you include the back of the leg. Do this a few times, then repeat the sequence as needed. Your partner can also tap her foot up and down to help her muscles push up the lymph. Afterwards, ask her to elevate her leg to assist the detox process.

Reflexology

According to reflexology, running through the body are ten zones that are reflected in the corresponding region of the foot. It's believed that by massaging certain points on the foot, you can help heal any imbalances.

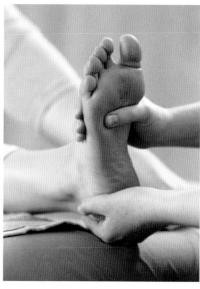

2 Holding the foot with one hand, the therapist works with the thumb of the other hand back and forth over the diaphragm line (refer to the diagram opposite) while the client breathes slowly and deeply. This technique is designed to help the receiver breathe more easily.

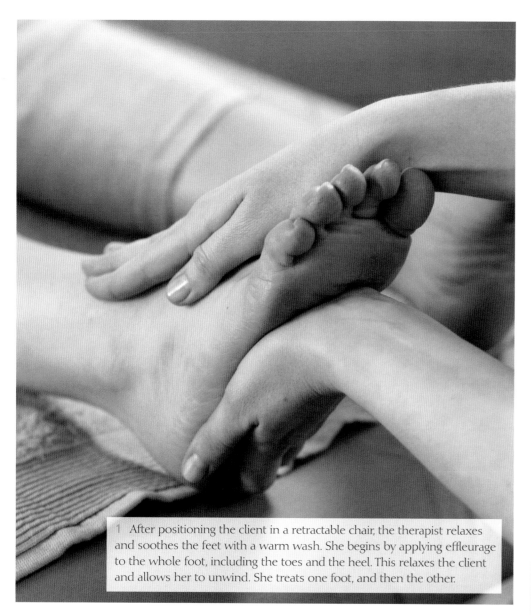

1 After positioning the client in a retractable chair, the therapist relaxes and soothes the feet with a warm wash. She begins by applying effleurage to the whole foot, including the toes and the heel. This relaxes the client and allows her to unwind. She treats one foot, and then the other.

KEY PRINCIPLES

● *Reflexology examines the relation between the areas of the feet or hands and the rest of the body via a reflex zone system. A qualified therapist will massage the feet, relaxing and rejuvenating them while working on the relevant areas of the body.*

● *Before the treatment the reflexologist will conduct a consultation, but it actually begins when she touches the feet, feeling for sore and restricted areas she will massage.*

● *Relaxation techniques are always used first before the reflexologist uses thumb and finger pressure in a rhythmical manner to stimulate and rejuvenate the different points. The treatment finishes with gentle stretching.*

CAUTIONS ● See 'Safety and cautions', page 134. ● Some points on the foot and also the plantar fascia might be very sensitive to touch, so a trained reflexologist will go in slowly and build up to more pressure over a few treatments.

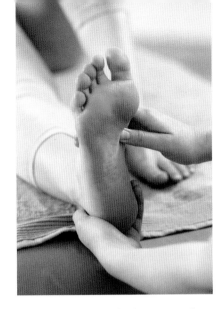

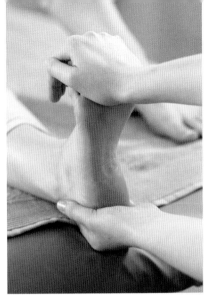

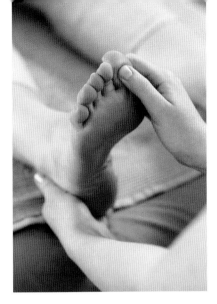

3 Beginning with the big toe and finishing at the heel, the therapist starts massaging the whole inside of the foot. As you can see in the diagram below, this area is said to relate to the spine. She presses the different points to assist with back, shoulder or neck pain.

4 Between movements, she uses effleurage moves to help keep the client in a blissful state. Then she applies massage to the heels, using a slow, even pressure from both palms, back and forth. She finishes with stretching out the ankle joint and the Achilles tendon.

5 Next, she massages the toes and works over calluses and any corresponding regions of the head, brain and sinus areas that need to be stimulated, including the tops of the toes for respiratory conditions. She finishes with a general foot massage and gentle stretching.

REFLEX POINTS ON THE FEET

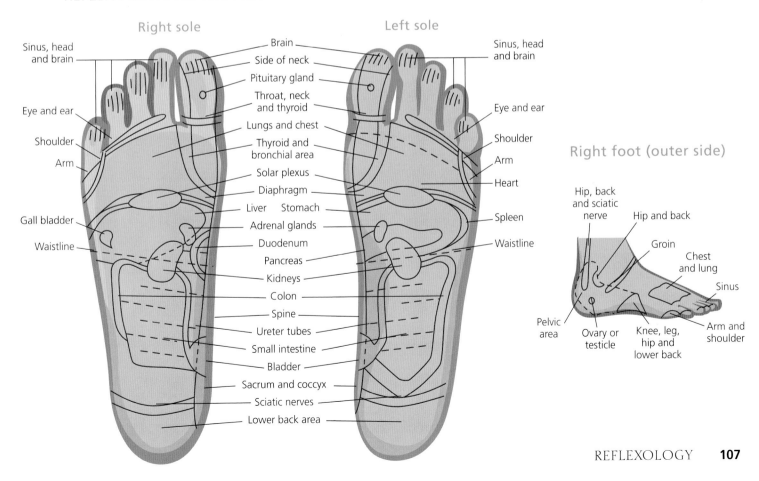

Right sole

Left sole

Sinus, head and brain
Brain
Side of neck
Pituitary gland
Sinus, head and brain

Eye and ear
Throat, neck and thyroid
Lungs and chest

Shoulder
Thyroid and bronchial area
Eye and ear

Arm
Solar plexus
Shoulder

Diaphragm
Arm

Liver   Stomach
Heart

Gall bladder
Adrenal glands
Spleen

Waistline
Duodenum
Pancreas
Waistline

Kidneys

Colon

Spine

Ureter tubes

Small intestine

Bladder

Sacrum and coccyx

Sciatic nerves

Lower back area

Right foot (outer side)

Hip, back and sciatic nerve
Hip and back
Groin
Chest and lung
Sinus

Pelvic area
Ovary or testicle
Knee, leg, hip and lower back
Arm and shoulder

Seated massage

All you need for a seated massage is a chair and a willing participant, but you can create a relaxed ambience with essential oils, candles and some soft music before trying this easy and efficient technique on a friend or loved one.

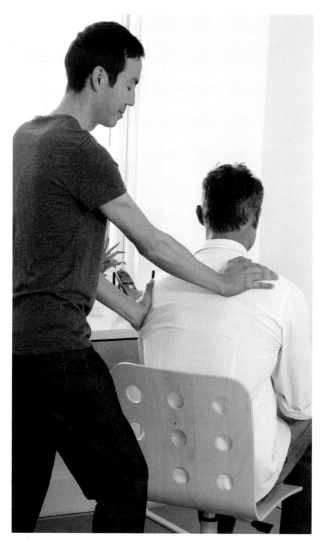

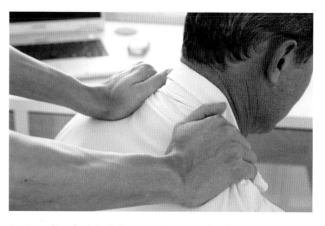

2 Standing behind the receiver, gently place your hands over the trapezius muscle and squeeze gently. This will allow blood to rush to the area, helping to release tension. Hold for 10–15 seconds, then release. Repeat this move up to 3 times.

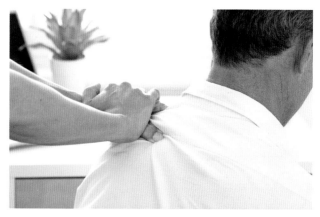

1 With the receiver facing forwards on a low chair, leaning on pillows, massage the back with your hands and palms. Make contact at the top of the hips, then warm the back muscles by applying pressure up the sides of the spine. Standing to one side, use your palms to push the muscles a little away from the spine on the side opposite to you. Repeat on the other side.

3 Kneading allows you to work into any knots in the shoulders. Start at the middle of the shoulder blades and, with your thumbs, use friction to massage into the muscles. Then knead into the tops of the shoulders. Repeat this up and down, up to 3 times.

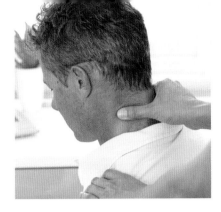

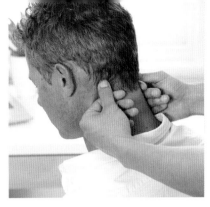

4 Standing alongside the receiver, massage into the neck. Use the inside of your thumb and index finger to gently knead from the shoulder to the base of the neck until the muscles start to soften.

5 Next, massage the base of the skull with both thumbs to help relieve tension. Working your way along the ridge, press in and hold for up to 15–20 seconds. If the receiver feels too much pain, stop.

CAUTIONS ● See 'Safety and cautions', page 134. ● Take care not to use too much pressure when massaging, especially in the neck area. ● Be careful not to work over the spine, which will be obscured by clothing. See page 134.

KEY PRINCIPLES

● *Seated massage allows perfect access to the shoulder, neck, back and head – the areas most affected by working at a computer. These areas include postural muscles that are involved in holding your body upright and preventing it from slouching. As they tire, your posture weakens, and that's when you can experience muscular problems.*

● *A lot of people hold their stress in the shoulders, so massaging them eases tension in the muscles and frees up the neck muscles, which are responsible for holding up the head. In their constant fight against gravity, these get tense from the considerable weight of the head. Seated massage assists the circulation of blood to the head by relaxing the neck muscles, which in turn allows more movement.*

● *The massage often starts with a back rub with the palms and then progresses onto the shoulders and neck. It can finish with a head massage, which stimulates circulation and blood flow, re-energising and refreshing the recipient.*

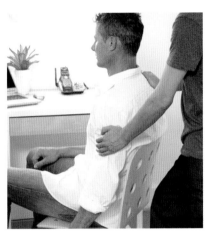

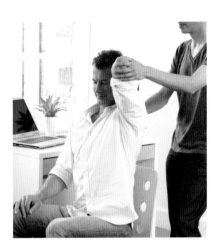

6 With the receiver's arms hanging down by his sides, massage into the arm muscles with holding and kneading techniques. Start at the upper arms and massage all the way down to the forearms. Do both sides.

7 Ask him to bend one arm back and try to touch his shoulder at the back. Place your hand on the elbow and gently stretch the arm back for up to 15 seconds. *Do not* try this if he has ever dislocated his shoulder.

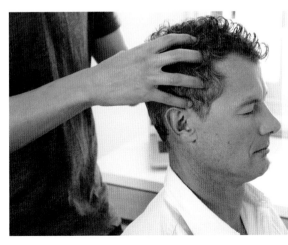

8 Using the pads of your fingers, finish the treatment with a relaxing, slow and rhythmical massage to the head and scalp. Massage the front of the scalp, then work your way over the whole head.

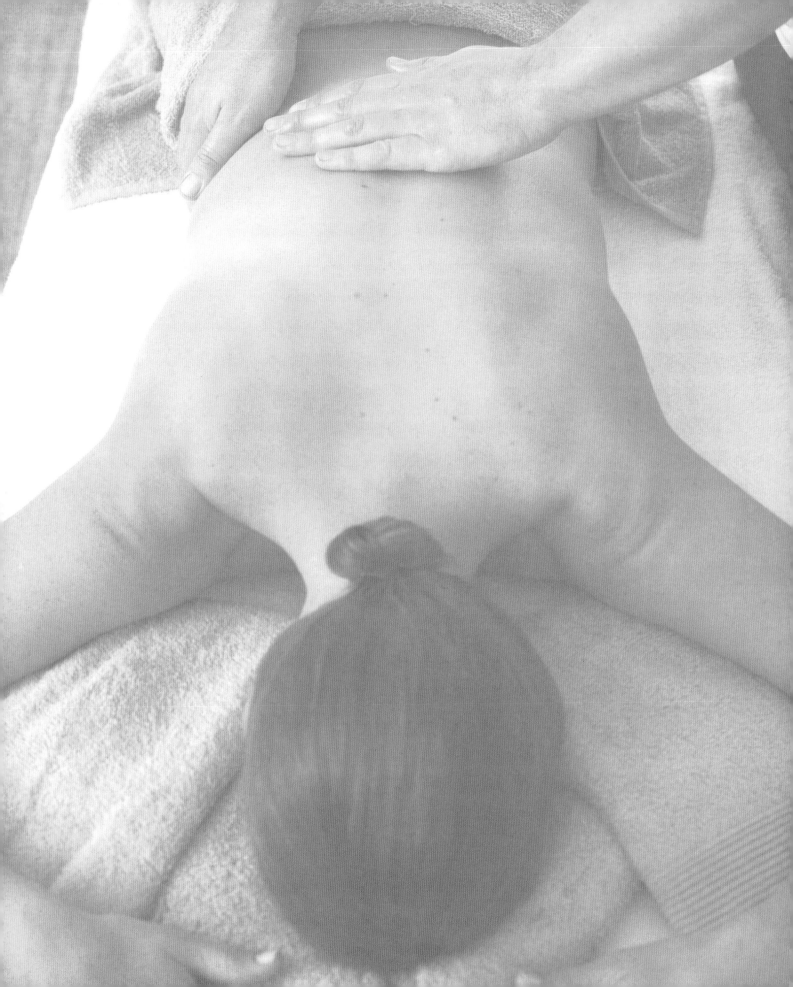

TECHNIQUES

Effleurage

A very relaxing technique that relies on soft touch combined with gentle gliding, effleurage is the simplest massage technique in aromatherapy/ Swedish massage. Use it with oil to warm up and soothe muscles during massage and also as a transition move from one area to another.

BENEFITS • Improves circulation by enhancing blood flow and assisting with waste and toxin removal.
• Relaxes, soothes and releases tight, tender muscles.

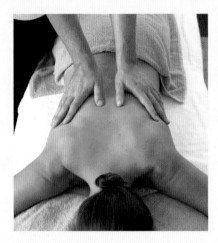

Rowing stroke
Apply slow, easy pressure up the back in a rhythmic sequence to the shoulders, then separate your hands and return them down the sides.

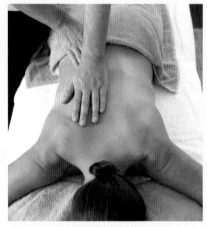

Hand after hand
Start with one hand moving up and the other following. After a short gliding move, lift one hand up as the other comes underneath it.

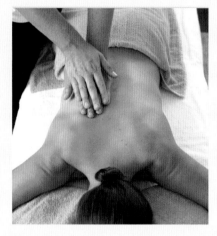

Supported hands
Place one hand palm down, the other on top, and apply slow, even pressure, working up the body. At the shoulders, use lighter pressure.

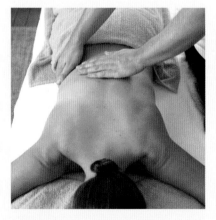

Side pulls
From the other side of the body, pull both hands towards the middle of the body in a rhythmic manner.

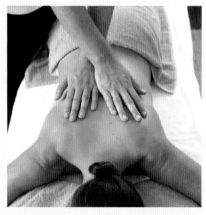

Figure-8
Glide your hands up both sides of the spine, across the shoulders and down, crossing hands in the middle.

The word 'effleurage' is derived from the French verb effleurer, meaning 'to brush against, to skim over or to touch lightly'.

➡ *'Swedish massage', page 86*
• *'Full body sequence', pages 136, 154*

Holding

Used to warm, relax and mobilise the muscle tissues, the holding technique involves grasping an area of the body, such as an arm or a leg, and holding it for a brief period. You can also use it to start and finish a massage treatment, or as a way to communicate empathy.

CAUTIONS
- See 'Safety and cautions', page 134.
- Do not apply too strong a pressure.
- Do not apply over a varicose vein.
- Do not apply over any bruising.

BENEFITS • The build-up and release of slight pressure results in improved circulation in that area.

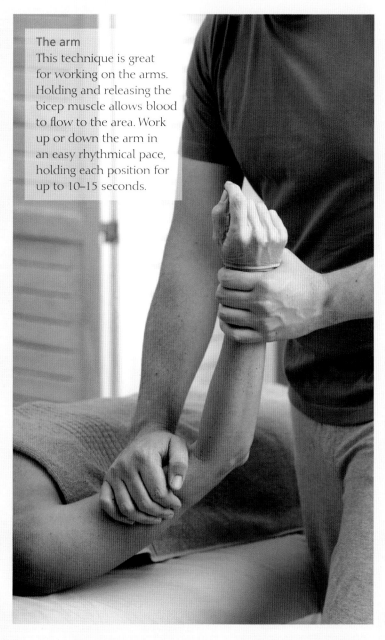

The arm
This technique is great for working on the arms. Holding and releasing the bicep muscle allows blood to flow to the area. Work up or down the arm in an easy rhythmical pace, holding each position for up to 10–15 seconds.

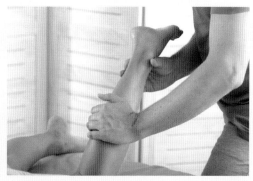

The leg
Holding is effective for relieving tension in the bigger muscle areas of the lower and upper legs. As with the arms, hold and release the legs, but use a slightly firmer pressure so you can reach the deeper layers.

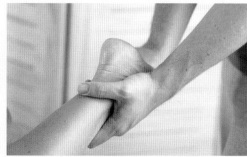

The foot
This technique is a basic move in reflexology or when massaging the feet – use it to hold the foot in place while you apply massage with the other hand. Hold the foot being massaged, compress a little and then release. This helps any tension to dissipate.

➜ 'Reflexology', page 106

Feathering

A lighter version of stroking, sometimes known as nerve stroking, feathering involves moving the fingers in a light, slow rhythm over the area. It can also be applied above the skin, thus moving energy in the energetic field surrounding the receiver. Some people may find it ticklish.

BENEFITS ● Stimulates the nerve endings on the surface of the skin.

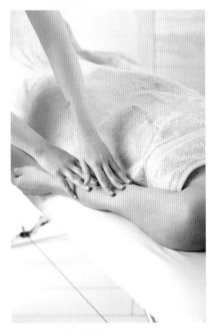 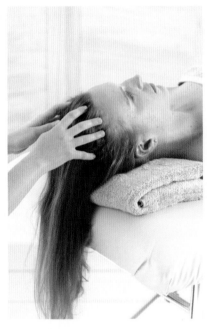 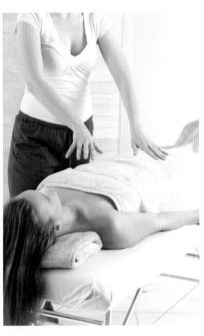

Any area of the body
Feathering can be used over any area of the body. Very lightly, just touching the skin, move your fingers across the body part. This will stimulate your partner's hair follicles and nerve endings. When reaching the end of the move, flick the fingers away, imagining that you're removing any tension or toxins from the body.

The head
You can also apply feathering over the head. Starting at the crown, gently move your fingers through the hair in a fanning movement. Slowly work up or down, moving your fingers through the hair as you go. This blissfully relaxing technique can make tension or stress drain away from the face and head.

The aura
Apply this feathering technique to any part. It will balance energies in the body and remove any excess or dense energy from the aura. Start by holding your fingers above the area – do not let them actually touch the skin. Then flick your wrists so your fingers move away from the area. Imagine as you do this that your partner's energy is moving freely underneath your fingers.

CAUTIONS ● Take care to ensure the receiver does not interpret this stroke as a sensual move.

Stroking

Use light, fluid stroking with your fingertips to finish off the massage of an area before applying percussion, or just as a relaxing technique over any part of the body. Best used after massaging an area, this is one of the most versatile massage techniques.

BENEFITS • Rhythmic and gentle stroking stimulates the superficial muscles and nerves and assists with blood flow.

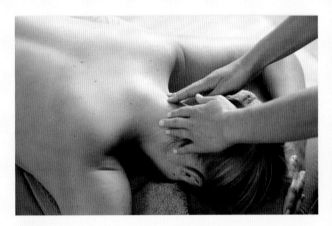

The back
Starting at the shoulders, with fingers and hands alternating, gently stroke the back, slowly working down towards the base of the spine, or start in the middle of the shoulders, and stroke towards the head and into the hair. Apply soft pressure with the fingertips, raking them softly across the skin.

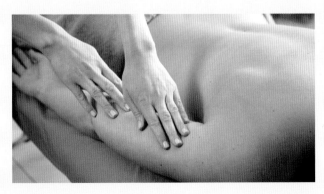

The arms
To stimulate blood flow to the fingertips, start at the top of the arms and gently stroke down towards the hands and fingers. You can also stroke in an upwards direction to stimulate and relax the arm muscles.

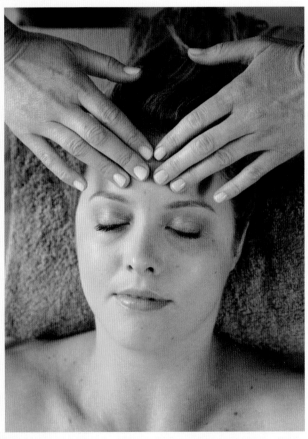

The face
When giving a facial or a lymphatic drainage massage, gently stroke the face and head. This wonderfully relaxing technique can help bring colour to the face. Start with the three middle fingers of each hand meeting at the forehead, then slowly stroke the fingers across and down, working past the temples to the bottom of the jaw. Finish by lifting and flicking off the face.

➡ *'Beauty or facial massage', page 102*
• *'Lymphatic massage', page 104*

Kneading

Kneading is always applied *after* effleurage in a Swedish treatment, once the muscles have been warmed. Applied by the thumbs, fingers or palms, this technique works on lifting, rolling, squeezing and moving around the soft tissue of the muscles to release tension.

BENEFITS • Best for working deeply on any area, kneading can increase blood flow to the muscles and skin, releasing tension in the muscles, and also assist the lymphatic system by removing waste and toxins.

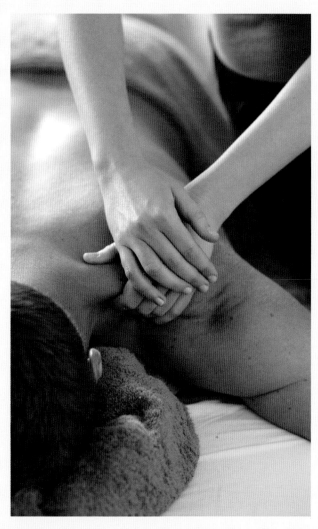

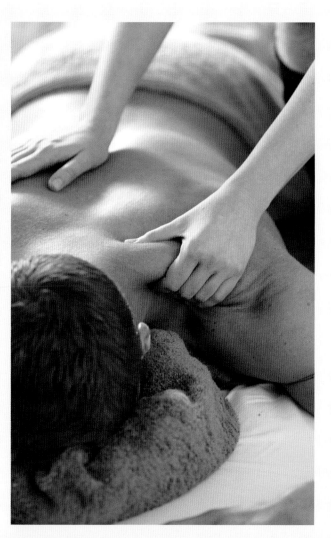

Thumb kneading
Often used on the trapezius muscle, this can also be used on the arms or legs. Apply it with one hand or two, alternately or together. Grasp the top of the shoulder with your hands, then roll your thumbs forwards and back – fantastic for releasing tension in the shoulders.

Palm kneading
This requires using your hands but applying pressure through your palms. Use it on the lower back/gluteal area, shoulders, arms and legs. Make contact with your fingertips, then lift them up as the palms of your hands come through. Continue the move up to your wrist.

Often applied over larger surface areas such as the back, shoulders or legs, this popular technique is also usually performed after effleurage. Hold both your hands in a C-position over the area to be worked. With your hands flowing in a relaxed, synchronised manner, start slow, rhythmical movements back and forth. Move your hands towards each other, then pull away. Once you can see the skin moving and stretching with your hands, you will know that the muscles underneath are loosening and relaxing, easing any tension in your partner's body.

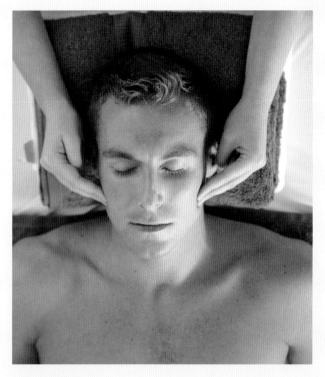

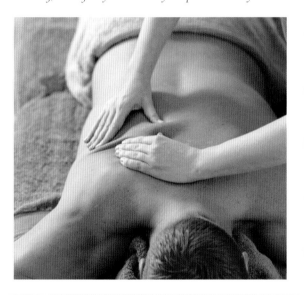

Finger kneading

Kneading with the fingers is a relaxing and rejuvenating way to massage the neck, arms, face, hands and fingers. Usually the first two fingers are used, although you can add the ring fingers as well. Gently work into the area to be massaged, moving the fingers back and forth to create a relaxing and sedative effect.

Pinching or pistol grip

Use this technique in facial massages and treatments. Bring your thumb and finger together to form a pistol grip. You can then work around the jaw line or the eyebrow areas, pinching and rolling as you go. This soothes and stretches the skin and fascia, relaxing the muscles underneath and allowing your partner to feel blissfully relaxed.

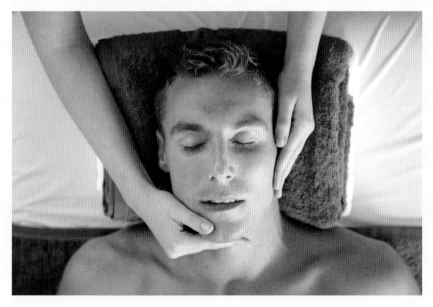

➡ *'Lymphatic massage'*, page 104

Frictions

This precise technique, which is used to move superficial muscles, fascia or skin over the bones, usually relies on small circular or straight movements over bony areas of the body. It is also a wonderfully relaxing and soothing technique when used on the temples.

BENEFITS • Best used for the hands and feet, the face and scalp or over bony areas such as the ankles and hips. • The effects include increased blood flow, reduced pain and the loosening of adhesions in the muscles.

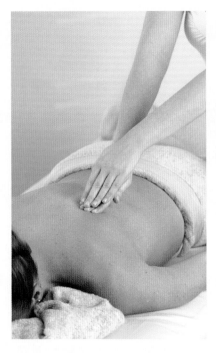 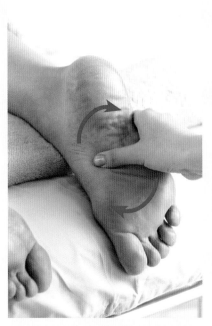 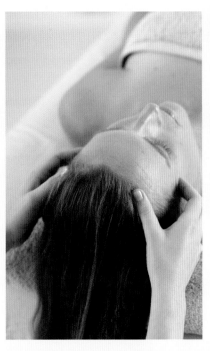

Linear or straight friction movements
Use this technique in a Swedish massage treatment to loosen up stiff back muscles. You can stand on either side of the body, but it is usually applied with reinforced hands – that is, with one hand on top of the other. Work up from the lower back to the shoulders with moderate pressure.

Circular frictions with the thumb
Frictions are beneficial for massaging the feet. Start with effleurage (see page 112), then massage into the soles of the feet with your thumbs or fingers. Circular movements applied to the front or back of the feet are very relaxing.

Circular frictions with the fingers
Use this technique on many parts of the body, including the arms, hands, feet and head. When massaging the temples, use very slow rhythmical frictions with the first two fingers to help ease the tension in the head and jaw area. When combined with essential oils, this technique can sometimes help alleviate a headache.

'Swedish massage', page 86 • 'Full body sequence', page 136

Vibrating

Vibrating is sometimes used to stir up or loosen any tension in the muscles or joints. Simply make contact with your fingers or palms and vibrate them, imagining as you do so that a wave is coming free from your hands.

BENEFITS • Vibrating is known to soothe irritated nerves, loosen scar tissue and relax muscles, but it should not be applied over vital areas such as the organs of the abdomen and lower back.

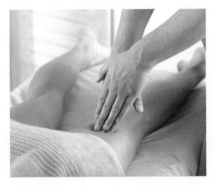

Vibration on muscle tightness
During the course of a Swedish massage, the therapist might use this technique on an area of restriction. Apply vibration by gently supporting your fingers and pressing down into the skin.

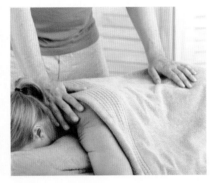

Rocking
A nurturing way to start and/or finish a massage sequence is to place your hands on the towel covering your partner, one hand on the shoulder/neck area and the other on the lower back. Very softly, apply a smooth but rhythmic rocking vibration to relax her.

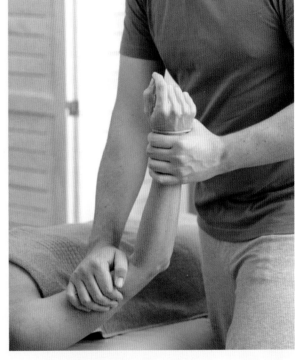

Vibrating the wrists
Use this movement at the end of the massage. Place your partner's wrist in your hand and ask her to relax her whole arm and hand. Then gently rotate your wrist back and forth, causing a vibration up the arm towards the shoulder. This relaxes the muscles and loosens the glenohumeral/shoulder joint. Repeat for the other wrist.

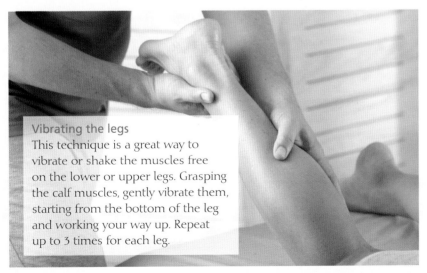

Vibrating the legs
This technique is a great way to vibrate or shake the muscles free on the lower or upper legs. Grasping the calf muscles, gently vibrate them, starting from the bottom of the leg and working your way up. Repeat up to 3 times for each leg.

➜ 'Swedish massage', page 86
• 'Full body sequence', page 136

Percussion

Used during or at the end of a Swedish/aromatherapy treatment, percussion features six techniques, all of which are applied by relaxed hands and fingers in a repeated, striking and rhythmical manner, which allows a rebound movement – a great way to bring the receiver out of a state of deep relaxation.

> **BENEFITS** • Stimulates muscle and nerve tissue.

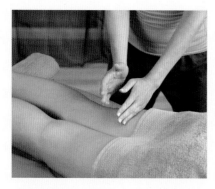

Hacking
Performed with both hands, this is a great way to stimulate your partner's muscles at the end of a treatment. Stand to the side and, with relaxed limp wrists, gently strike the large back, shoulder and leg areas in a fast chopping manner.

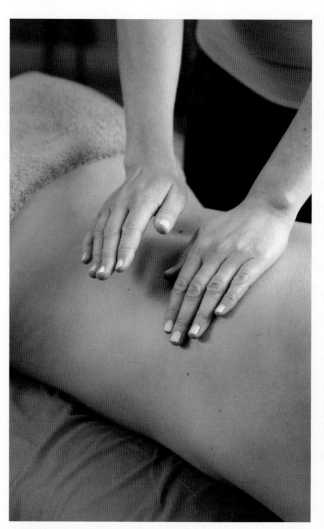

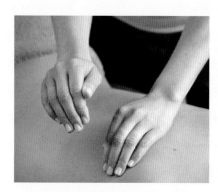

Cupping
Cupping your hands in a C-shape creates a vacuum effect that has been known to loosen and dislodge mucous build-up in the respiratory system and lung area.

Striking
This version of the percussion move can be used between cupping and pummelling. Bring both open palms down to make contact with your partner's body. This creates a slapping sound, so you may prefer to apply it through a towel or clothing.

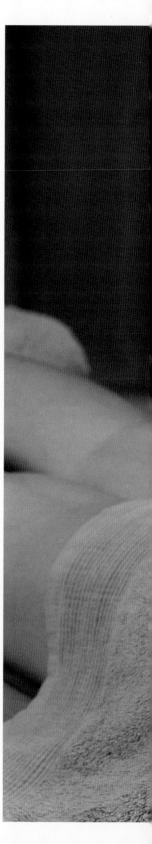

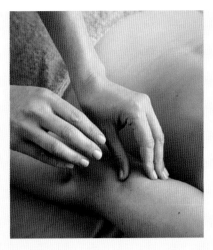

Plucking

Use this technique, which involves gently plucking or pulling at the skin, in areas where the skin is pliable, such as the legs. Pick up the superficial skin and tissues with your thumbs and first two fingers, and gently pull and release them in a relaxed and rhythmic manner.

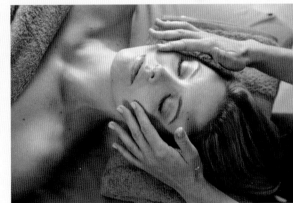

Finger tapping

Often used in aromatherapy and Swedish treatments on the face, chest or arms, this technique can be further enhanced by using alternate fingers on both sides. Slightly bend your fingers and gently tap over the area of the body you are massaging. This is the lightest of the percussion techniques and a nice way to finish.

➜ 'Aromatherapy massage', page 84
 • 'Swedish massage', page 86
 • 'Eastern or Chinese massage', page 92
 • 'Full body sequence', pages 136, 154

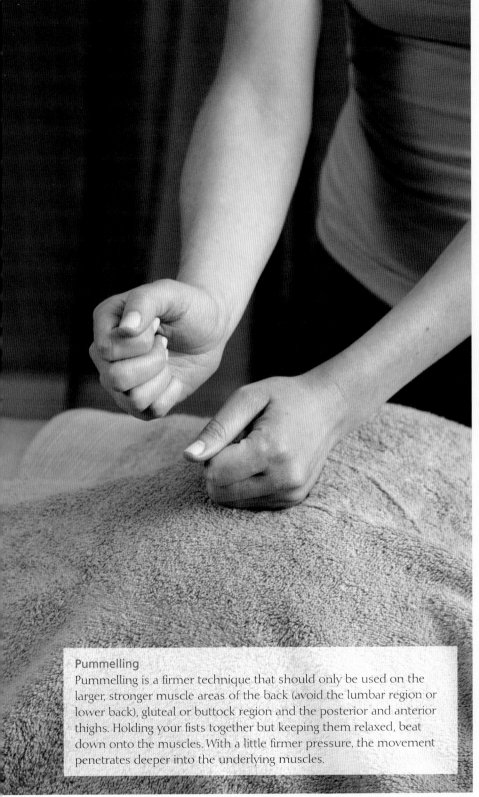

Pummelling

Pummelling is a firmer technique that should only be used on the larger, stronger muscle areas of the back (avoid the lumbar region or lower back), gluteal or buttock region and the posterior and anterior thighs. Holding your fists together but keeping them relaxed, beat down onto the muscles. With a little firmer pressure, the movement penetrates deeper into the underlying muscles.

Acupressure

This technique involves pressing down the thumbs, fingers or hands on certain points of the body for a specific effect. These points are part of an energy system that runs through the body in channels called meridians, and each meridian relates to an organ or section of the body.

> **BENEFITS** ● Best for stimulating energy points on meridian lines, which can have a flow-on effect within the body.
> ● Fantastic for relieving stress and anxiety and unblocking sinus congestion.

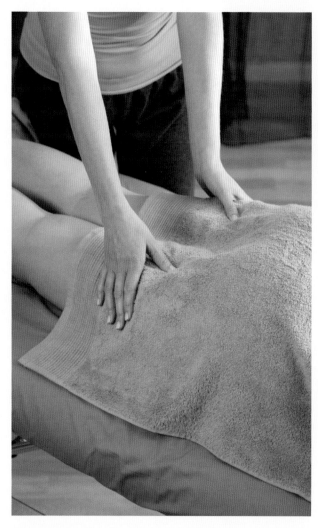

Thumb acupressure
Applied directly onto the acupressure points, this is often used in aromatherapy massage on the body, and in Swedish on the face or head. Keep your thumb as straight as possible, press the point, hold and then release. This will stimulate a particular meridian.

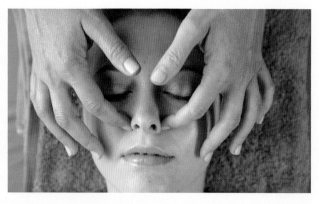

Finger acupressure
As with thumb acupressure, use the fingers on the acupressure points. This is especially useful and beneficial when working on the face, scalp and hands.

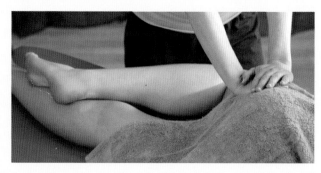

Palm pressure
To use palm or hand pressure, stand over the area you want to massage and then press down with your hands. This technique is often used over the larger areas of the body, such as the buttocks and legs, where a broader pressure is needed.

➔ 'Aromatherapy massage', page 84
● 'Swedish massage', page 86 ● 'Eastern or Chinese massage', page 92 ● 'Full body sequence', pages 136, 154

Stretching

Best given after a full massage, when the area is warm and relaxed, the stretching technique is a great way to lengthen muscle fibres so they can return to normal function. As always, only stretch within your partner's comfort level.

> **BENEFITS** • Can increase the range of motion in the joints and free the body for greater movement.

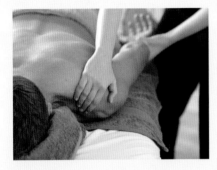

Shoulders

This technique helps to stretch the trapezius, one of the main shoulder muscles. Standing on the left side of the body, place your right hand on the left shoulder. With your other hand, gently grasp the left arm and simultaneously pull it down, stretching the shoulders and neck as you do so. Repeat on the other side.

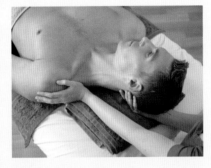

Neck

Ask your partner to lie face up. With your right hand, gently support the head and lift it up slowly; don't go too far. Place your other hand on the left shoulder and, at the same time, push the shoulder down and stretch the neck to the right. Don't try this stretch if he has disc problems in the neck or a recent whiplash injury. Repeat on the other side.

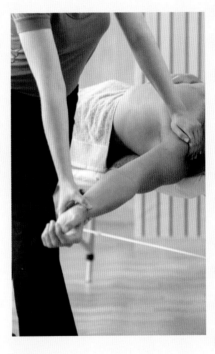

Chest

The chest is always a good area to stretch — when it tightens up, it can cause pain in the thoracic area of the upper back due to that area being pulled on excessively. Start by grasping your partner's wrist, then stretch it out at a 90-degree angle. You may need to ask your partner to move closer to the side of the table. Repeat on both sides.

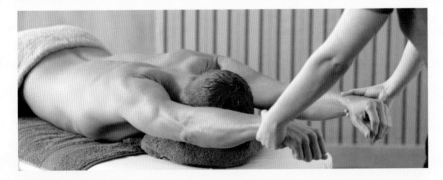

Back stretch

This is a great way to stretch through the lower and middle back area. Gently grasping your partner's wrist, lift his arms above his head, stretching them as far as is comfortable.

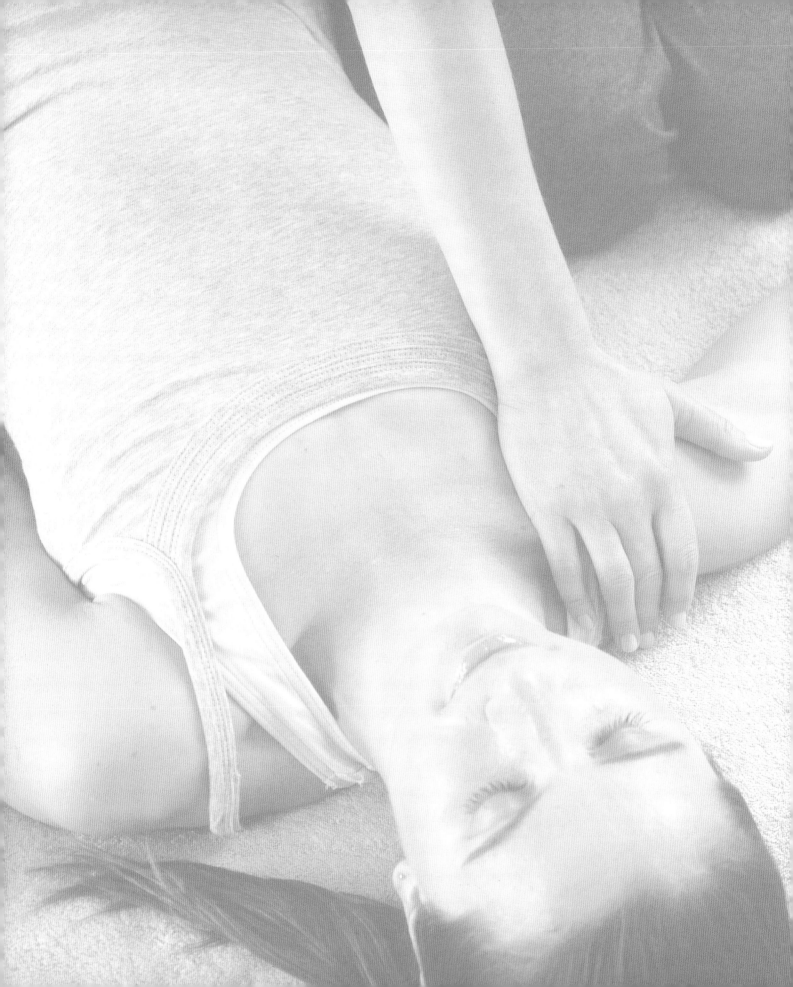

Full body
MASSAGE

Before you start

Your partner must be able to relax and unwind in order to experience the benefits of massage, so make sure you create the right mood, with muted lighting, soothing ambient music and a comfortably warm temperature.

Healing via touch and smell

With or without essential oils, massage is an evolved form of our innate instinct to offer healing via touch — seen at its simplest in a mother's attempt to 'rub it better'. With time and practice, you will develop an understanding of which essential oils and techniques work best for your partner, or for the part of your own body you're massaging.

Each practitioner of aromatherapy massage will develop their own style of giving and receiving massage. Some may prefer more vigorous strokes, such as Swedish massage (see page 86) or deep tissue massage (page 88); others may find that different systems of touch that stimulate the body, such as reflexology (page 106) or Shiatsu (page 90), have a more powerful effect on energy levels and general wellbeing.

Create the right mood

Choose a clean, uncluttered, warm and quiet room for the massage. Warmth is essential, as massage usually makes the receiver's blood pressure drop. Have a blanket, heater or extra

TOWELS AND PILLOWS

You'll need towels for draping, comfort and warmth. Be sure to choose the colour carefully, as it will contribute to the relaxing ambience of the room. One or two nice fluffy bath sheets are best, plus some normal bath towels for setting the table or massage area and covering the pillows and props. It's a good idea to have two to three pillows or boosters on hand for back, ankle, knee and head support.

towels on hand in case more heat is needed. Make sure the room is well ventilated, and add a humidifier if the air is a little stuffy or stale. Soft lighting, provided by dimmer lights or scented candles; gentle background music; and burning a few drops of a nurturing, comforting essential oil in a vaporiser will all help create a more relaxing atmosphere.

A special massage table, with a hole for the face, eases the strain on the therapist's back, and is more comfortable for the receiver. Another option is to use a large, firm table, and secure several folded blankets on top of it. Massage can also be given on a single bed, but only if it has

a firm mattress. For seated massage, use a comfortable chair.

However, for aromatherapy massage treatments at home, place a padded yoga or gym mat on the floor and cover it with a couple of large towels and a cotton bed sheet. To reduce the strain on your back, always administer the massage from a kneeling position, rather than bend from the waist.

What to wear

Freshly showered, and with your nails clipped short, wear loose, comfortable clothing and flat-heeled shoes (or go barefoot), and take off any jewellery so you won't scratch your partner.

Ask your partner to remove her clothing, glasses and jewellery, but to leave on a pair of underpants if she wishes. To keep her warm and comfortable, and also to encourage the absorption of the oil, cover with towels any parts of her body on which you are not working. Have on hand plenty of tissues and also some antibacterial wipes or spray so you can clean her feet before massaging them.

Begin the massage

Before starting the massage, warm a little aromatherapy oil that suits your partner's skin type in your hands. The amount of oil required will depend on the area to be massaged, as well as on the area

Being cold during a massage triggers the release of adrenalin, a stress hormone, which causes the muscles to stiffen and contract.

Always ask the person receiving the massage if the pressure is too firm, or too light, and stop if she indicates any pain or discomfort.

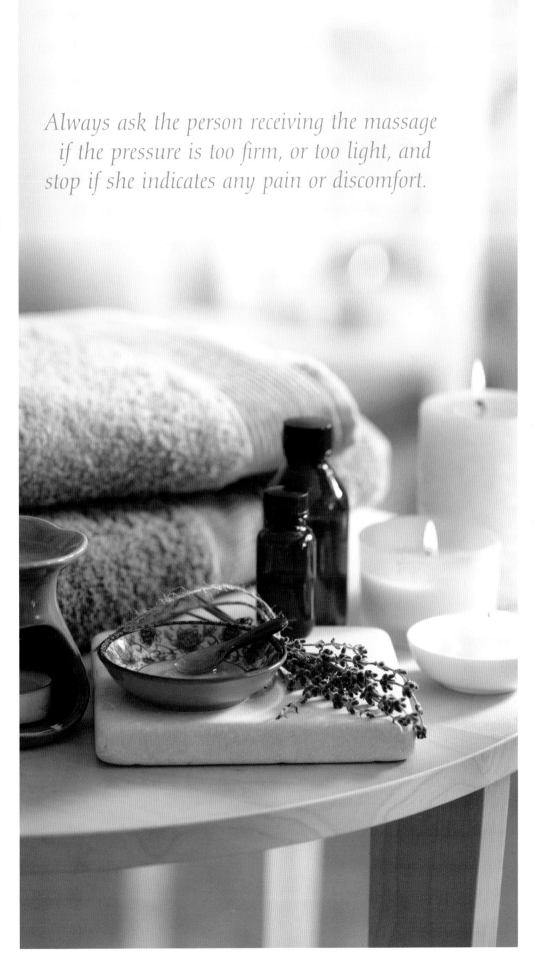

Before the massage begins, avoid eating a large meal or taking alcohol or caffeine or other stimulants; also empty your bladder. Ideally, do not watch television, listen to the radio or drive a car before the massage, and turn off your mobile phone, so you can focus your full awareness on the massage. During or just after a massage, some people may feel a little dizzy; others may even fall asleep. Drink plenty of water after the session.

of your partner's skin, whether it's hairy, or dry or oily. Start with about 1 teaspoon of oil and add more: beginning with too much oil, before it is absorbed, will make the area too slippery, while too little will drag the skin.

As you finish one stage and move around her body, gently run your hands along her limbs until you start the next stage of the massage. Use a variety of techniques to create interest and provide maximum thera-peutic benefit. Use your whole body, not just your hands — for example, when you're massaging her back, lean in with your whole body weight.

While you are massaging, aim for a relaxed and positive frame of mind, and practise deep, steady breathing so you communicate neither stress nor tension. Both you and your partner should remain quiet during the massage.

Circulatory system

The circulatory system is responsible for the movement of blood, oxygen and nutrients through the body. Various conditions contribute to a slow, sluggish circulatory system and the build-up of toxins, but massage can assist greatly.

How the system works

The whole body is dependent on blood, which carries what you need to survive. Pumped around the body by the heart through cardiac muscle contraction, the blood travels from the heart to the lungs, where it picks up oxygen, then returns to the heart.

The blood is then carried throughout the body in arteries, which have thick muscular walls. The arteries are dependent on pressure from the heart to work, but smoking, poor diet, lack of exercise and various other factors can lead to thickening of the arteries, causing the pressure to increase.

Along the way, the blood picks up nutrients from the digestive tract as well as hormones from various glands in specific locations. The heart pushes the blood out to the organs, bones, ligaments and muscles through smaller arteries called arterioles, and then through capillaries, the smallest vessels, which in turn deliver nutrients and oxygen to the cells.

An exchange occurs, producing waste and carbon dioxide, which must be filtered or eliminated from the body.

Once the blood has been exchanged, it must then return to the heart, which pumps it to the lungs. Here the blood filters the carbon dioxide out through the lungs and takes on fresh oxygen needed by the body. Finally, it is returned to the heart, and the cycle continues.

On its way back from the cells, blood is transported first through venules and then through veins up to the venae cavae. These are not as strong as the arteries, arterioles and capillaries, and are not subject to the same pressure. Instead they rely on muscle movement to move the blood back to the heart.

Veins have a non-return valve, which prevents blood from flowing backwards, but over time, and due to certain lifestyle factors, these can become built up with deposits of calcium. The result is poor circulation.

Massage is fantastic for moving the blood to the arms, hands, legs and feet, which are furthest from the heart.

CIRCULATORY SYSTEM

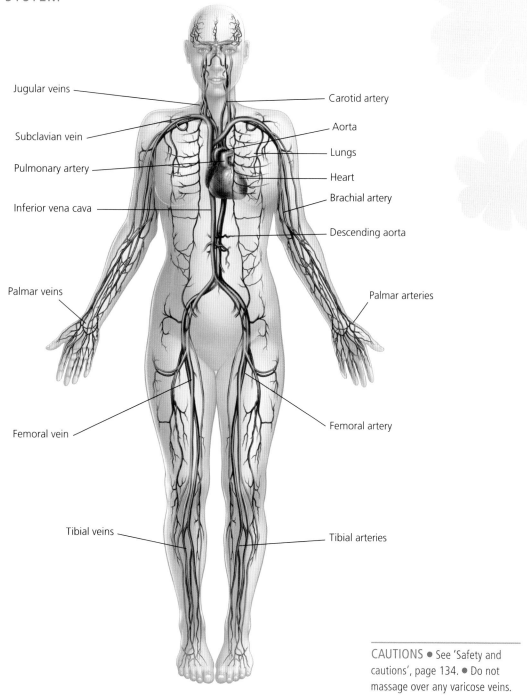

Jugular veins

Subclavian vein

Pulmonary artery

Inferior vena cava

Palmar veins

Femoral vein

Tibial veins

Carotid artery

Aorta

Lungs

Heart

Brachial artery

Descending aorta

Palmar arteries

Femoral artery

Tibial arteries

CAUTIONS • See 'Safety and cautions', page 134. • Do not massage over any varicose veins.

See also the following topics in 'For health and vitality', starting on page 176: 'Anxiety and stress', 'Arms and hands', 'Back pain', 'Brain boosters', 'Circulatory problems', 'Coughs and colds', 'Cramps', 'Digestive disorders', 'Face and scalp', 'Fatigue', 'Headaches', 'Joint pain', 'Legs and feet', 'Neck and shoulders', 'Sinus congestion', 'Sports injuries' and 'Getting older'

Muscles and joints

Regular massage and exercise both help the muscles and joints by strengthening and toning the muscles and also by increasing the range of joint movements, thus improving your body's flexibility and allowing you to move freely.

Bones

In an adult, 206 bones form the skeleton, support the body's weight, allow movement and protect the vital organs. Most muscles are skeletal muscles, which help keep your bones in position. Bones also store important bone marrow, which contains red blood cells – these are needed throughout the body.

Joints

Where a bone meets another bone, a joint is formed. Most of these have some movement, but how much depends on the type of joint. Joints can be held together by connective tissue, cartilage or a capsule that is supported by ligaments.

When muscles become tight or over-contract for long periods, preventing full movement, joint function can become limited. Old age, poor diet, bad circulation and inflammation all contribute.

Muscles

The 650 muscles are the body's movers, and skeletal muscles allow a wide range of movement. Muscles also protect the body's organs; regulate organ volume; produce heat by shivering and contracting; and pump lymph and deoxygenated blood through the blood and lymph vessels.

In order to work efficiently, each muscle needs a supply of blood rich with oxygen, fresh

The facial muscles move the skin, so massaging them helps to smooth out lines or wrinkles, thus creating a healthier, rejuvenated look.

nutrients and hormones. These are supplied in the capillaries of blood vessels when a muscle relaxes, allowing the muscle to fire or contract. This in turn causes the muscle to move by pulling on the tendons and bringing the bones together.

As muscle fibres contract, they push out the deoxygenated blood through the vein walls. They also assist with moving lymph flow. The cardiac muscle in the heart is always contracting to allow blood movement.

Contraction produces waste and natural chemical toxins. If the muscles use more oxygen than can be supplied by the blood, as in the case of an extended period of exercise, then waste products can build up. Massage is great for moving them through the body to be reabsorbed or eliminated. Use slow pressure with kneading techniques for the best effect.

Posture

Postural muscles support our bodies in an upright position. In modern society they can easily become overworked, as we tend to do things repetitively, such as

clicking a computer mouse. When a muscle is overworked, it begins to become hard, then tightens up. This can cause pain, so the surrounding muscles start to compensate. Thus the body can actually change in appearance, as with rounded shoulders.

Massage smoothes out the muscles, helping them soften and return to normal length and function. Stretching is also important.

Fatigue

Muscles can become weak and fatigued due to stress, tension and overuse, when the circulation of blood and oxygen to the muscle becomes restricted and the removal of lymph, waste or toxins becomes less efficient.

Using the techniques of effleurage, kneading and frictions can assist this immensely by moving the blood and oxygen flow into the muscles, thus helping to remove the stagnant waste that has built up.

CAUTIONS ● See 'Safety and cautions', page 134.

MUSCLES USED IN SWEDISH AND AROMATHERAPY MASSAGE

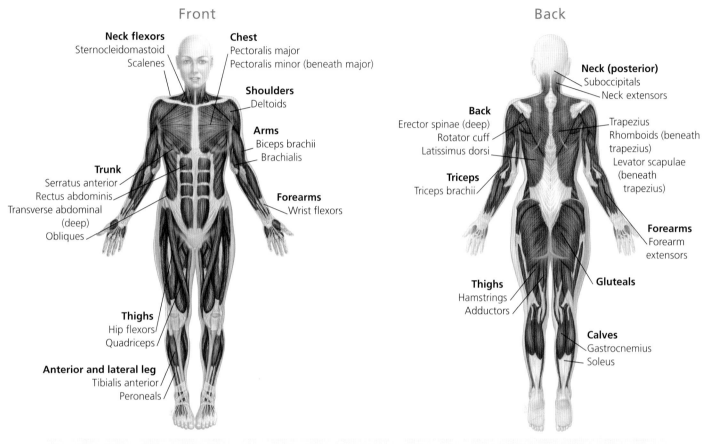

Front

Neck flexors
Sternocleidomastoid
Scalenes

Chest
Pectoralis major
Pectoralis minor (beneath major)

Shoulders
Deltoids

Arms
Biceps brachii
Brachialis

Trunk
Serratus anterior
Rectus abdominis
Transverse abdominal
(deep)
Obliques

Forearms
Wrist flexors

Thighs
Hip flexors
Quadriceps

Anterior and lateral leg
Tibialis anterior
Peroneals

Back

Neck (posterior)
Suboccipitals
Neck extensors

Back
Erector spinae (deep)
Rotator cuff
Latissimus dorsi

Trapezius
Rhomboids (beneath
trapezius)
Levator scapulae
(beneath
trapezius)

Triceps
Triceps brachii

Forearms
Forearm
extensors

Thighs
Hamstrings
Adductors

Gluteals

Calves
Gastrocnemius
Soleus

Benefits of massage for muscles, bones and joints

The benefits of massaging these parts of the body include:

1 Breaking down the adhesions that have built up through overuse with the frictions technique; the resulting improved circulation removes them.

2 Allowing lymph and venous blood to return or move through the body more efficiently – massage enhances this natural process.

3 Lengthening muscle tissue – especially beneficial for short, contracted muscles.

4 Bringing heat and friction to the tissues that speed up the body's natural chemical processes, allowing a faster recovery after exercise or sickness. It also allows the massage to gain access to the deeper layers as the superficial muscles relax.

5 Helping to remove excess fluid from the receiver's inflamed joints and limbs.

6 Improving joint mobility and movement by facilitating increased blood circulation, allowing the muscles attached to the joint to relax and taking pressure off the joint.

7 Assisting the movement of the endorphins, the 'feel good' hormones, through the body.

8 Giving the receiver of a massage an increased awareness of their body, so they become more adept at recognising tense muscles and relaxing them.

➜ *See also the following topics in 'Full body massage': 'Back sequence' (page 138) and 'Abdomen and chest sequence' (page 148); and in 'For health and vitality', starting on page 178: 'Arms and hands', 'Back pain', 'Cellulite', 'Computer-related ailments', 'Cramps', 'Eye strain', 'Face and scalp', 'Fatigue', 'Headaches', 'Insomnia', 'Joint pain', 'Legs and feet', 'Neck and shoulders', 'Posture', 'Sports injuries', 'Getting older' and 'Pregnancy'*

Lymphatic system

The lymphatic system, which fights disease or sickness, is responsible for the body's immune function as well as the transport of fats, lipids and vitamins. Massage greatly assists the lymphatic system before or after an illness.

Lymph flow

Lymph flow is a lot like blood flow – both move through the body in vessels, and both have an important role in maintaining homeostasis, or equilibrium, in the body. Lymph flow is also similar to venous blood flow, as they both need muscle movement and contraction to move around the body and back to the heart.

Lymph is collected from the excess fluid between tissue cells, where it is pushed out to the awaiting lymph capillaries. In this way the lymphatic system acts as a drainage network, especially for excess plasma proteins from cells. Up to 3 litres of excess fluid can be filtered by the body in one day. It is then transported from the capillaries to the lymphatic vessels, which carry the lymph fluid to the lymph nodes.

Lymph nodes

Lymph nodes are small bean-like, oval-shaped organs, which usually cluster together. These little nodes filter the lymph from pathogens and waste, and when you are suffering an illness, they can become sore and enlarged.

For example, when you have a sore throat, the lymph nodes in your neck will be painful and tender due to the accumulation of immune cells and dead germs. This shows that your body is fighting the viruses or bacteria that are threatening it.

These nodes can be found throughout the body, and within them are special white blood cells, called leukocytes, which can destroy invading viruses or bacteria. These cells gather, divide and then attach or destroy the threat. So the lymphatic system is the cleanser and rescuer of the body.

Once viruses or bacteria have entered the body, and the defence lines, such as the stomach, skin or mucus, cannot deal with them, it is the lymphatic system's job to begin the response. It also produces the antibodies needed to counterbalance the threat.

Lymphatic network

After filtering, the lymph proceeds along the lymphatic network, as it is pushes up through the vessels, eventually returning to the venous system via the left and right thoracic duct, which is located in the chest area. It will then return to the heart.

The other role of the lymphatic system is to transport lipids or fats and vitamins that are absorbed by the gastrointestinal tract and move them through to the blood. In a slow or sluggish immune system, toxins, waste and fluid can build up, leading to an overall feeling of being run-down and lacking energy and vitality.

This can also lead to sickness, fatigue, coughs and colds, flu, headaches, congestion (especially of the head and face, resulting in sinus problems), headaches and puffiness around the eyes.

Various factors assist the lymphatic system, including a good diet, adequate rest and sleep, and also adequate activity, which includes exercise. The lymphatic system relies on muscle movement rather than the heart to push it around the body, so exercise will greatly assist with this. In addition, drinking enough water will help flush out the system.

However, problems can occur when too much fluid remains in the body, as can happen after treatment for breast cancer, when lymph nodes may be removed in the axillary or armpit region to prevent the spread of cancer cells. This can then lead to oedema or swelling in the arms, as the fluid cannot be drained or filtered as efficiently.

CAUTIONS ● See 'Safety and cautions', page 134.

Benefits of lymphatic massage

The benefits of general massage or specific lymphatic massage for the lymphatic system include:

1   Removing metabolic wastes, which are produced by movement of the muscles, from the cells and tissues – massage helps move this waste more quickly.

2   Assisting with removing excess fluid from cells, which helps in cases of oedema or swelling. Any leftover swelling from inflammation (not acute) can be massaged into the system.

3   After a sickness, helping to move leftover toxins as well as transport fresh nutrients to a particular area.

4   Helping to move excess proteins from the cells and back into the bloodstream.

5   Assisting the body to provide immunity by preventing the build-up of toxins in one area and helping them to be moved and filtered by the lymph nodes.

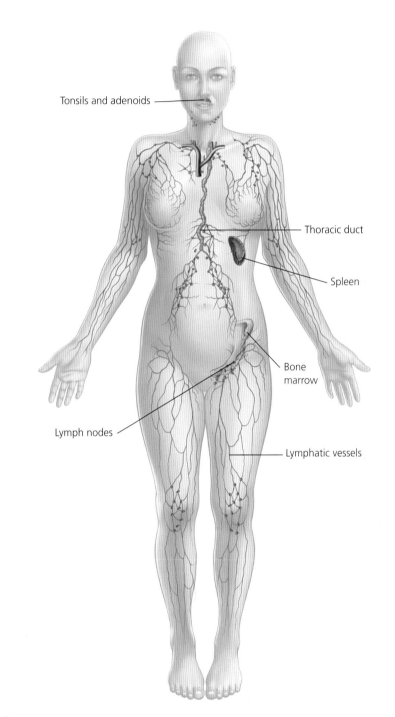

Tonsils and adenoids

Thoracic duct

Spleen

Bone marrow

Lymph nodes

Lymphatic vessels

See also the following topics in the 'For health and vitality' section, starting on page 184: 'Cellulite', 'Circulatory problems', 'Coughs and colds', 'Cramps', 'Detox', 'Digestive disorders', 'Face and scalp', 'Fatigue', 'Hangover', 'Joint pain', 'Legs and feet', 'Sinus congestion', 'Sports injuries' and 'Travel ailments'

Safety and cautions

A professional therapist will ask for details of a patient's medical history, lifestyle, diet, and mental and emotional state to find out if the treatment is likely to have any adverse effects, so follow these guidelines as best you can.

When massaging

The general rule of thumb for a massage treatment is *do no harm*, either to yourself or to the person whom you are massaging. We have provided step-by-step photographs and captions for safe, proven techniques, but at times you might want to change them a bit to suit your own body type, or just to experiment a little.

In a Swedish massage, always keep the pressure light to moderate and within the receiver's comfort level. Whenever you're in doubt, reduce the pressure or avoid doing the movement.

Food and drink

Drink plenty of water beforehand, and make sure you eat before you start, as giving a massage can be quite physical and make you very hungry. Avoid big meals so you don't feel sluggish — light snacks such as fruit or muesli bars should provide you with all the energy you need.

Practice

Give yourself time to build up to giving massage treatments. Possibly start with a limited period, such as 30 minutes, then gradually extend it. Remember to have fun. A good way to massage is to apply the techniques you'd like to be massaged with.

Always encourage feedback — this will prevent you from hurting your partner and also allow you to change what you're doing if it's not right.

Posture and breathing

It is very important to maintain a good posture throughout the treatment, otherwise you might become tired and sore, and be the one needing a massage!

Always try to keep a straight back. This will not only encourage you to use more of your body weight but will also stop you from leaning too far forwards with your neck. To encourage this, try to hold in your stomach so you activate the core muscles. Also try to use your leg muscles, not just your arms and hands, to push. This is a great way to maintain your energy levels.

Keeping your hands, wrists and shoulders as relaxed as you can will allow good transfer of force, otherwise your hands and arms might get sore. Some stretching before and after you give your partner a massage will help you stay flexible.

Maintain a good breathing pattern throughout the massage and encourage your partner to do the same. Before the massage, sit still and take three big, deep breaths, allowing the breath to reach all parts of your body. If you are tense or stressed, your partner might not be able to relax during the treatment, so always check that you are breathing well.

Try to match your breath with your partner's. This will allow you to be in synchrony with him, making it easier to perceive what is going on in his body and helping you give a better massage.

Contraindications

Whenever you're in doubt about any possible adverse effects of massage, check with a health professional. Sometimes there are local contraindications, such as inflammation to a joint or a break in the leg — that is, only one area of the body that should not be massaged.

Here are some specific contraindications to keep in mind.
- **Arthritis or rheumatism** Avoid applying strong pressure directly over the spine and joints. In particular, avoid using strong pressure on joints that are swollen or inflamed by arthritis or rheumatism.
- **Breaks and fractures** Do not massage over a break or fracture. It will not only be painful but may also cause further damage. Wait until the area has healed. In most cases, you can massage the rest of the body.
- **Cancer** If your partner is undergoing treatment for cancer, the increased lymph and blood flow resulting from massage may spread cancerous cells from the infected site. If your partner is in remission, ask their doctor if you can administer a massage.

To support the flow of blood to the heart, use firmer strokes from the extremities towards the centre of the body, but use lighter strokes when moving outwards.

- **Diabetes** Diabetics often have circulatory problems, which sometimes result in a lack of sensation in certain parts of the body, such as the legs and feet, so they may not be able to fully interpret the pressure you're applying. Have them seek advice from their doctor first, and always apply massage cautiously.
- **The elderly** Massaging the elderly is a great way to treat muscular aches and pains. The increased lymph flow also assists their circulation and immunity. However, in cases of osteoporosis, chronic arthritis and brittle or weak bones, massage is generally contraindicated. Check with your partner first before using some very light techniques.
- **Fever or flu** Avoid full body aromatherapy massage on people who are suffering from fever or flu; in these cases, other aromatherapy applications, such as baths or compresses (see page 26), may be more suitable.
- **Headaches and migraines** Never apply massage if your partner has a migraine, as you might make the symptoms worse. A headache may be the result of chemical or hormonal causes, or tense or tight muscles. In the latter case, gentle massage might help, but check with your partner first.
- **Heart problems** With any heart problems, always seek advice first: with some types of medications, a massage can be contraindicated.

- **Inflammation** Never massage over acute inflammation, as the massage will bring more blood to the area, often making the injury more painful. Massaging the affected area after it has stopped swelling and is no longer inflamed can sometimes be beneficial, as it assists in removing toxins and wastes that have remained during the healing process.
- **Pregnancy** Massage is generally contraindicated during the first trimester, as the foetus has not yet settled in the womb. However, gentle massage may be given by a trained practitioner, who will avoid certain acupressure points and massage over the sacrum. (See 'During pregnancy', page 14, and 'Pregnancy', page 232.)
- **Recent injuries** Do not massage over areas of recent injury such as whiplash and muscle sprains.
- **Recent surgery** If your partner is recovering from surgery, massaging over the scars may not only be painful but may also cause further damage. They should always check with their doctor first.
- **Serious illness** Before you massage any person suffering from a serious illness, seek professional medical advice.
- **Skin conditions** Avoid massaging directly over sensitive or contagious skin conditions, such as rashes, allergies, ulcers, boils, cuts and abrasions, bites, bruises, healing scars, sunburn, burns or wounds. Massage can irritate

and/or spread the condition, making it worse or possibly rendering you vulnerable to catching it. If in doubt, wear rubber gloves.
- **Systemic infections** If your partner has the flu, fever or rheumatoid arthritis, giving her a massage will make it worse by spreading the affected cells around her body. You may also risk catching the infection yourself. Never massage your partner if either of you has any of these conditions.
- **Thrombosis** If your partner has a circulatory problem such as deep vein thrombosis (DVT), avoid massage, as you run the risk of dislodging a clot or causing an embolism that could travel to the heart or brain. Common symptoms of DVT include sore calves, swollen feet, a lump or bruise in the leg and pain on dorsi-flexion (lifting of the foot).
- **Varicose veins** Do not massage directly below, or over the top of, varicose veins. If the veins are not too weak, you can apply very light pressure with essential oils, but check with your doctor first.

➔ *'During pregnancy', page 14*
  • *'Before you start', page 126*
    • *'Pregnancy', page 232*

Full body sequence for Swedish massage

This full body sequence usually takes an hour, but you can vary the length of the session to suit you and your partner's needs. The massage should be fun for both of you, so relax and use only the techniques you find comfortable.

CAUTIONS ● See 'Safety and cautions', page 134. ● Avoid massaging over the spine at all times, and be careful when working close to bony landmarks such as the shoulders and hips.

Preparation

Before you begin a Swedish or massage, make sure everything is ready (see 'Before you start', page 126). Next, conduct a consultation with your partner to make sure there are no contraindications to massage. Remember the rule for massage – *do no harm* (page 134).

If everything is OK, then you can begin the massage. Here's a guide to a popular sequence (see the step-by-step photographs on pages 138–53).

Ask your partner to undress and lie down, covered, on the table, then leave the room while she does so. Wash your hands and then return. You may need to reset the towels so she is covered properly. Cover her whole body and check that she is comfortable.

Encourage verbal feedback during the treatment so you can be sure you're applying suitable pressure and your partner is enjoying the massage.

Back

Begin the back sequence by placing one hand on the shoulder area and the other on the lower back. Then apply a gentle rocking movement. This technique will help to relax her.

Next, uncover the back area and tuck the towel into her underwear. You can then begin to palpate into the muscles so you can feel for any restrictions.

Now you can begin the massage. Use effleurage in rhythmical strokes on the entire back area, keeping your hands soft. These moves are best applied towards the heart, but they can be used in any direction.

Shoulders

Next, apply effleurage and then kneading to the shoulders. Take your time to knead any tension in the muscles. Apply the techniques to both sides. By this stage you should have spent 15–20 minutes of a one-hour massage.

Neck and head

Now use a scooping movement to apply effleurage to the neck muscles. Check that the pressure is comfortable for your partner, and keep doing so throughout the massage.

Keep massaging the neck with the different techniques, then move your hands up to the head and scalp and massage with pressure-point techniques and small, slow frictions with the fingers.

If your partner does not want oil in her hair, place a small towel over the hair and head while you massage. This also prevents you from pulling on the hair.

Percussion to the back

Once you have finished, cover your partner with the towel and apply percussion techniques – including hacking, cupping and pummelling – to the whole back area. By this stage, 25 minutes should have elapsed.

Back of legs and feet

Move down to the bottom of the table and clean the feet with an antibacterial wipe or spray before beginning to massage the feet and legs. Most people who are not ticklish love their feet being massaged, so spend a little longer on them if required.

Warm your partner's feet first, then use your thumbs to massage into the muscles and loosen them up. It is usually best to massage one side of each foot first, continuing up onto the leg, before massaging the other side.

Apply effleurage and petrissage to the lower and upper legs, always ensuring you're moving towards the heart.

When you have finished, wipe off the oil with the towel, pulling it down to redrape the area you have just worked on. Then apply the same techniques to the other foot and leg. It doesn't matter which side you massage first. About 10 minutes on each leg is recommended.

Front of the legs

Continue the treatment by turning your partner over. Place a pillow under the knees for lower back support, and also a towel or small pillow under the neck. Apply the same techniques to both sides of the fronts of the legs, then drape them with towels and move up to the abdomen.

Abdomen and chest

Always apply massage on the abdomen in a clockwise direction to assist with digestion. Apply the oil and massage in circles slowly, first with one hand and then two. If, at any point, the receiver feels uncomfortable, stop massaging. Drape the abdomen and move up to the chest area. Draping is very important here, so tuck the towel in tightly to make sure it won't fall down while you're massaging.

Arms and hands

Apply effleurage to the arms and hands, finishing with gentle stretching on the fingers.

Face

To finish off the treatment, sit on a stool or kneel so you're above your partner's head, ready to massage the face. You might want to wash or wipe your hands before continuing, as up to this point you have massaged the rest of the body, including the feet. Wipe off any excess makeup, then apply minimal amounts of oil before massaging.

The techniques used on the face should be very slow and relaxing. The face is also a small, defined area, so movements should be more precise and specific. When using effleurage movements on the face, try to bring your hands down towards the jaw, as this helps to drain away any toxins and waste. Finish the full treatment with light finger tapping on the face and/or stroking to the hair.

Ending the treatment

Let your partner know that the massage has ended and you'll be leaving to wash your hands while she gets dressed. Help her off the table if necessary, and encourage her to drink a lot of water to help flush any toxins from the body. Advise her to avoid strenuous activity, and ask for feedback, as that is the best way to learn. Clean the area, and note how it went so you can adjust the treatment next time, if necessary.

Touch is an ancient healing art, and the more you practise massage, the better you will become.

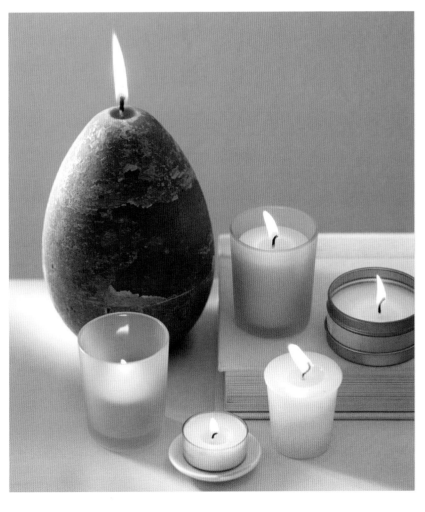

Back sequence

A Swedish massage sequence will often start on the back, where the therapist spends most of the massage time. The movements should be rhythmical, even and smooth and, because the back muscles are big, broad strokes are best.

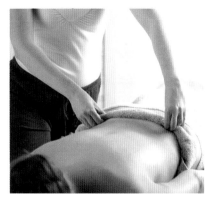

1 Undrape your partner so you can begin the treatment on the back. Pull down the towel and tuck it neatly into the top of her underwear to protect it from the oil. Begin by palpating to determine if there is any tension in the area to be massaged.

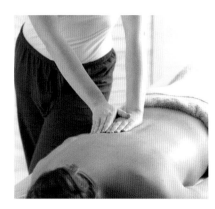

2 Warm the oil in your hands before applying it to the entire back area. Begin by applying effleurage with both hands alongside the spine to the tops of the shoulders, then knead and return along the sides of the trunk.

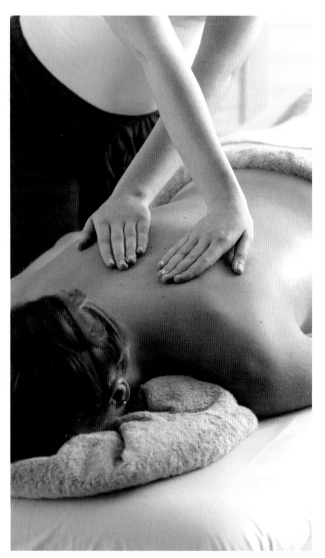

3 This next move uses both hands to apply effleurage up to the shoulders. When you reach the top, bring your hands around in a circle and cross them over so they are on the other side. Then bring them back to the other side, thus forming a figure-8. Finish with effleurage down to the pelvis and start again. Repeat this sequence 4–5 times.

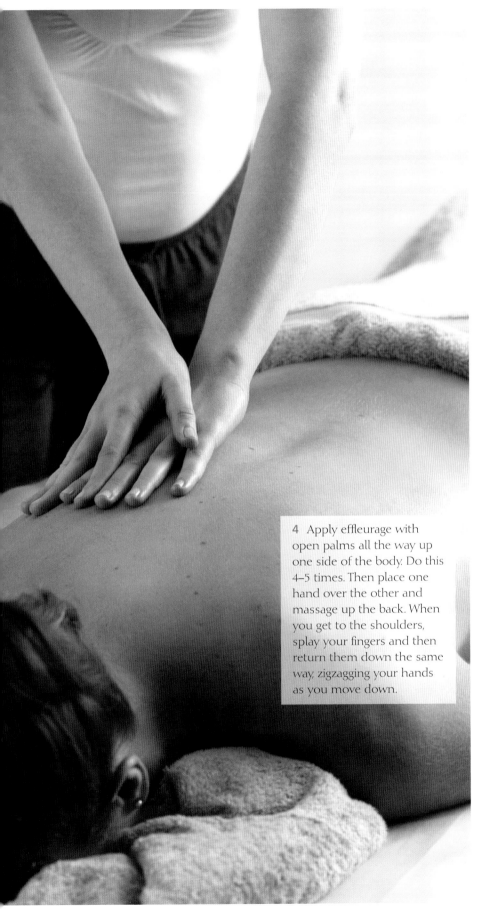

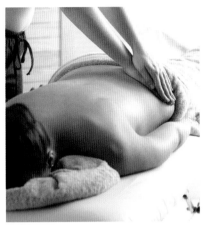

5 Now that the muscles are warm, you can apply kneading. Standing on one side, use your fingers and then your palms to massage across the top of the pelvis in a slow, smooth manner. Start close to your partner's spine and work out towards the edge of the hip.

4 Apply effleurage with open palms all the way up one side of the body. Do this 4–5 times. Then place one hand over the other and massage up the back. When you get to the shoulders, splay your fingers and then return them down the same way, zigzagging your hands as you move down.

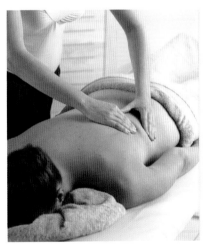

6 Finally, apply kneading to the whole back area. Place both hands down on the back and in a rhythmic sequence bring them together, gently lifting and moving the muscle tissues. This is very effective for releasing tension. When you're finished, apply steps 4–6 on the other side.

Shoulder sequence

Many of us hold tension and stress from both work and life in our shoulders, so they often need massaging. Use techniques such as effleurage to warm up the muscles, and kneading, frictions and holding to loosen them.

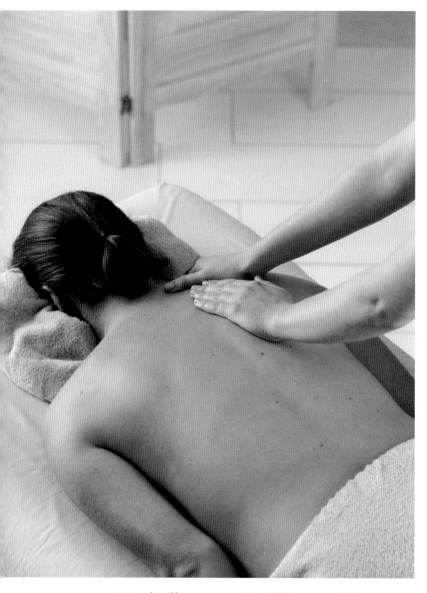

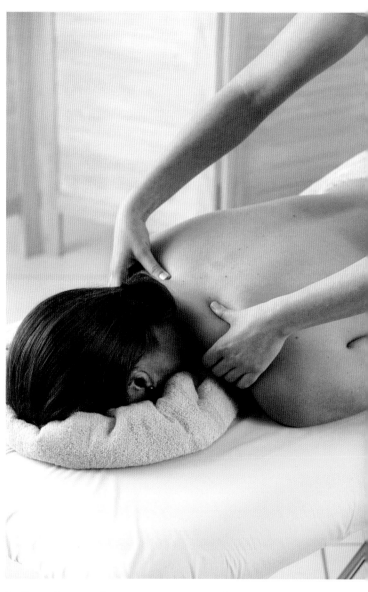

1 Apply effleurage over the whole area, making sure you cover all the shoulder muscles. First massage both sides of the spine at the same time, then use both hands, one on top of the other, to work on each side.

2 Once the muscles are warm, start working into the tops of the shoulders, a hand on each side. This is like kneading pizza dough. Then massage into the area with your thumbs, moving them through in an easy manner.

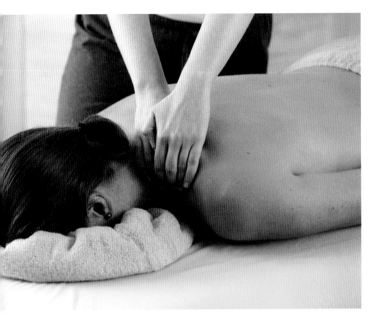

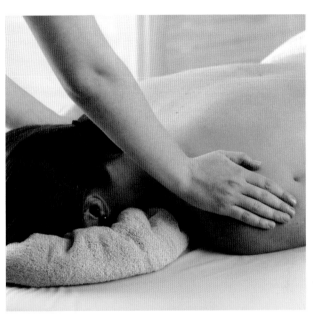

3 Stand on one side of the body so you can use both hands to lightly pull back the trapezius muscle on the other side. Repeat this a few times, alternating it with effleurage. Then gently take hold of the muscle and squeeze, releasing slowly. Repeat on the other side.

4 Position yourself at the end of the table so that you are looking down your partner's body. Place your hands palm down on the tops of the shoulders and move them out to the edge. Then roll them around so they end up on the backs of the shoulders.

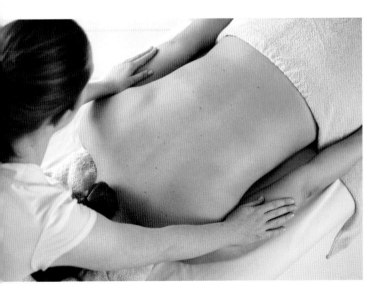

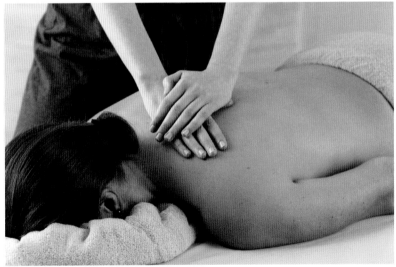

5 Continue massaging down the back on either side, then use effleurage to return up the back. Then move back across the shoulders and down the arms to the hands, which should be lying along your partner's sides. Bring your hands back up. Repeat this move a few times.

6 Place your thumb between the shoulder blades, then place your other hand over the top and move them both up along the spine to the top near the neck. Swap hands so the other thumb is down, then massage down alongside the spine.

Neck and head sequence

The weight of the head puts the neck muscles under a lot of strain, but massage can alleviate and relax the area. Massaging the head is just as soothing, and you can work on the pressure points here to great effect.

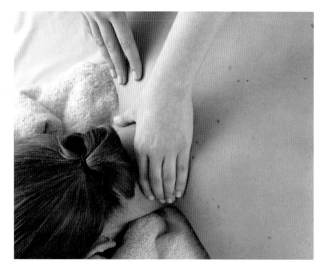

1 To avoid getting a lot of oil in the hair, start the neck massage with only a little. Place one hand in a C-scoop position on the back of the neck, then complete the move with effleurage, using your fingers to work gently into the muscles towards the base of the skull and back.

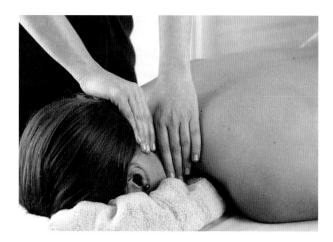

2 With the other hand also in a C-scoop position, scoop with alternate hands in a rhythmical fashion, massaging the whole length of the neck. Apply moderate pressure, and ask your partner for feedback.

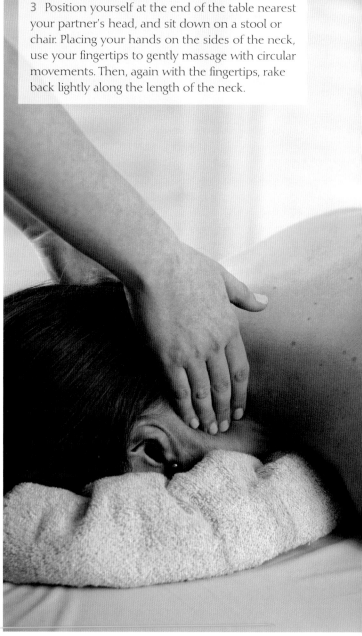

3 Position yourself at the end of the table nearest your partner's head, and sit down on a stool or chair. Placing your hands on the sides of the neck, use your fingertips to gently massage with circular movements. Then, again with the fingertips, rake back lightly along the length of the neck.

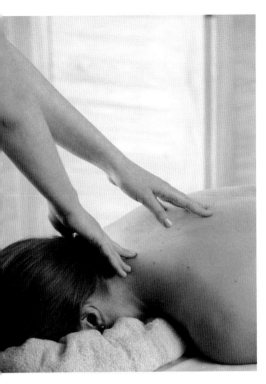

4 Start between the shoulder blades and gently stroke your fingertips up towards the neck, moving them alternately in a light and rhythmic motion. You can also start at the base of the neck and work downwards. This has a relaxing and soothing effect on the body.

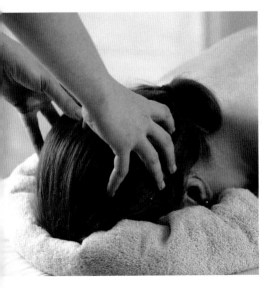

5 Using your fingertips, gently move the scalp around, soothing the skin and hair follicles. Then place your thumbs at the top of the crown and massage back towards the neck on the meridian line.

6 Pull the towel up so it covers the shoulders, and apply percussion to the back and shoulder area with hacking, cupping and pummelling before moving on to massage the legs and feet.

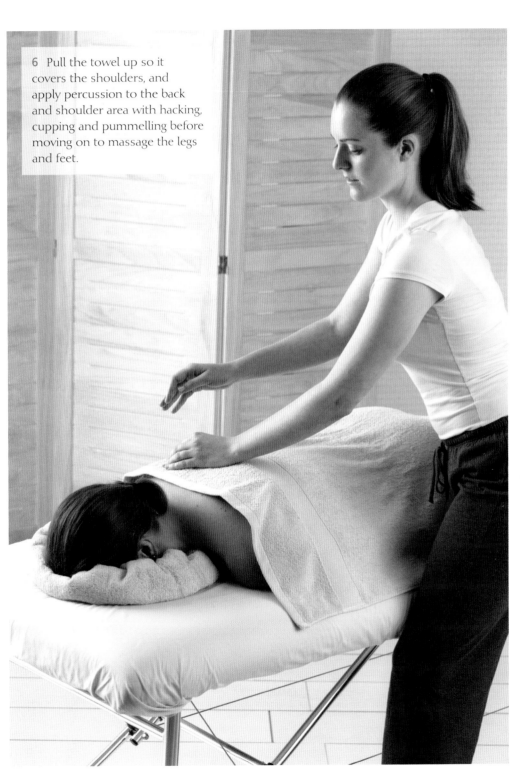

➔ 'The meridians', page 93

NECK AND HEAD SEQUENCE   **143**

Back of legs and feet sequence

To complete the massage sequence for the back of the body, move down to the legs and feet. Once you've cleaned the feet, you can massage them before moving on to the lower legs and then the bottom of the pelvis.

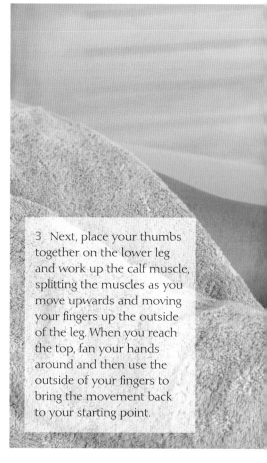

3 Next, place your thumbs together on the lower leg and work up the calf muscle, splitting the muscles as you move upwards and moving your fingers up the outside of the leg. When you reach the top, fan your hands around and then use the outside of your fingers to bring the movement back to your starting point.

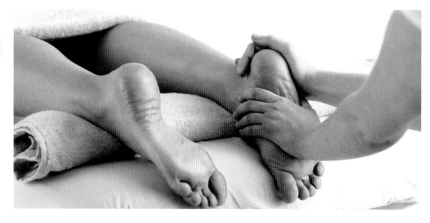

1 Remove the towel draping to uncover the feet, then apply oil to one foot with effleurage (the other foot will be massaged after you have completed one leg). Make sure you massage the whole foot, working slowly on each toe as well as the heel and the front of the foot. If your partner is ticklish, you may have to adjust your pressure.

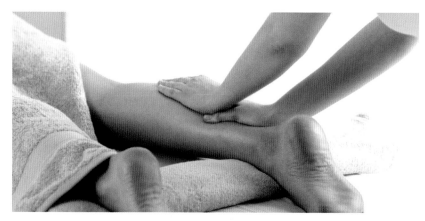

2 Redrape the towel so that only the leg being massaged is showing. Begin by applying oil, and then effleurage, up the calf muscle. Smooth, broad strokes are best here, starting above the heel and continuing up to below the back of the knee. Move your hands back slowly and lightly, and repeat this movement up to 7 times.

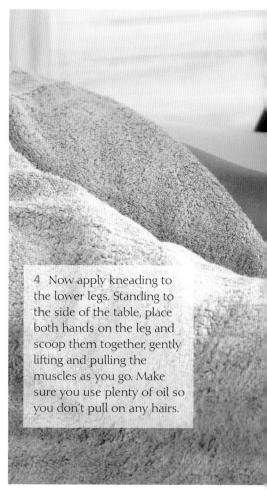

4 Now apply kneading to the lower legs. Standing to the side of the table, place both hands on the leg and scoop them together, gently lifting and pulling the muscles as you go. Make sure you use plenty of oil so you don't pull on any hairs.

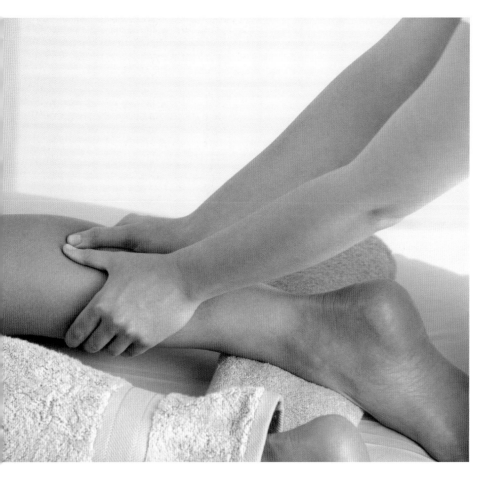

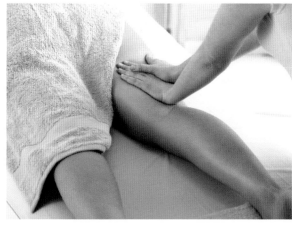

5 Moving up to the posterior thighs, apply effleurage with both hands to this area. The hamstring muscles are very strong, so a firmer pressure can be applied. Place one hand over the other and massage up from above the back of the knee to the bottom of the pelvis. Forearms can also be used.

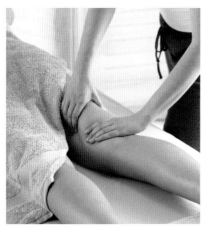

6 Once you have warmed up the muscles, apply kneading with a wringing technique. Standing to the side, place both hands on the leg and move them back and forth across the muscles, moving up and down the length of the whole leg as you go. Repeat all the moves on the other leg, and finish with percussion.

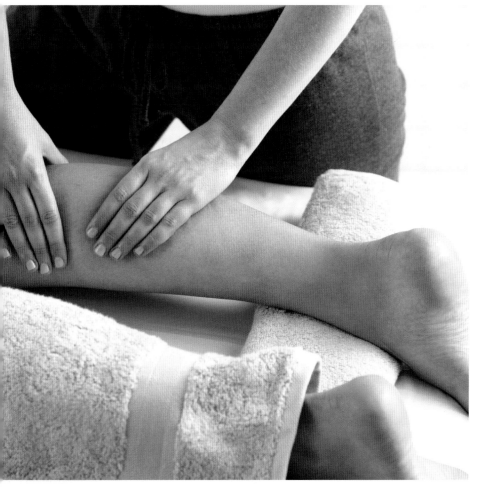

145

Front of legs sequence

Continue the sequence on the front of the legs, massaging one side, then the other. When turning over your partner, preserve her modesty at all times by taking care with the draping. You can also massage the feet in this position.

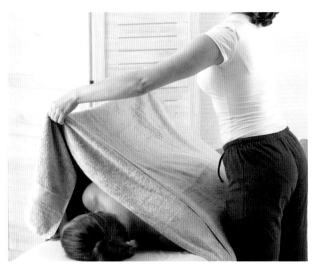

1 Before asking your partner to turn over, pull up the towels and hold them against the edge of the table with your knees. Once she is lying on her back, redrape the towel, and place a folded towel or bolster under her knees.

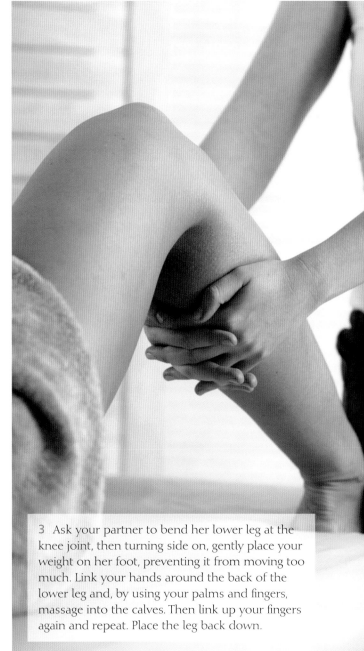

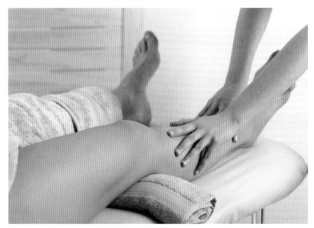

2 Warm oil in your hands and apply effleurage up the lower legs. With the lower extremities, it's always a good idea to work in an upwards direction to assist with venous blood return. A few passes will be enough.

3 Ask your partner to bend her lower leg at the knee joint, then turning side on, gently place your weight on her foot, preventing it from moving too much. Link your hands around the back of the lower leg and, by using your palms and fingers, massage into the calves. Then link up your fingers again and repeat. Place the leg back down.

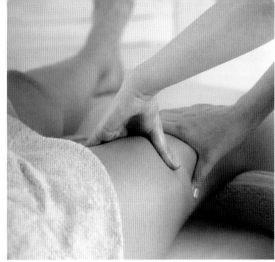

5 Knead this area – wringing across the muscles is great, as is petrissage. Apply one technique and then the other, loosening up any tension in the quadriceps muscles. Vibration is also useful here. Apply supported chiselled fingers, and vibrate them slowly on the leg below.

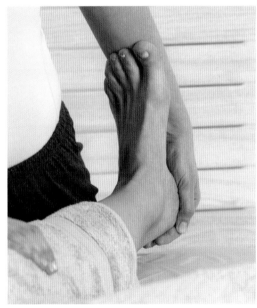

6 Finish the movements on the front of the leg with some stretching and percussion. Grasp the sole of the foot and the toes, and pull them back towards the rest of the body to stretch the calves and hamstrings. Lightly apply the hacking technique to the lower leg, then more strongly to the upper thigh. Repeat all the sequences on the other side of the leg.

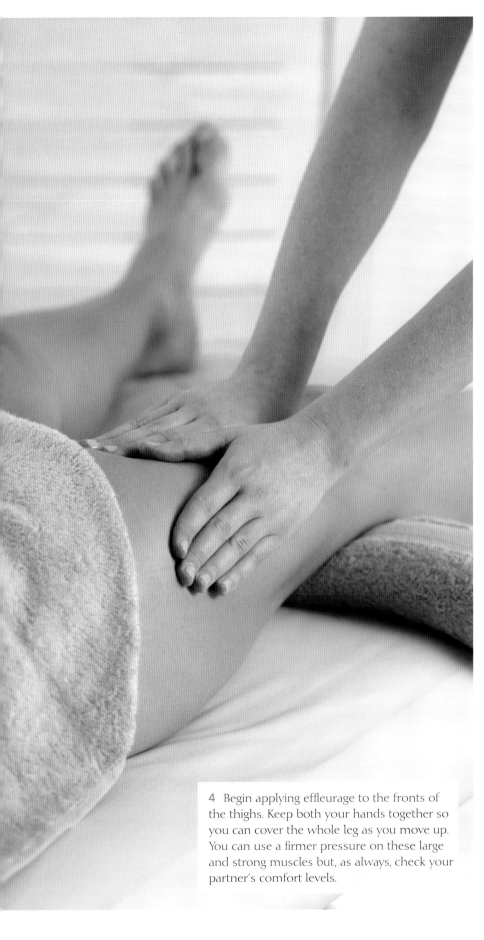

4 Begin applying effleurage to the fronts of the thighs. Keep both your hands together so you can cover the whole leg as you move up. You can use a firmer pressure on these large and strong muscles but, as always, check your partner's comfort levels.

Abdomen and chest sequence

When massaging the abdomen, the movements should be slow and smooth, always in a clockwise direction. Treatments that include the chest area are also beneficial, and assist the flow of the massage on to the arms and hands.

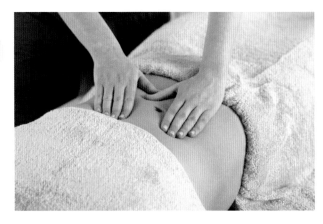

1 Begin the massage of the abdomen with palpation. Make contact with the skin and gently press in around the area with the fingertips of both hands. Be careful not to apply too much pressure. The aim of this technique is to get your partner used to you working in this area, as some people can feel uncomfortable about it.

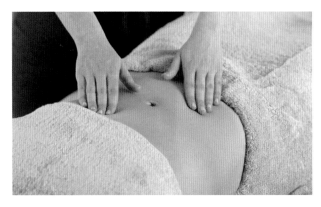

2 Start on the bottom left side of the abdomen. Using one hand, start moving in a clockwise direction, then follow it with the other hand. Do this a few times before using both hands at the same time. Keep your hands relaxed and the pressure flowing rather than direct.

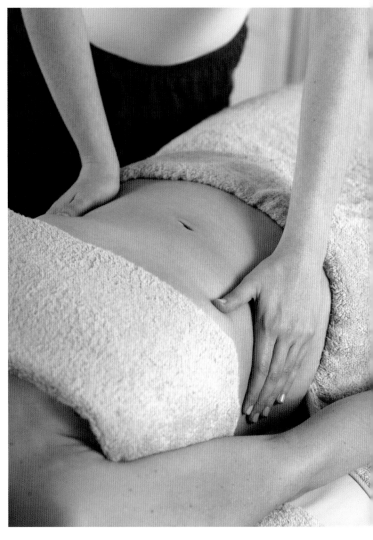

3 Place your thumbs alongside the bottom of the ribs with your fingers on the outside of the abdomen. Slide your hands around to the back area until they link, then bring them back towards the front. This beautiful move is very relaxing.

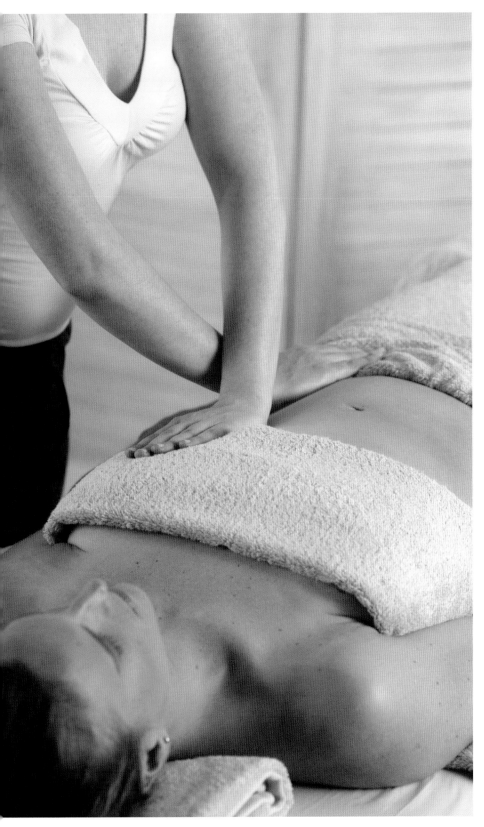

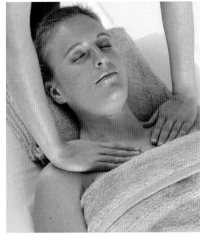

5 Drape the abdomen and slowly pull down the towel covering the chest. Tuck the towel tightly behind the back. Sitting at your partner's head, starting with the flats of your hands in the middle of the chest, move out to the shoulders, rolling your hands underneath, then move up to the neck.

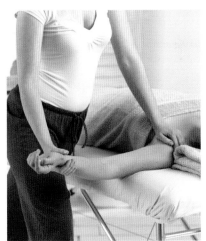

6 Stand on your partner's left side and gently pull out her left arm with your right hand. Begin effleurage with your left hand over the chest area; as you move out towards the shoulders, include your palms. Move your hand back slowly and repeat before moving onto the arms.

4 Stand on one side of the body. Place your left hand at the bottom of the ribs, and the right on top of the bony prominence of the hip. Gently apply pressure either way, stretching the abdominal muscles, then repeat on the other side.

Arms and hands sequence

Being massaged on the arms and hands is delightful, and everyone can benefit from treatment to this area, as we use our hands for so many tasks every day and consequently the muscles can tighten up over a period.

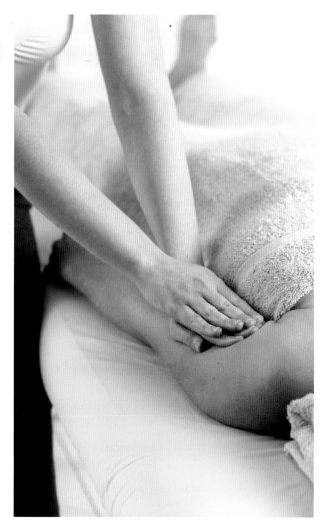

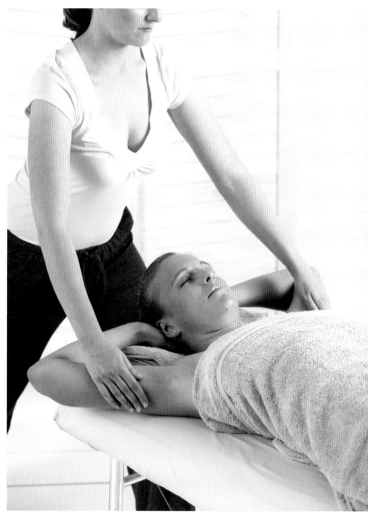

1 Place your partner's arms alongside her body, and begin by applying effleurage to the upper arm with one hand. The strokes should go the full length of the arm. Once you reach the top of the arm, massage into the shoulder and move your hands back down the arm lightly.

2 Grasp your partner's hands and place her palms under her head. Making sure she is comfortable, massage slowly and gently along the length of the backs of the arms. Repeat this move 4–5 times, then stretch the arms out, and hold, before returning her arms to her sides.

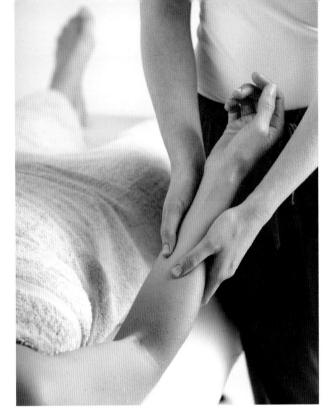

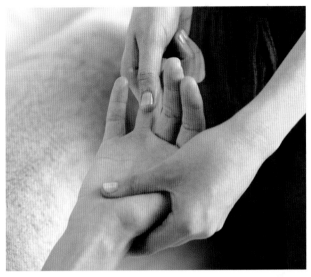

3 Next, bend one arm at the elbow and massage the forearm with both hands. Then knead in with your thumbs, starting at the wrist and working from the inside outwards until you reach the bottom of the elbow. Repeat the whole sequence on both sides of the arm.

4 Massage into the hand by using both your ring and little fingers to spread out your partner's palm. Then use your thumbs to knead slowly into the palm, taking your time to work up and down along the tendons. Finish by applying effleurage to each finger; as you go, stretch the finger and wrist forward and back.

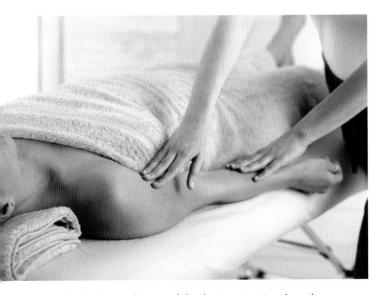

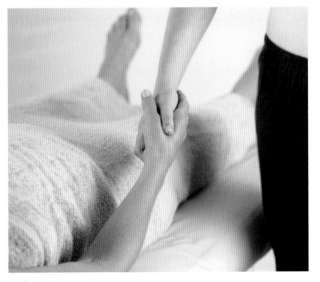

5 Apply stroking and feathering to stimulate the nerve endings of the skin, which assists circulation and relaxation. Starting at the top of the shoulder, stroke your fingers down the length of the arm to the hand. Then, starting at the bottom, feather up to the top.

6 To complete the arm sequence, take hold of your partner's hand as if you are going to shake it. Making sure the pressure is soft, rotate your wrist back and forth so the whole arm shakes, freeing up any left-over tension and assisting with range of motion of the shoulder. Repeat all moves (steps 1–6) on the other arm.

ARMS AND HANDS SEQUENCE   **151**

Face sequence

A Swedish massage sequence often finishes with the face, leaving the receiver in a state of total relaxation and bliss. If your partner is wearing any makeup, it's a good idea to remove it first, so you don't spread it across her face.

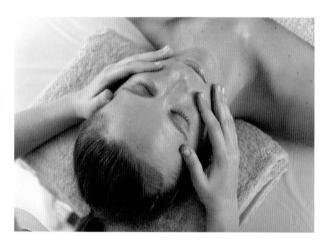

1 Starting at the middle of the forehead, and with a minimal amount of essential oil, use long strokes across the forehead, then continue down to the chin. Repeat this sequence a few times before using your index fingers to massage down the bridge of the nose and across the cheeks.

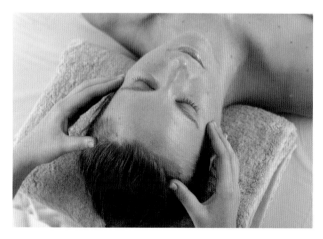

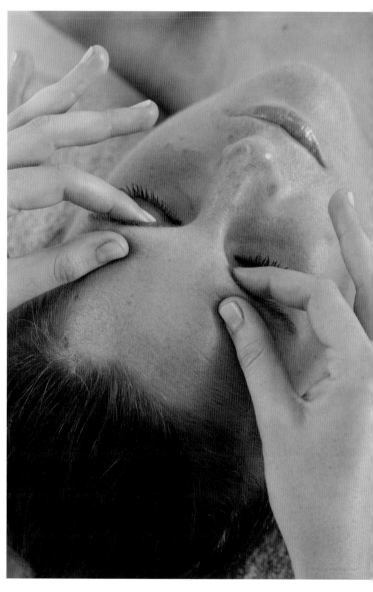

2 Using your fingertips, massage with circular frictions on both temples. Work slowly, applying pressure on one side and then the other so your partner experiences a rhythmic effect. Continue this technique by massaging down into the cheek and jaw area.

3 Place your index finger and thumb together on your partner's eyebrows and gently roll the skin back and forth, relaxing any puffiness in this area. Then bend your index fingers and place them below the eyebrow line, pressing into the tops of the eye sockets.

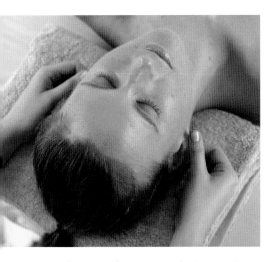

4 Using the same technique as in step 3, massage along the chin and jaw. Start in the middle and work your way up along the length of the jaw, rolling as you go. Continue on the ears, starting at the bottom and moving up to the top of the ears and back.

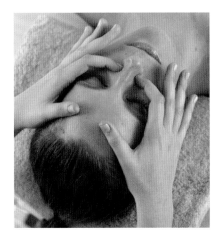

5 Place your fingertips between the eyebrows and press into the acupressure points to clear the sinuses. Continue this on the point where the eyes meet the nose and where the bridge meets the nostrils. Add some effleurage over the face to clear any toxins that might have been released.

6 Massage into the scalp with your fingers, then gently tug on the hair, taking care not to pull too hard. Let your partner know you are finished, offer water and leave her alone to get dressed.

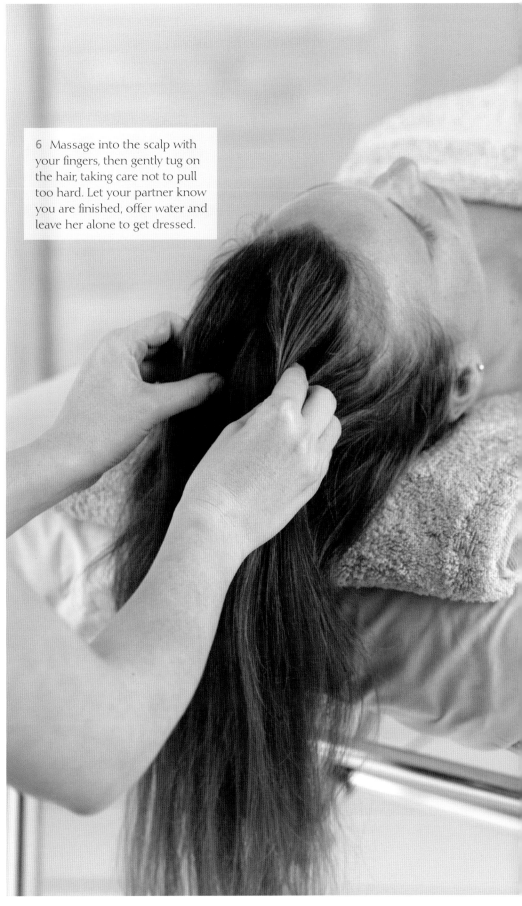

Full body sequence for aromatherapy massage

Each move of this wonderful aromatherapy massage sequence should be repeated 3 to 5 times. With your partner lying face down, warmly covered, a pillow under her feet and ankles, start the massage on the back.

About this treatment

This holistic treatment, developed by Micheline Arcier, involves a combination of relaxing yet healing natural therapies.

These include: effleurage (Swedish massage); kneading; stimulating acupressure points, based on Traditional Chinese Medicine's concept of meridians; lymphatic drainage techniques, which help to remove toxins, aid fluid retention and stimulate the immune system; reflexology of the hands, feet and face, where various points correspond to particular organs and parts of the body; and finally, polarity therapy, where the practitioner always stands on the receiver's right side – it is believed that each part of the body has both a positive and a negative charge, so the therapist's own electromagnetic field rebalances the receiver's body.

Polarity balance

The first move on the back involves polarity therapy, which allows you to establish contact with your partner. Place your left hand around the base of the skull and hold it for a few seconds. Leave it there while you place your right hand between the shoulder blades for a few seconds, then in the middle of the back and, lastly, on the lower back.

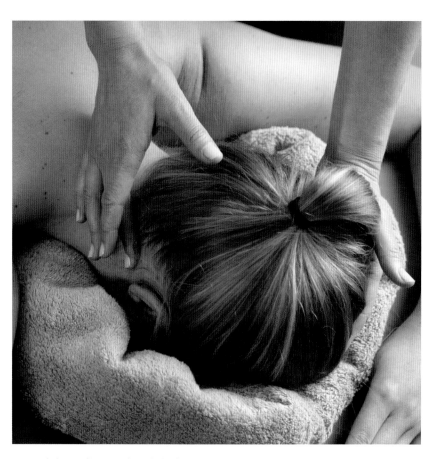

1 Neck kneading and occipital pressure
With your hands, gently knead the neck in an upward direction and then across the base of the head. Holding the right side of the head with your left hand, apply pressure with your right thumb to the base of the skull, starting close to the ear. When you reach the spine, swap hands and use the middle finger of your right hand to apply pressure to the right side of the cranium. This move loosens tight muscles in that area.

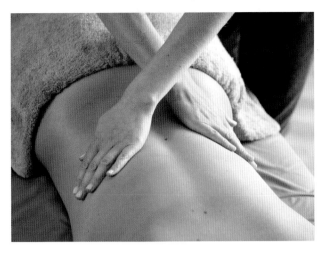

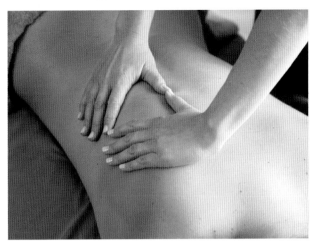

2 Figure-8

Using smooth, long strokes, apply oil over the whole back. Place both hands on the lower back and sweep up the spine, across the shoulder then down the back. When you reach the mid-back, cross your hands over and finish off by gently pulling on the sides of the hips. This move can be done any time in the back sequence, as it adds to the continuity of the treatment.

3 Spinal gutter pressures

Starting at the base of the spine, lay both your thumbs flat along the back and move them up in a press, release and slide motion. Work all the way up to the neck, then commence the move on the other side of the spine. Massage each side of the spine alternately 5 times. This move, which follows the Bladder Meridian in Traditional Chinese Medicine (see page 91), stimulates the sympathetic nervous system.

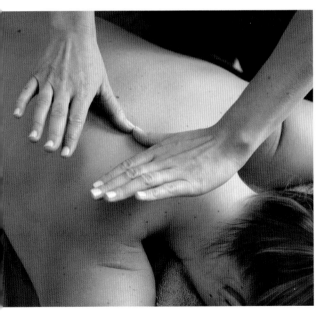

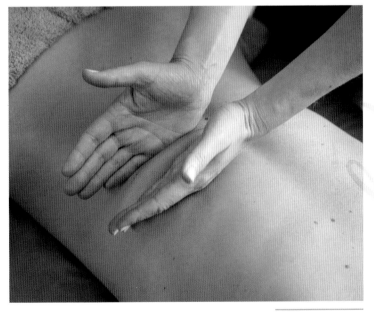

4 Lymph sweeps

For the next move, perform lymphatic sweeps. Start just above the buttocks, with touching thumbs, and lightly slide up the sides of the spine, using one long sweep and two short ones to finish at the neck. Lymphatic drainage helps to improve the flow of lymph (see also page 104).

5 Scooping and piano moves

Scooping the skin with both hands is a great decongesting move for the back muscles, and also promotes blood and lymph flow. Beginning at the lower back, scoop the skin up to the neck. Work both sides of the spine alternately. Then run your fingers and hands down the side of the body. Use this technique all the way up to the shoulders, then step back and bend your knees to work the other side of the spine.

CAUTIONS
• See 'Safety and cautions', page 134.

Lower back and arms

Aromatherapy massage improves blood and lymph flow, so it can aid the lower back area – often prone to aches and tightness – while applying gentle techniques to the arms and hands relieves general tightness.

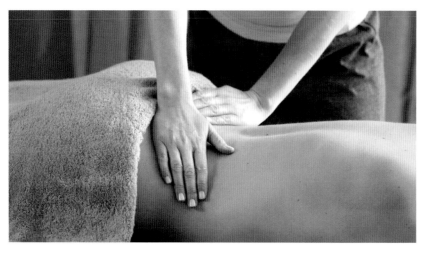

1 Figure-8
The figure-8 move over the hip area is a great effleurage technique for oil application and warming up the muscles. Place both hands on the right hip, then bring your left hand towards you as you let the right hand follow, massaging in the figure-8 pattern.

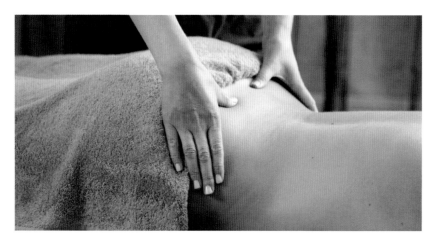

2 Circular moves and fanning
Beginning at the top of the sacrum, move the thumbs over the hip bone in a circular motion, then slide them over the same area in a fan-like movement. These movements will loosen up the muscles of the buttocks.

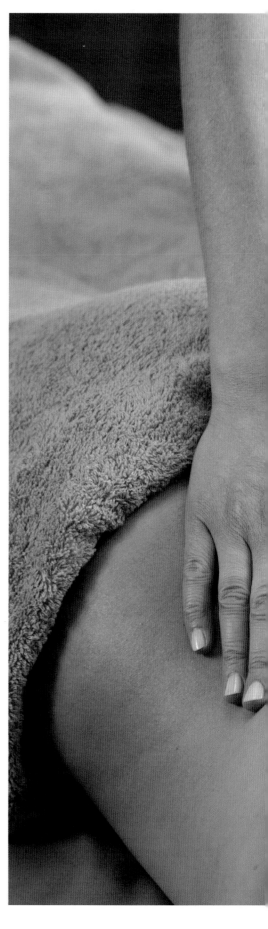

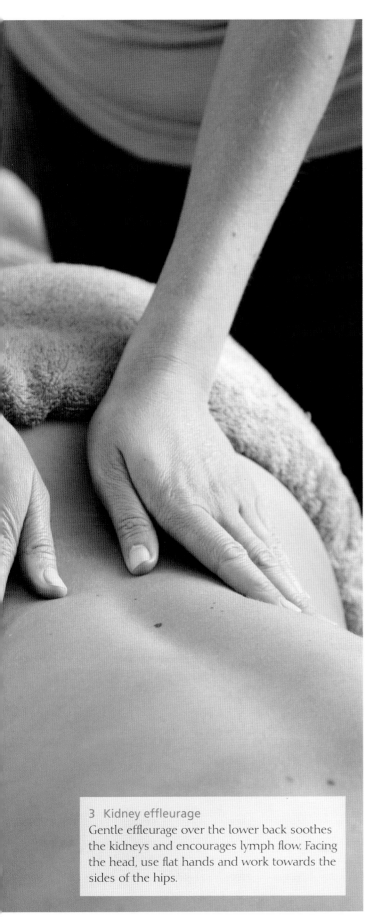

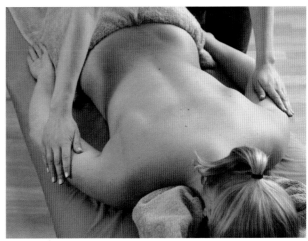

4 Effleurage on the arms

Use effleurage techniques to apply essential oil over the arms. Commence the arm massage at the lower back, then slide up over the shoulders and down the arms, finishing by gently pulling the fingers. At this point you can massage each hand if you wish, or involve the pressure points, as on page 91.

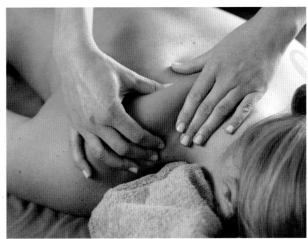

5 Back kneading

To complete the back sequence, use gentle kneading and effleurage techniques to massage the whole area. Your partner will be particularly grateful for the extra attention around the shoulders and neck, where tension is usually held. Finish with a soft stroke through the hair, then cover the whole back with a towel.

3 Kidney effleurage

Gentle effleurage over the lower back soothes the kidneys and encourages lymph flow. Facing the head, use flat hands and work towards the sides of the hips.

Back of legs

This nurturing leg massage relaxes and energises, and also improves the circulation of blood and lymph, helping to ease tension and tired, heavy legs. Using soft lymphatic techniques may also reduce swelling around the ankles.

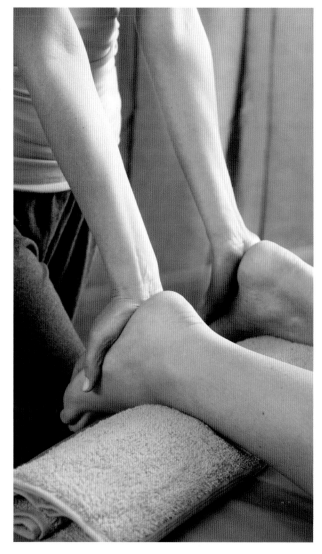

1 Swedish techniques
Standing at the end of the massage table, place your hands on the soles of both feet and hold for a few seconds. Apply oil over both legs with soft effleurage and kneading techniques. Massage both legs at the same time.

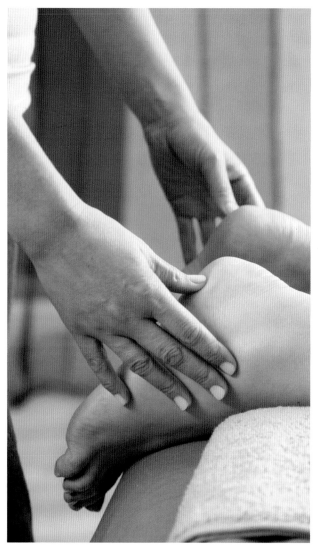

2 Circular friction to the soles
Starting at the top of the heel, use your thumbs to apply circular and sliding movements over the soles of the feet. Apply pressure with your body weight. This move is part of foot reflexology, which holds that particular points on the feet correspond to certain organs and parts of the body.

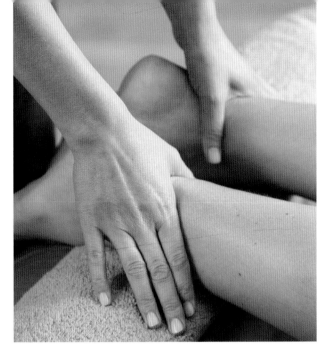

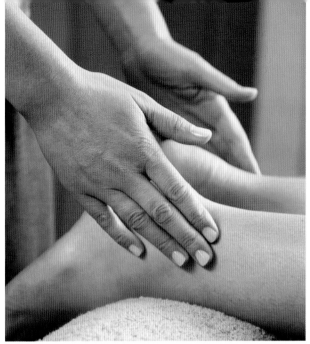

3 Achilles tendon stretch
Use the webbing between your thumb and index finger to stretch the Achilles tendon as you slide your hands up and down a couple of times. This move may alleviate tension in the lower leg.

4 Ankle circles
This light pressure technique will help draw fluid away from swollen ankles. First, turn your hands and use your fingers to circle the lateral ankles, then turn your hands again and circle the middle ankles.

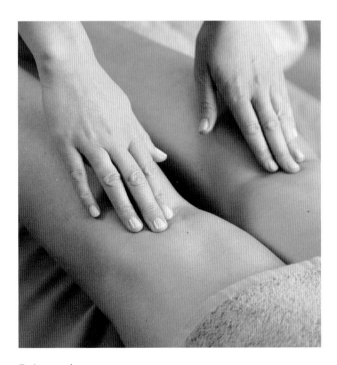

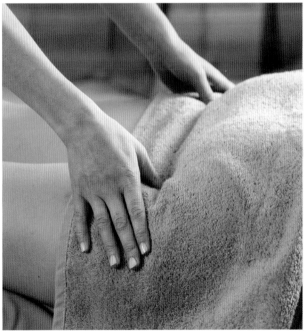

5 Lower leg
Run your hands up the lower legs, then use your finger-tips to gently press the Bladder 40 acupressure point for 2 seconds. This point, behind the knees between the tendons, is useful for acute lower back pain relief. It also moves the blood in the lower leg, making it beneficial for treating varicose veins.

6 Upper leg
Continue to slide your hands up the legs to just below the buttocks and press the Bladder 36 point in the middle of the thigh for 2 seconds. Finish by resting your hands on the feet, then help your partner to turn over and move the pillow to behind the knees. Wash your hands before the next move.

Scalp, face and chest

Aromatherapy scalp and face massage is wonderful, helping to rebalance the skin, improve the circulation and relieve tension, especially with headaches, while chest massage is great for cough relief and stiff shoulders.

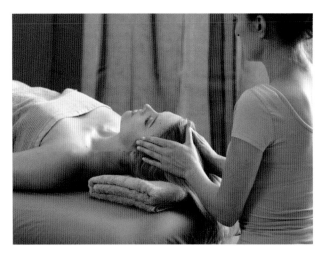

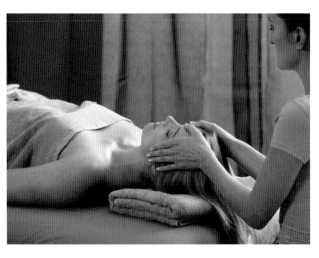

1 Scalp massage
With dry hands, place one thumb on top of the other, then press on the middle of the head, starting at the hairline and moving over the scalp. Then spread your fingers and massage all over the scalp. This will loosen the fascia, increase the blood flow and relieve head tension. Finish by raking your fingers through the hair and gently pulling it.

2 Forehead
Apply a small amount of oil onto your palms and spread it around the face in an upward stroking movement. Next, treat the forehead above the eyebrows by working towards the temples with the press and slide movement. Finally, commencing at the root of the nose, use alternating thumbs to slide up to the hairline. This will soothe away any frowning wrinkles.

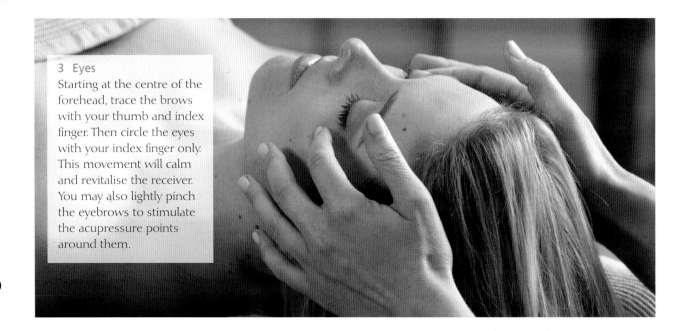

3 Eyes
Starting at the centre of the forehead, trace the brows with your thumb and index finger. Then circle the eyes with your index finger only. This movement will calm and revitalise the receiver. You may also lightly pinch the eyebrows to stimulate the acupressure points around them.

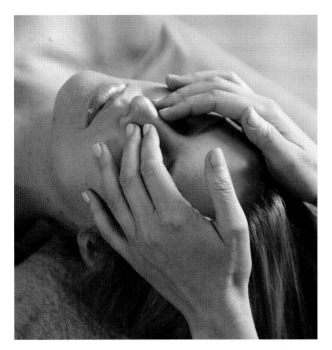

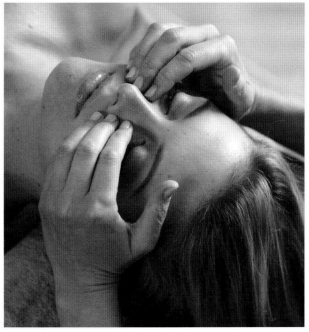

4 Nose

With two fingers on each side and working upwards, gently circle the nose. Continue the move by running your fingers up the forehead to the hairline; this technique relieves congestion in the nose. You can use a draining technique here by sliding your fingers down the sides of the nose.

5 Cheeks, jaw and ears

Place your fingers on each side of the nose and spread them over the cheeks, raking towards the ears. With the index fingers, press the Colon 20 acupuncture point on the sides of the nostrils and hold for a few seconds. Continue this movement by sweeping across the cheekbones with all fingers. These techniques will help to clear nasal obstruction and blocked sinuses. Knead the jaw outwards with your thumb and index finger, finishing with a relaxing ear massage.

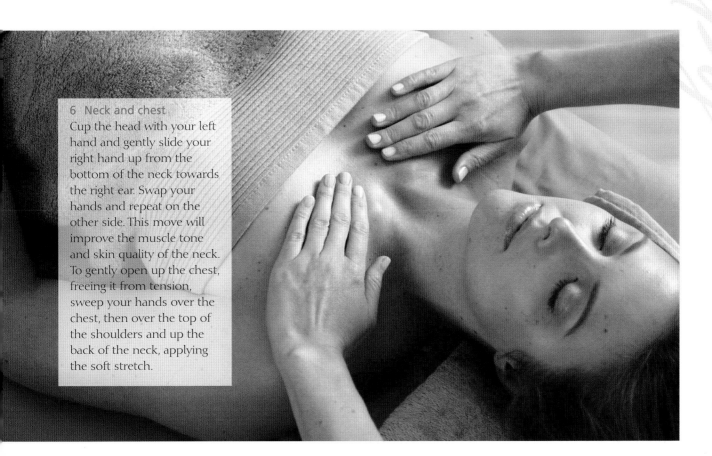

6 Neck and chest

Cup the head with your left hand and gently slide your right hand up from the bottom of the neck towards the right ear. Swap your hands and repeat on the other side. This move will improve the muscle tone and skin quality of the neck. To gently open up the chest, freeing it from tension, sweep your hands over the chest, then over the top of the shoulders and up the back of the neck, applying the soft stretch.

Abdomen

During abdominal massage, which stimulates the digestive system, your partner may experience an emotional release, such as crying, laughing or nausea, so provide assurance if necessary. Always check if she has any injuries in this area.

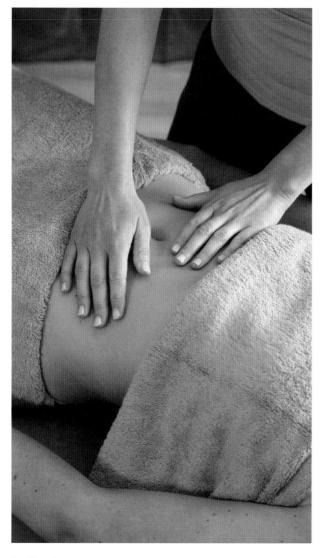

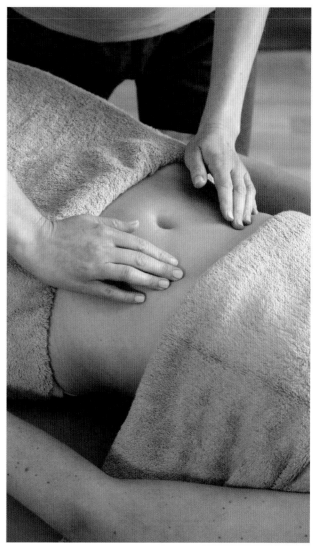

1 Circular movement

Apply a small amount of oil to your right hand, then place it softly between the navel and the breastbone and hold it there for a few moments to familiarise your partner with your touch. Circle the abdomen in a clockwise motion – this movement should feel soothing and relaxing.

2 Ribs

Using your fingers only, trace down the ribcage, sliding underneath the sides as far as possible, then pull back, finishing off at the front of the hips. This area often feels tight and tense, so check the pressure with your partner.

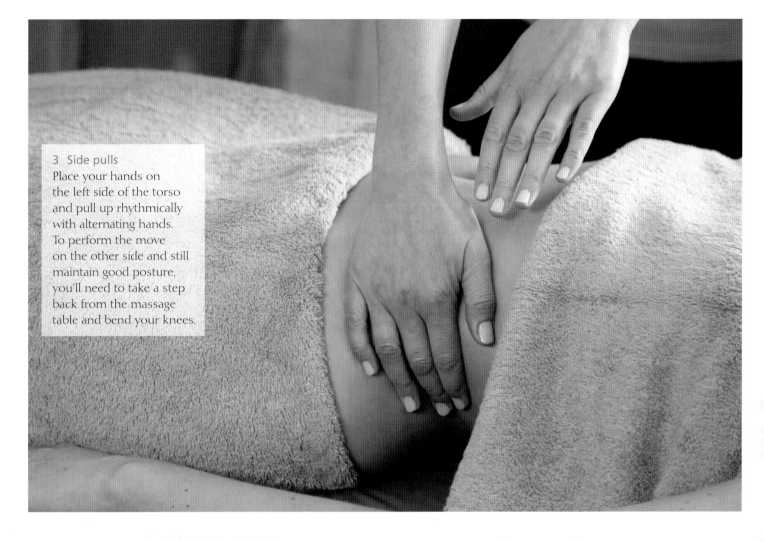

3 Side pulls
Place your hands on the left side of the torso and pull up rhythmically with alternating hands. To perform the move on the other side and still maintain good posture, you'll need to take a step back from the massage table and bend your knees.

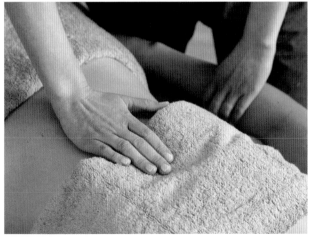

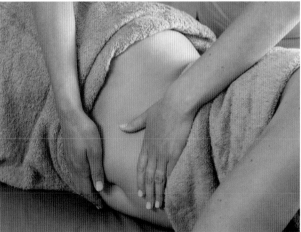

4 Vibrations
Rest your left hand on the right arm, then place your right hand on the solar plexus, between the navel and breastbone. Ask her to breathe in. On the out breath, gently press down and vibrate the abdomen muscles to release any tension. Apply pressure softly and then, if possible, sink your hands deeper.

IF THE RECEIVER IS PREGNANT

After the first trimester, apply abdominal massage while the woman lies on her side. Using the tender hold, massage the abdomen in clockwise circles. Gentle touch can relax the mother and help calm the baby, and from the seventh month, the use of essential oils will help prevent stretch marks. (See 'During pregnancy', page 14, and 'Pregnancy', page 232.)

Front of legs

To complete the massage, these beautiful techniques will encourage blood and lymph flow, reducing any tightness and swelling of the legs. You can add gentle stretches and ankle rotations at the end of the treatment.

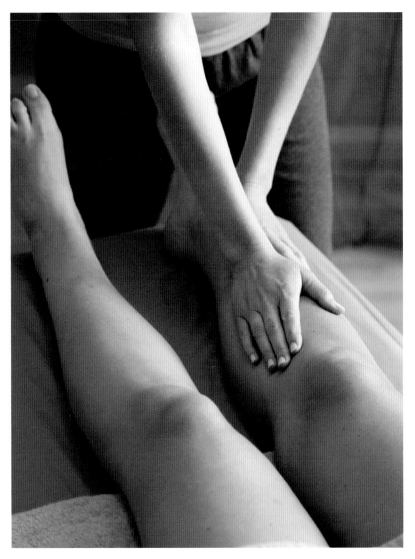

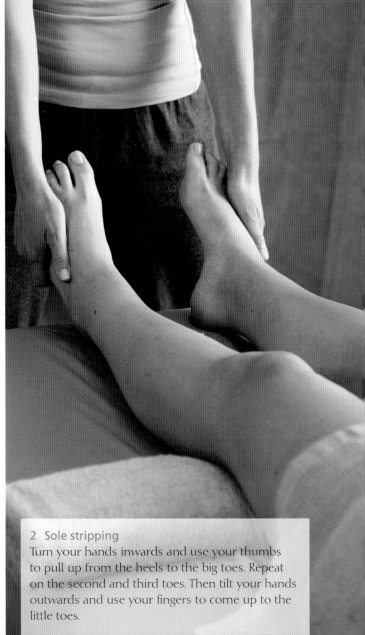

1 Effleurage to the legs
Begin the massage by placing the flats of your hands on the soles of the feet for a few seconds, then commence effleurage movements over the whole of each leg. The sliding technique is the best way to apply the essential oil and generally warm up your partner. It is easier to massage one leg at a time.

2 Sole stripping
Turn your hands inwards and use your thumbs to pull up from the heels to the big toes. Repeat on the second and third toes. Then tilt your hands outwards and use your fingers to come up to the little toes.

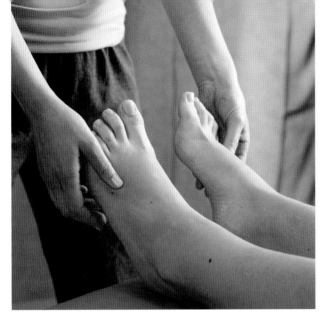

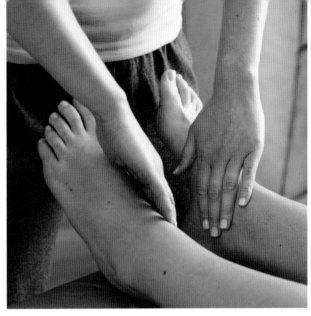

3 Lymph drainage
Lightly stroke the feet between the metatarsals, starting between the big and second toes, then moving towards the lateral ankles. Always sweep in the direction of the knees, where the lymph nodes are located. This drainage technique will help promote lymph flow.

4 Ankle circles
Circle both ankles with your fingers. Start on the outside of the ankles and then progress to the inside.

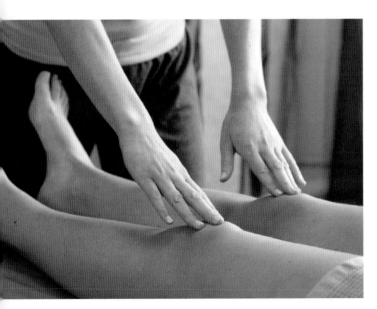

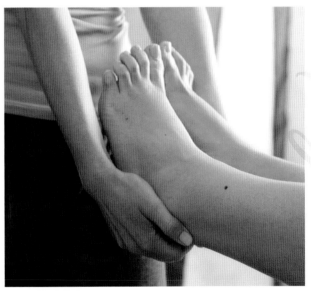

5 Leg massage
To stimulate the lymph nodes located at the back of the knees, slide your hands up to the kneecaps and rest them there for a few seconds. Then move up towards the groin area, and press gently in the middle of the thigh to stimulate the inguinal lymph nodes there.

6 Leg lift and shake
Place the palms of your hands on the soles of the feet and hold for a few seconds. This move rebalances the flow of energy at the end of the treatment. Raise the legs slightly by cupping the heels and give them a soft shake. Advise your partner that you have finished the massage, then drape her with the towel and leave her to dress.

➡ *'Aromatherapy blends', page 78*

Full body sequence for pressure point massage

The pressure point techniques, used in Shiatsu and Eastern or Chinese massage, can be applied through clothing, with your partner lying down. These easy techniques involve compressions with parts of your hands and forearms.

Back sequence

The Shiatsu back routine, part of which is shown here, is a terrific unwinding treatment that builds from gentle to firmer pressure.

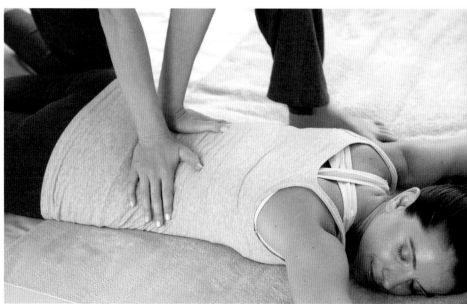

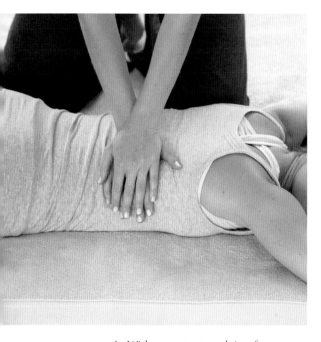

2 Position yourself so that you're kneeling on one knee. Place both palms on either side of the lower back, starting on the gluteals (buttocks), trying to apply even pressure on both sides. Slowly move your way up the back, applying more pressure as you go but avoiding the spine. Repeat 3–5 times.

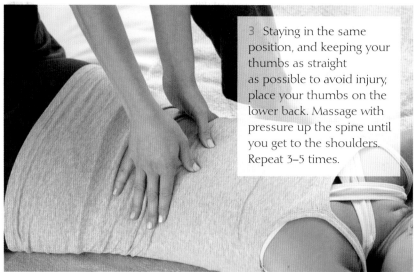

1 With your partner lying face down, her arms by her sides or above her head, kneel next to her and place one hand on her sacrum for a few seconds, trying to sync your breathing with hers. Place both palms on the other side of the back. Pushing slowly away from the spine, massage up to the shoulders. Repeat this move 3–5 times, then repeat on the other side.

3 Staying in the same position, and keeping your thumbs as straight as possible to avoid injury, place your thumbs on the lower back. Massage with pressure up the spine until you get to the shoulders. Repeat 3–5 times.

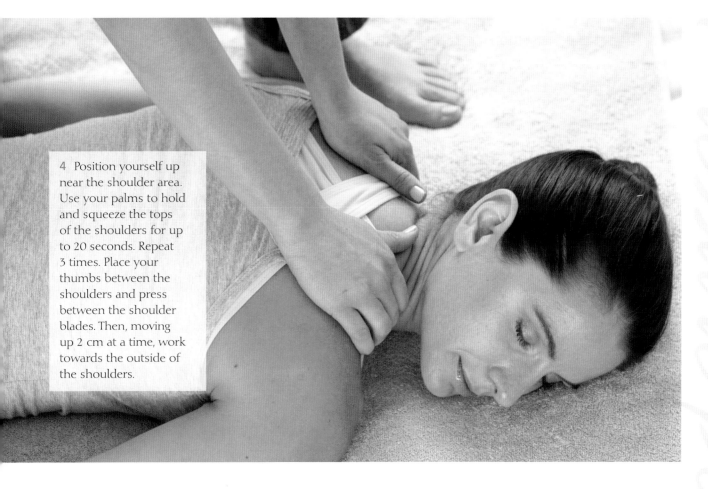

4 Position yourself up near the shoulder area. Use your palms to hold and squeeze the tops of the shoulders for up to 20 seconds. Repeat 3 times. Place your thumbs between the shoulders and press between the shoulder blades. Then, moving up 2 cm at a time, work towards the outside of the shoulders.

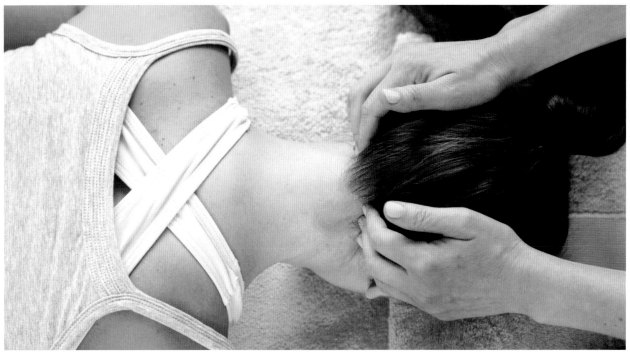

5 Sitting comfortably at your partner's head, place a small towel under her forehead. Apply rhythmic pressure to the neck muscles with your fingers and thumbs, massaging between the shoulders and the base of the skull. Then, with your thumbs together, apply pressure in a line over the scalp. Repeat this a few times.

Legs and hips sequence

This easy six-step sequence for pressure point massage to the legs and hips will rejuvenate tired and weary legs.

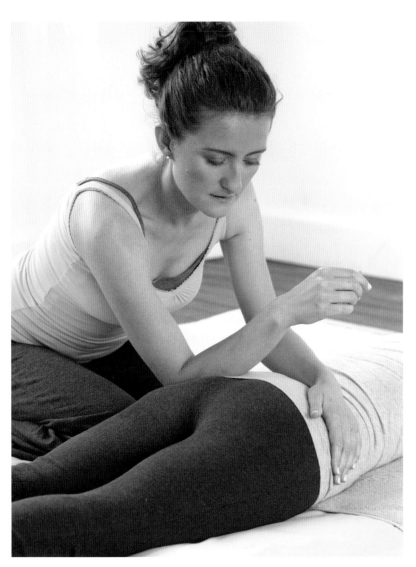

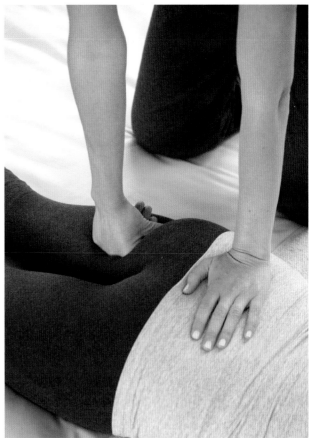

2 Staying on the same side of the body, gently make a fist with your hand and apply pressure to the backs of the thighs. Start at the top of the back of the knee and slowly apply pressure to the hamstring muscles. As you go, try to gently roll your wrist so that the muscles move under your hand. For stronger pressure, use two fists or your knees.

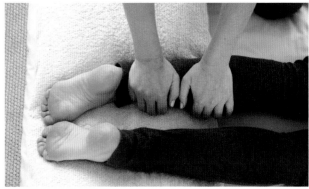

1 Kneeling to the side of your partner, place your forearm on the tops of the buttocks and slowly begin to apply pressure into these thick, strong muscles. Start at the top of the hip and move your way down, covering the whole area. If your partner is strong, use your knees and elbows to apply more pressure. Repeat 3–5 times, then apply to the other side of the body.

3 Position yourself alongside the lower leg and place a pillow under both legs. With your palms, apply gentle pressure, starting at the heel of the foot and moving up to below the back of the knee. This move is great for warming up the calf muscles. Apply pressure from the outside, pushing towards the middle. Repeat 3–5 times.

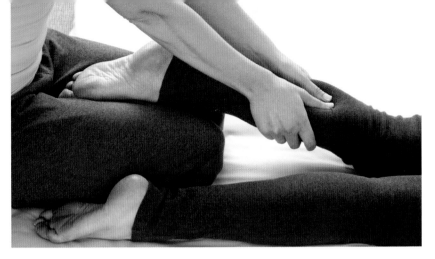

4 Kneel in line with your partner. Place her foot on top of your thigh, towards your knee. With your thumbs, apply medium pressure all the way along the lower leg. When you get to the upper part of the calf muscle, try to gently and slowly separate the muscles. Repeat 3–5 times.

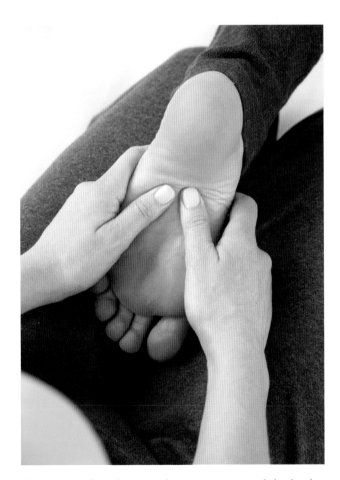

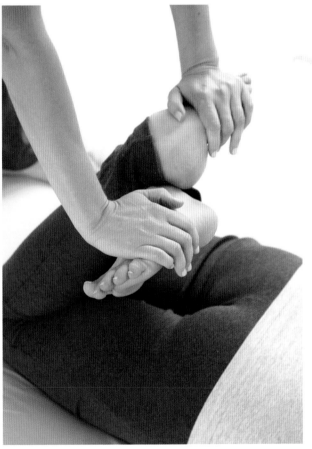

5 Use your thumbs to apply pressure around the heel, and massage in lines down the length of the foot to the toes. Next, apply pressure over the sole of the foot with your fist. Finish by applying pressure along the inside of the foot, which relates to the spine in reflexology. Repeat all these moves on the other side of the legs and feet.

6 Now finish off the leg sequence by bending the lower legs and crossing them so each foot is on the opposite buttock. The ankles should be crossed over each other. Put gentle pressure on the feet so that the receiver feels a stretch at the front of the legs. Cross the feet over and then apply pressure again, holding for up to 10 seconds.

Front of body sequence

This wonderful pressure point massage sequence finishes on the front of the body.

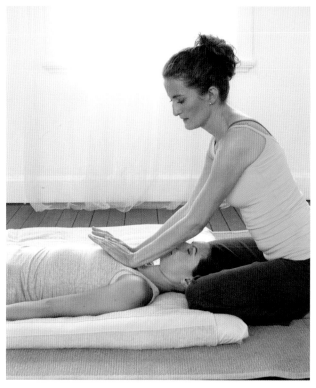

2 Kneel comfortably above your partner's head, looking down her body. Place your palms on either side of the chest, then start in the middle and slowly apply pressure to both sides so that the chest is gently stretched. Keep applying pressure out and over the shoulders. Repeat this move 3–5 times, increasing the pressure each time.

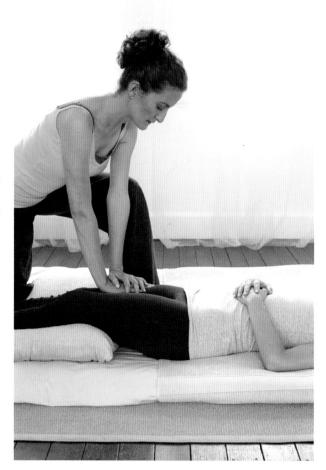

1 Ask your partner to lie on her back, then place a pillow under her knees. Kneel to one side of one leg, then place your palms on the lower leg. With easy pressure, palm all the way up to the top of the hips. As you go over the fronts of the thighs, where the muscles are stronger, apply more pressure. Repeat slowly 3–5 times, then repeat on the other leg.

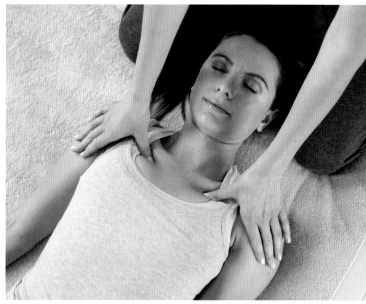

3 Kneeling in the same position, place your thumbs in the middle of the chest at the sternum. Slowly apply pressure with your thumbs alongside the clavicle (collar bone) on both sides until you get to the shoulders. Repeat this move 7–10 times.

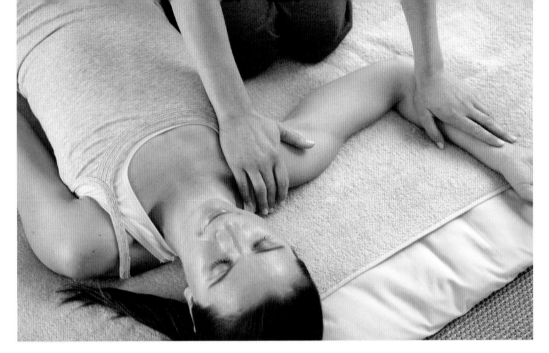

4 Move yourself around so you're at the side of the body. Place her arm at a 90-degree angle to her body, with the hand facing up, and apply pressure with your palms over the chest. Continue this move up the insides of the arms and along the forearms. Repeat 3–5 times.

➜ 'Shiatsu', page 90 • 'Eastern or Chinese massage', page 92

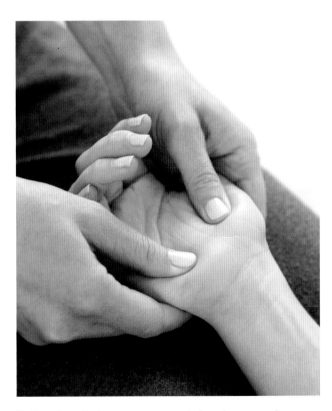

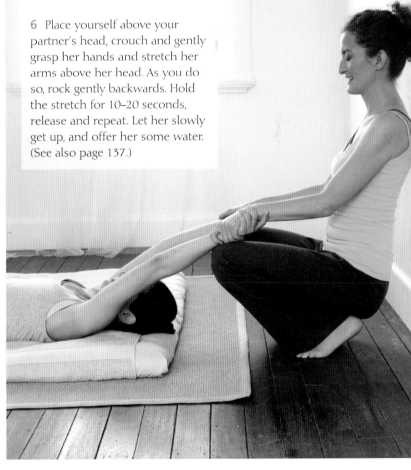

6 Place yourself above your partner's head, crouch and gently grasp her hands and stretch her arms above her head. As you do so, rock gently backwards. Hold the stretch for 10–20 seconds, release and repeat. Let her slowly get up, and offer her some water. (See also page 137.)

5 Kneel, and place your partner's hand on your lap. With both thumbs, apply pressure below the elbow joint and massage down to the wrist. Repeat. Then massage the palms of the hands and the fingers. Repeat these two moves on the other side.

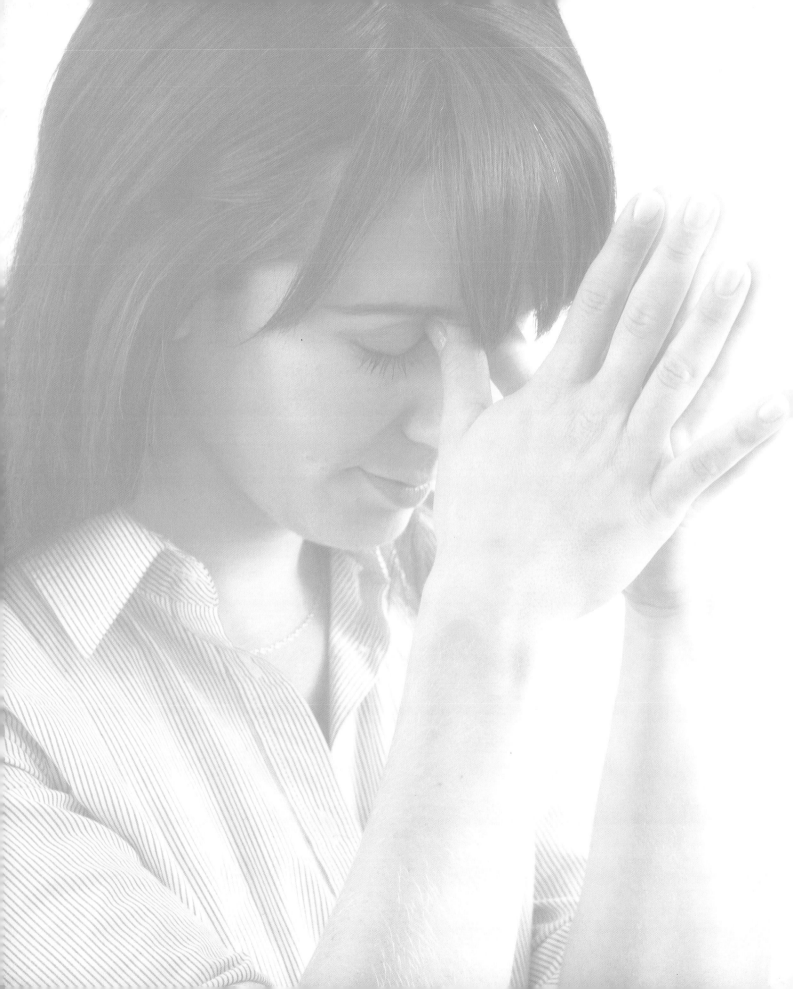

for
HEALTH
&VITALITY

Massage for ailments and conditions

The application of aromatherapy via massage combines the benefits of touch with the therapeutic properties of essential oils, creating a powerful combination for dealing with a wide range of health ailments.

Stress relief

The most obvious benefit of aromatherapy massage is in healing the physical body. For example, aromatherapy massage can help to improve circulation; ease aches, pains and stiffness; and heal muscular strains and sprains. But one of its most important benefits is stress relief – not only can the fragrances help you relax, but this therapy has also been scientifically shown to reduce hypertension (high blood pressure) and help regulate breathing and heart rate.

Particular calming essential oils, notably chamomile and rose, help to dissolve emotional and physical stress, helping with a short-term goal, such as having a good night's sleep, as well as defusing ongoing nervous tension before it conveys habitual discomfort and long-term negativity to the mind.

Thus the body is able to both restore and rebalance itself, rather than establish a vicious cycle of anxiety and depression. The use of essential oils with euphoric properties in aromatherapy massage, such as ylang ylang and lavender, has been shown to have antidepressant, uplifting and soothing effects on the mind as well as the body, with the release of physical tension also easing mental and emotional tension.

SELF-MASSAGE

People who regularly practise self-massage invariably report feeling relaxed and energised, and also being more alert to their own body's signals when it is stressed or strained. Self-massage will make you more aware of your body, and help you to exercise more control over how it functions, changes and reacts.

In the following pages, wherever it's appropriate, we have included self-massage techniques for treating various ailments and conditions.

Common health problems

Profoundly stimulating, calming and relaxing, depending on the massage style selected, aromatherapy massage is highly beneficial for easing digestive disturbances, such as bloating, and respiratory ailments, especially influenza, colds, sinusitis and hay fever. It may be used to combat many minor and irritating health complaints without having to resort to prescription drugs, which could have side effects.

Several essential oils – such as lemon balm, tea tree and lemongrass – have been scientifically proven to stimulate the immune system and to have antiviral, antifungal and antibacterial properties. Also, when essential oils with specific regenerative qualities, such as frankincense, are used in aromatherapy massage, that particular treatment can help to nourish skin on the face and body, and prevent age-related dryness, inflammation and the appearance of fine wrinkles.

Many of the benefits of aromatherapy massage work on more subtle, even energetic levels. For example, including particular essential oils such as juniper and cypress in individual massage treatments will help to detoxify the body, stimulating circulation and promoting lymphatic drainage, which in turn speeds the elimination of tissue waste.

The use of other circulation-promoting essential oils, such as rosemary and pine, will relax tight muscles as well as penetrate beneath the skin, allowing the therapeutic effects to reach the muscles, bloodstream and internal organs. This benefit applies to all essential oils used in aromatherapy, as the skin offers us the largest and most effective means of absorbing the oils into the body.

Time out

Perhaps the most important benefit of aromatherapy massage is the fact that it provides such a restorative break from the hectic demands of 21st century life. The

Over time, the regular use of aromatherapy massage can help you to become more in tune with your body and its needs. It is an inexpensive and effective way to learn to heal yourself and others. Along with eating a balanced and healthy diet, drinking plenty of fresh, clean water, and exercising, aromatherapy massage is a way to be creative as well as practical about your health.

When used between partners, aromatherapy massage helps to foster a more intimate understanding of each other's bodies and needs.

profound calm delivered by this modality relieves mental and emotional burnout and improves overall quality of life, helping you to realise your fullest potential in mind, body and spirit.

The beautiful fragrances have great potential to encourage your personal development, enhance your wellbeing, improve your attention and memory, aid your concentration, and even overcome fears and phobias.

The power of touch

In a world driven by technology, we tend to use our eyes and ears to seek and absorb information far more than our ancestors, who would have used their sense of touch at least equally.

Research shows that those who are not regularly hugged or stroked by others, such as older people in nursing homes, suffer from a higher than average incidence of depression, while babies and toddlers who do not receive regular, loving touch will experience emotional distress.

With aromatherapy massage you can reintroduce the power of touch into your life – your health, and the health of those you care about, is literally in your hands.

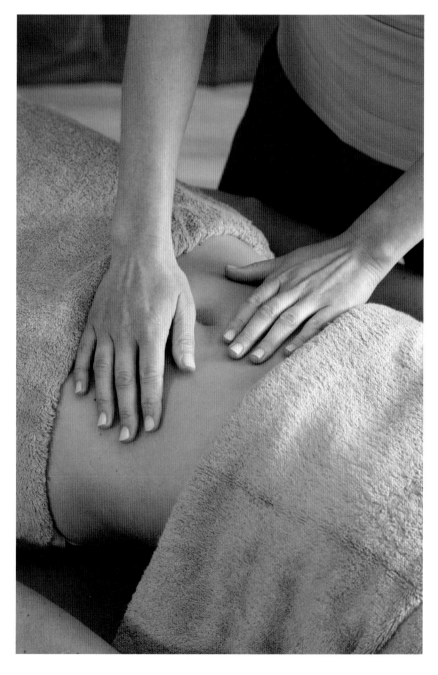

Anxiety and stress

Stress and anxiety can have an impact on your mental and social health, reducing your quality of life. Not only can stress increase your blood pressure and reduce your body's immune function, it has also been linked to chronic health conditions such as heart disease and diabetes.

Relaxing essential oils

Massage can help reduce stress and anxiety levels by releasing tension in the muscles, clearing metabolic waste and creating a space for healing.

There are many essential oils that help to reduce stress and anxiety. For anxiety, try essential oils with sedative properties, such as chamomile, jasmine, marjoram, melissa, neroli and rose. For stress, use essential oils with relaxing properties, such as Roman chamomile, rosewood, sweet marjoram, sweet orange and tangerine.

The process of the massage itself can help reduce stress and tension as the receiver takes time out of their busy lifestyle to relax. You can ask your partner to follow the Swedish massage routine demonstrated on pages 136–53, or the aromatherapy sequence, described on pages 154–65. You could also try the tennis ball technique on page 180.

In the work environment, stress and anxiety can become overwhelming. The following massage and self-massage techniques, which are convenient and easy to administer, can be performed by you or a colleague while you are at your desk.

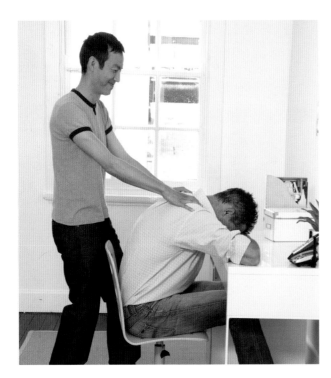

Desk massage to the shoulders
Ask your massage partner to rest his head on his arms, which can be crossed on the desk in front of him. Apply kneading massage to the shoulder region.

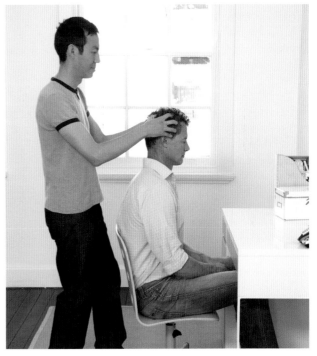

Desk massage to the head and temples
With your partner sitting comfortably upright in the chair, gently perform slow circular frictions around the temple and scalp region. Be sure not to press too firmly in the centre of the temple region.

When you're anxious or nervous about an upcoming event, your sympathetic nervous system is stimulated, increasing your heart rate and breathing rate, and pumping the body with adrenaline. You can tense your muscles, and may even experience stomach upsets. Here are some useful tips for preparing for a stressful event.

1 Slow down your breathing rate *Take 10 deep breaths, counting to 5 as you breathe in, then hold the breath for a few seconds and take 5 more counts to release the breath. Having a few drops of a relaxing essential oil such as lavender on a handkerchief can assist this technique.*

2 Neck and shoulders self-massage *Using one hand, squeeze through the shoulder and neck muscles of the opposite side to release built up tension. Repeat on the other side.*

3 Visualisation *This technique can prepare you to conquer the stressful event. Find a quiet place, shut your eyes and visualise yourself successfully completing your task.*

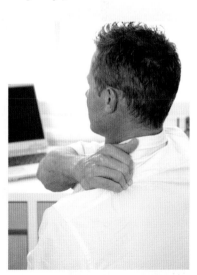

Bergamot, frankincense, lavender, sandalwood and ylang ylang essential oils help alleviate both stress and anxiety.

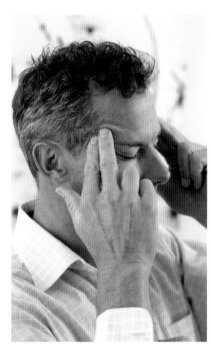

Self-massage to the temples
You can perform self-massage techniques to relieve stress and anxiety. Sitting comfortably in a chair, perform gentle, slow circular frictions around your temple and scalp region.

CAUTIONS ● See 'Safety and cautions', page 134.

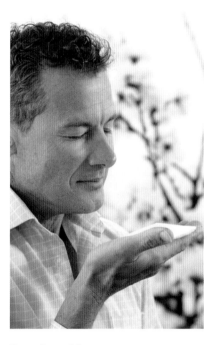

Deep breathing
Taking 10 deep breaths can be enough to calm you down after a stressful situation. Make sure you breathe deeply into your diaphragm, allowing your ribs to expand slowly. You can combine this technique with inhaling from a handkerchief 2–3 drops (in total) of one or more of the essential oils mentioned opposite.

➜ *'Aromatherapy blends', page 74*

Arms and hands

When your arms and hands become a little overworked, try some massage, which can assist with conditions such as repetitive strain or stress injury (RSI), carpal tunnel syndrome, arthritis and dry skin.

Arthritis massage

Black pepper, German chamomile, ginger, lavender, rosemary and thyme essential oils are known to help ease inflammation of the joints. If you suffer from arthritis, dilute a few drops of one or two of the oils in 20–30 ml of a carrier oil, then slowly and gently rub over the affected area, finishing with a nice massage to the fingers.

Repetitive strain injury

Repetitive strain injury and carpal tunnel syndrome can occur in the wrist as a result of repeated work-related actions – such as clicking a computer mouse – although carpal tunnel can also result from other causes. Check with your doctor first. Massage and stretching can help loosen the arm muscles, which tighten up due to overuse, inflaming the tendons of the arm. For relief, follow this five-step massage and stretching sequence.

CAUTIONS ● See 'Safety and cautions', page 134.

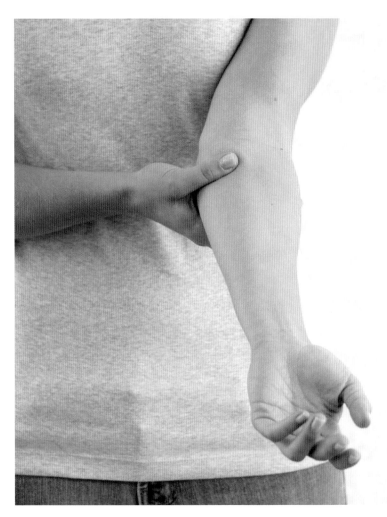

1 Massage your forearm. Place your arm down on a table, if one is handy, then use frictions with your thumbs or fingers to work into the muscles. Slow, easy pressure is best. Take your time to work around the bone on the inside of the elbow, as this is where the muscles attach.

For dry hands, soak your hands in a bowl of lukewarm water containing a few drops of ylang ylang essential oil.

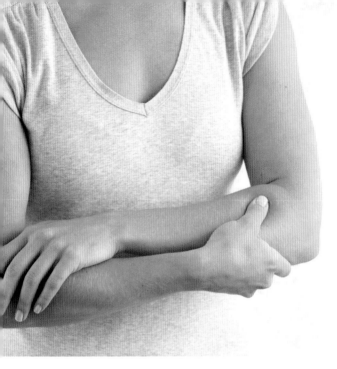

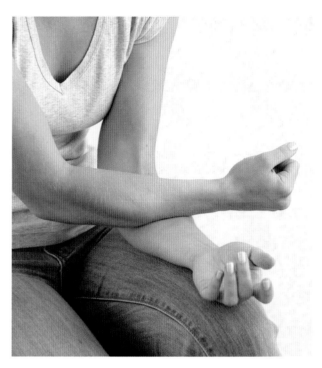

2 Turn your arm over and massage the other side of your forearm, mainly using your thumbs, as there is not as much muscle here. Wriggle your thumb back and forth as you move up and down.

3 Another option is to place your arm down on your leg and massage the arm with your other forearm. Start above the elbow crease and massage up and down, while rotating the arm, massaging back and forth. Apply a little oil to assist with the movement if you like.

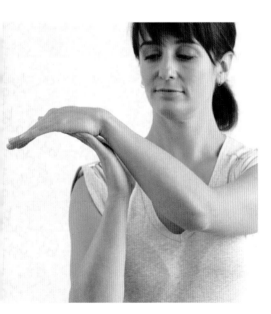

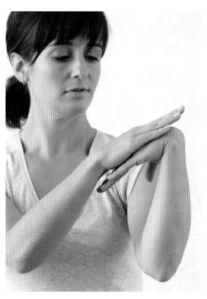

COLD HANDS AND FINGERS

Massage can assist people with poor circulation, who often have cold hands and fingers, but first check with your doctor that the condition is not caused by something serious. To assist with circulation and to also help promote stronger, healthier nails, apply general massage all over the fingers, taking the time to massage each finger separately.

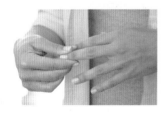

4 Hold the affected hand up straight, then place the palm of your other hand over the fingers and push back the wrist. Hold this position for 10–15 seconds, then release and repeat. If you experience any shooting pain during the stretch, stop.

5 This stretch focuses on the extensor muscles, which are affected by RSI. Start with your hand facing up and then bring it down to a 90-degree angle. With your other hand facing palm down, push down, enabling an efficient stretch. Hold for 10–15 seconds, then release and repeat.

➔ *'Aromatherapy massage', page 84*

Back pain

This extremely common problem can range from a small ache to severe, debilitating pain, and can last for a day or for years. The causes may include nerve and disc problems, musculoskeletal damage and muscular imbalance.

Relieving lower back pain

The back is greatly affected by your posture and daily activities. Refer to the section on posture (page 222), as this may be causing your back pain. Massage can help to relieve sore and fatigued back muscles, reducing pain and improving function. Any of the lower back techniques from the Swedish routine (see page 138) will stimulate blood to the area.

For added benefit, use some aromatherapy essential oils, such as arnica, black pepper, eucalyptus, ginger, lavender, peppermint and pine, all of which can assist in relieving back pain.

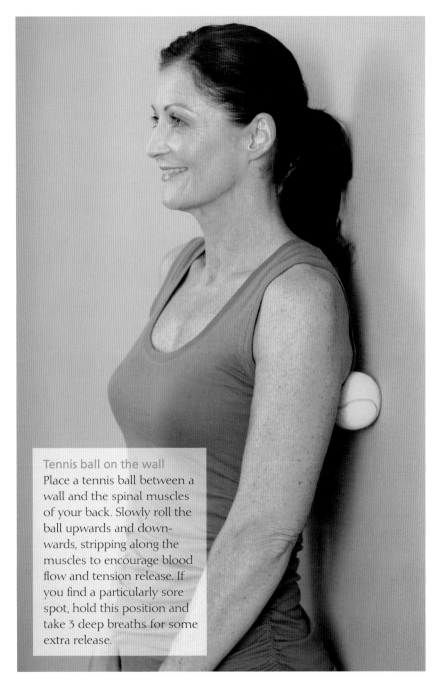

Tennis ball on the wall
Place a tennis ball between a wall and the spinal muscles of your back. Slowly roll the ball upwards and down-wards, stripping along the muscles to encourage blood flow and tension release. If you find a particularly sore spot, hold this position and take 3 deep breaths for some extra release.

➔ 'Back sequence', page 138
• 'Posture', page 222

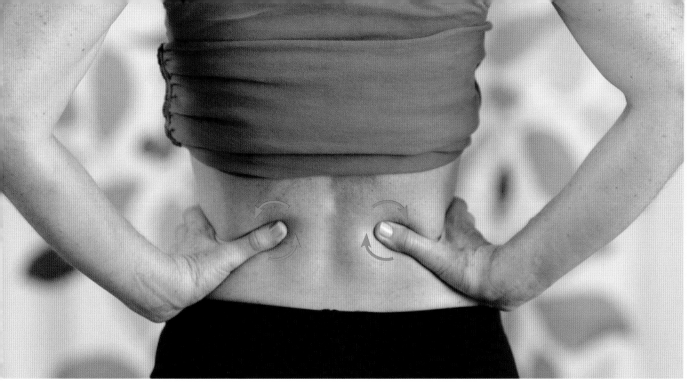

Spinal circles

Using some of the oils listed opposite, massage your lower back spinal muscles by performing small circular frictions with your thumbs.

CAUTIONS ● See 'Safety and cautions', page 134.

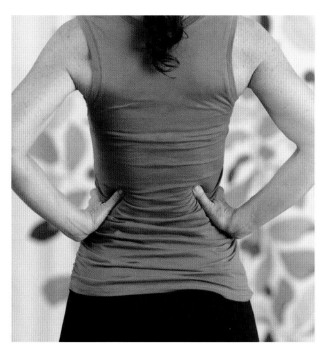

Spinal muscle release with breath work

This technique is excellent for releasing the quadratus lumborum, or spinal muscle, which often gets tight and sore. Place your thumbs in the space just below your last rib and press in to the muscle. Take 3 deep breaths, feeling the muscles press out against your thumbs.

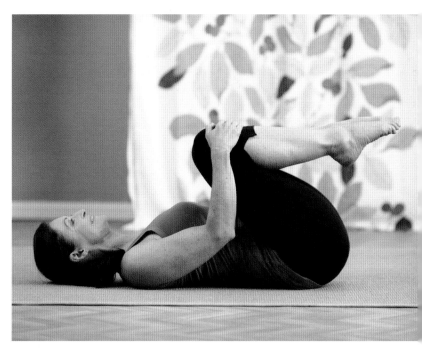

Lower back tuck stretch with small circles

Lie on the floor, then bring your knees to your chest and hold them with your hands. Take 3 deep breaths, and begin slowly circling your knees in one direction 5 times, then in the opposite direction 5 times. Repeat these circles 3 times.

Brain boosters

The brain needs blood and nutrients, but the supply can be inhibited by poor posture and tension in the neck muscles and scalp. Both massage and stretching can improve this nutrient-rich supply, enhancing mental alertness.

Improving your focus

Enhance your concentration by following these tips.

Maintain your hydration levels by drinking plenty of water throughout the day. Your body comprises mostly water, so you need to keep up a good water intake to ensure your brain and muscles have enough to function at their best. The elderly are often dehydrated, as they don't drink enough water. Try drinking water that is not too cold, as it is better absorbed by the body. Consider increasing your vitamin C intake by adding a piece of lemon or lime to the water.

If you can, go for a short walk during the day, especially at lunch or afternoon teatime. Take the stairs instead of the lift, and avoid using email with a co-worker if you just need to deliver a simple message – instead, walk to their desk, even if it's on another floor.

The caffeine in coffee and tea contains diuretics, which help move fluid out of the body. Try drinking water before you drink a cup of tea or coffee, and try to limit how many you have per day.

Sweets such as chocolate and cakes offer short-term energy and concentration boosts, but the downside is that they result in a lull after about 30–60 minutes. Try drinking a peppermint tea instead.

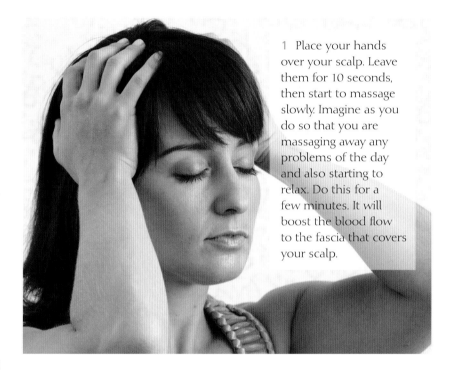

1 Place your hands over your scalp. Leave them for 10 seconds, then start to massage slowly. Imagine as you do so that you are massaging away any problems of the day and also starting to relax. Do this for a few minutes. It will boost the blood flow to the fascia that covers your scalp.

If you don't want to mess up your hair, try massaging through a small towel.

Pick-me-up routine

Here's an easy five-step, 10-minute sequence to boost blood circulation to your scalp, maintain your concentration levels and mental alertness, and also stop you reaching for that morning or afternoon pick-me-up. You can do each step either standing or sitting.

IMPROVE YOUR FOCUS

Improve your concentration by first closing your eyes and imagining a line running through your body into the earth. Imagine anchoring this line, and that it's running straight up, out of your head. Imagine your body is as straight as this line. Take 3 big, deep, slow breaths, visualising after each breath that you are more and more present in your body. When you open your eyes, you should be more focused.

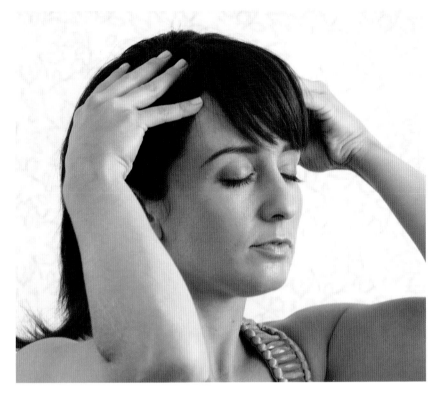

LUNCHTIME EXERCISE

A lot of workplaces have exercise or yoga programs during the lunch break – a great way to maintain your concentration levels and mental alertness. Exercise promotes blood flow and also produces endorphins, the body's 'feel-good' hormones. It will also give your mind a break, allowing it to focus on something else, so that when you do go back to work, you will feel fresher and mentally rejuvenated.

CAUTIONS • See 'Safety and cautions', page 134.

2 Continuing with the pads of your fingertips, massage over the same area. Try to feel for any tightness or restriction in your scalp that might be blocking blood flow. Working in little circles, cover the whole scalp.

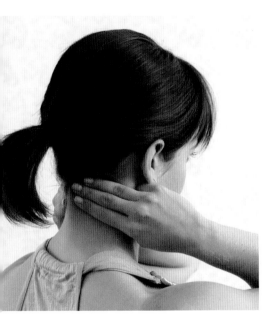

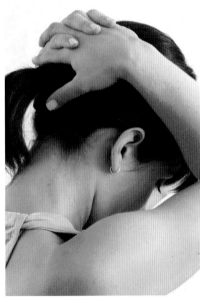

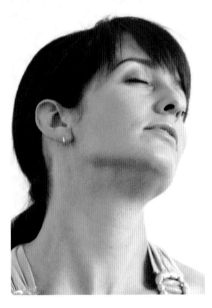

3 Next, place your three middle fingers at the back of your neck and head. At the base of the skull, rub them back and forth, warming them up and allowing the muscles to relax. This will assist with getting blood through to the brain. Do this for up to a minute.

4 Place all your fingers on the back of the head, lock them together and then slowly start to push your head forward. Keep doing this stretch as long as is comfortable and/or until you feel a stretch at the back of the neck. Hold this for 20–30 seconds. Repeat the sequence.

5 Slowly roll your head around on your shoulders in an anticlockwise circle. After 3 rolls, switch direction and roll your head the other way. This should take about a minute.

➔ *'Aromatherapy blends', page 64*

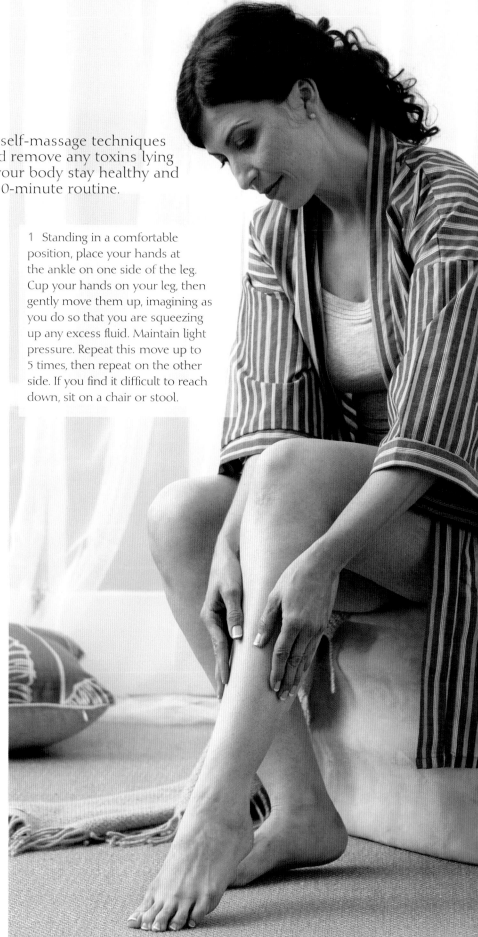

Cellulite

When applied regularly, these self-massage techniques can help tone the muscles and remove any toxins lying dormant in the skin. To help your body stay healthy and supple, make them part of a 10-minute routine.

Lymphatic massage

Lymphatic massage can assist with the natural ageing processes that can cause cellulite. Try this two-step routine, which assists the removal of waste and toxins that may be stored in your legs and muscles. Lymphatic massage should always be slow and gentle, as too much pressure will be ineffective. To enhance the effect, wear a skin-brushing glove, as shown in step 2.

DETOXIFYING OIL TREATMENT

Essential oils are great for cellulite, as they assist with detoxification, stimulating lymph flow and also moving fluid with diuretic properties. After a shower, apply a few drops each of cypress, grapefruit, geranium, lemon, juniper berry and/or rosemary essential oils to 3 tablespoons of 20–30 ml of a carrier oil to the skin. This will remove any dead surface skin cells, and allow the oils to soak through the pores and release their therapeutic properties. Alternatively, you could add the oils to a bath and have a relaxing soak.

CAUTIONS • See 'Safety and cautions', page 134.

1 Standing in a comfortable position, place your hands at the ankle on one side of the leg. Cup your hands on your leg, then gently move them up, imagining as you do so that you are squeezing up any excess fluid. Maintain light pressure. Repeat this move up to 5 times, then repeat on the other side. If you find it difficult to reach down, sit on a chair or stool.

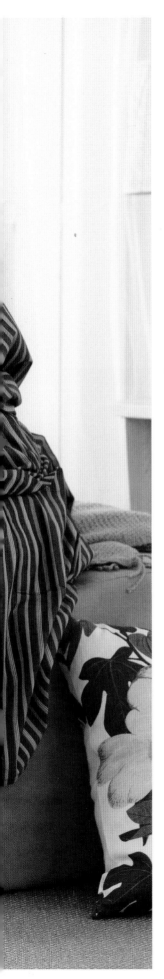

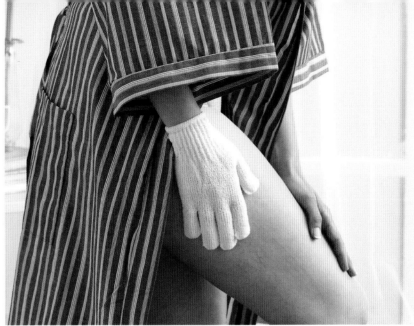

2 Place your hands on your upper thighs and move them around slowly in a clockwise direction. Try to cover the whole thigh area, including the front, back and sides. Next, move up to the buttocks and apply the same moves, either directly on the skin or through your clothes. This process will assist the lymphatic system. Repeat on both sides, taking up to 4–5 minutes on each.

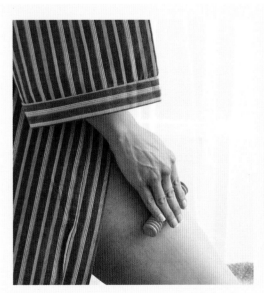

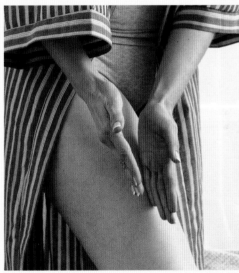

Self-massage
Self-massage to the legs helps keep the muscles loose and relaxed. You can also massage over your legs with a wooden roller, which smooths the skin and helps remove toxins. Move the roller back and forth over your legs for up to 3 minutes, repeating on all parts of both thighs.

Percussion
This stimulates the nerve endings in the skin and helps to maintain muscle tone, which in turn helps maintain suppleness in cellulite-prone thighs. After warming your muscles in a shower, apply quick rhythmical percussion movements up and down the legs for up to a minute, paying special attention to the cellulite-prone areas. Repeat on both sides of each leg.

Circulatory problems

A variety of conditions cause circulatory problems, but when the problem is not serious, use these techniques to help boost your circulation, especially when the weather is colder or when you start to become less active.

The benefits of massage

A lot of circulatory problems end up affecting the body's extremities – the legs and feet, arms and hands. This is the body's way of conserving blood for the areas where it is needed for survival – the brain and organs. If you have a circulation problem, you can improve it with exercise, which pumps blood around the body and helps tone the muscles, which in turn help push the blood back to the heart through more efficient contraction.

Massage also assists greatly by moving blood through the body, and helping bring blood to the extremities – the hands and feet. In addition, it generates heat, which allows the muscles to function more efficiently. Regular massage might help prevent varicose veins, as it assists with pushing venous blood through the veins (see also the box on 'Varicose veins', page 128).

Poor-fitting and tight shoes and clothing can also cause circulatory problems by restricting muscles, tendons and the skin, and not allowing the free flow of blood. This can be a problem if the restriction is focused on certain areas over a long period of time.

CAUTIONS ● See 'Safety and cautions', page 134. ● Do not massage over any varicose veins.

Massaging children from an early age can go a long way towards preventing circulatory problems later in life.

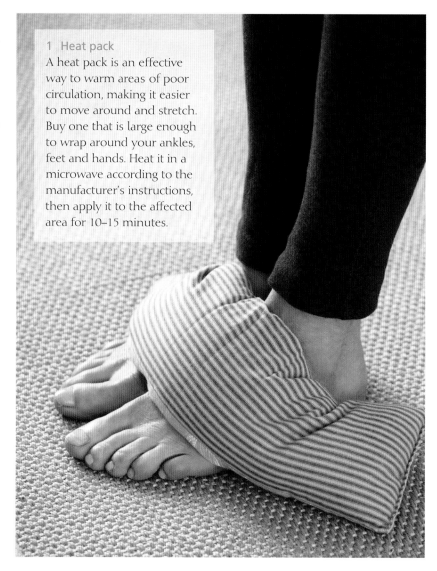

1 Heat pack
A heat pack is an effective way to warm areas of poor circulation, making it easier to move around and stretch. Buy one that is large enough to wrap around your ankles, feet and hands. Heat it in a microwave according to the manufacturer's instructions, then apply it to the affected area for 10–15 minutes.

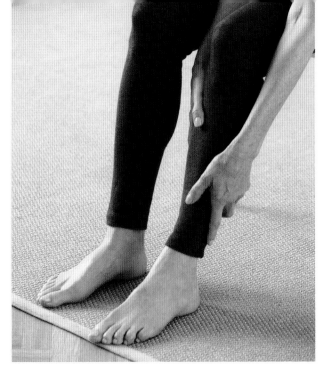

Massaging with a carrier oil containing a few drops of ginger, black pepper or rosemary essential oil helps warm up cold fingers and toes and stimulate the circulation.

2 Self-massage to the legs
Sitting down in a comfortable position, start at your ankles, using both hands to massage up to the knees. Work up the leg quite quickly, as if you were milking a cow, then return down to the ankles to start again.

➔ *'Aromatherapy blends', page 68*

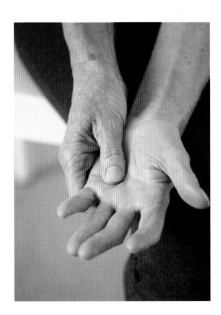

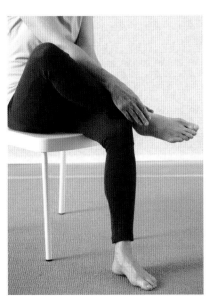

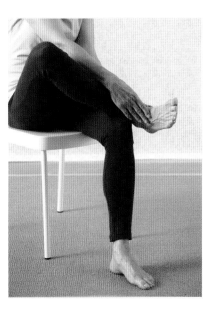

3 Self-massage to the hands
Starting at the base of the knuckle on your little finger, apply pressure with the index finger and thumb of your other hand until you reach the fingertip. Repeat twice before doing each of the other fingers, then repeat the sequence on the other hand.

4 Stretching the feet and toes
Cross your right leg over your left and grasp your foot. Rub your hands over the ankle, then point your foot forwards. Bring your foot back up towards your leg. Hold your toes to assist the stretch. Repeat up to 10 times. Repeat on the other foot.

5 Stretching the ankles
Now that your muscles are warm and your ankle joint has moved a little, roll your right foot around in circles, first clockwise, then anti-clockwise. Do this in both directions a couple of times each, then stretch the other foot.

Computer-related ailments

If you sit at a computer for long periods, try these easy techniques with the essential oils of warming black pepper and ginger and relaxing German chamomile and lavender – great for massaging your arms, neck and shoulders.

The price of poor posture

If your posture at the keyboard is typically slumped forward, with rounded shoulders, a curved back and an extended neck, it will place a lot of strain on the structures of the back, neck and shoulders, which can lead to problems in these areas. The glare from the computer and the closeness of the screen can cause eye strain and headaches. And when you sit for long periods of time, the hamstring muscles can shorten, which may lead to structural problems and knee or back pain.

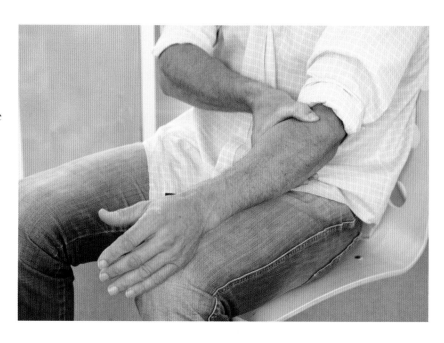

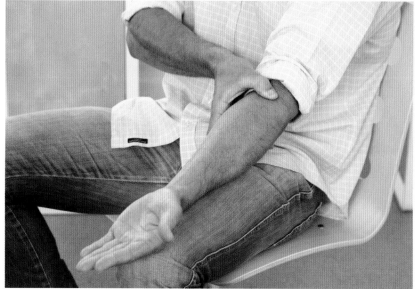

Wrist, elbow and hands

With the thumb and fingers of your right hand, hold onto the muscle bulk just below your left elbow where the wrist flexors and extensors attach. Keeping your right hand still, rotate your left arm backwards and forwards, feeling the muscles beneath being massaged. Repeat on the other arm.

CAUTIONS ● See 'Safety and cautions', page 134.

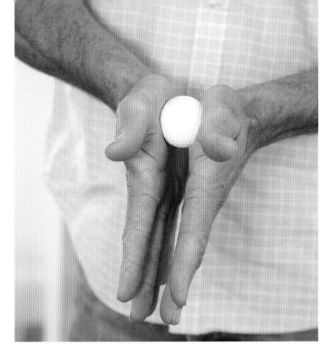

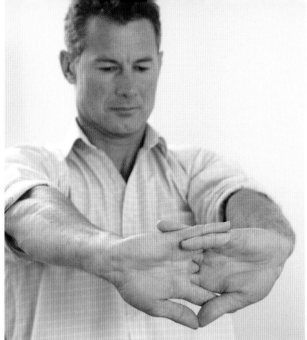

Hand massage
Place a golf ball between the palms of your hands. To release the muscles from tension, press slightly inwards and perform slow circles around the hand. Pay special attention to the muscles of the thumb, which get overworked.

Hand stretch
Finish with a stretch through your hands and fingers. Interlock your fingers and press your palms outwards, extending your arms until you feel a stretch. Hold for 15 seconds. Repeat 2–3 times.

COMPUTER WORK STATION

A poorly set up work station can result in unnecessary aches and pains.
- *Avoid neck and eye strain by setting your computer screen at eye level.*
- *Avoid excessive twisting of the back and torso by positioning your chair in the middle of the screen.*
- *Prevent back, hip and knee strain by keeping your knees at 90 degrees.*
- *Reduce the risk of conditions such as repetitive strain injury (RSI) by making sure your wrist is supported at the mouse.*

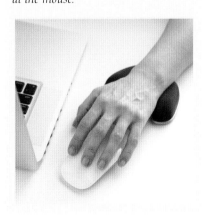

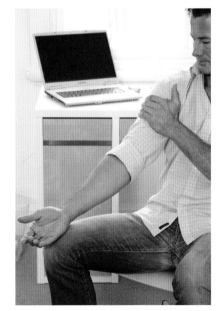

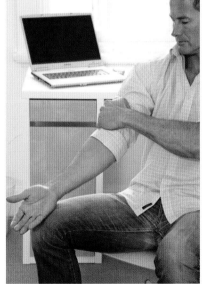

Quick shoulder release
Using your left hand, grasp the shoulder of the right. Place pressure on the arm with the palm of the hand and move the muscle outwards, creating a stretch on the muscle. Work down the arm and back up to the shoulder. Repeat the routine 3 times.

➔ *'Arms and hands sequence', page 150*
• *'Eye strain', page 200*

Convalescence

While you're recovering from an illness or injury, take great care not to stress your body, as stress lowers the immune function and the body will take longer to repair. Massage and aromatherapy can help restore you to full health.

Healing massage

If illness has led to long periods of bed rest, the muscles may be stiff and weak. The key to massage in convalescence is being gentle and promoting a healing space for the body. A few drops of relaxing essential oils such as bergamot, lavender, neroli and rose added to 20–30 ml of a carrier oil are good to use while you're recovering from an illness.

REFLEXOLOGY POINTS

Depending on the original ailment, you can use the specific reflexology points to promote a healing space for specific areas and organs of the body. Massage to the hands and feet can stimulate reflex points and help to give the whole body a treatment.

CAUTIONS ● See 'Safety and cautions', page 134.

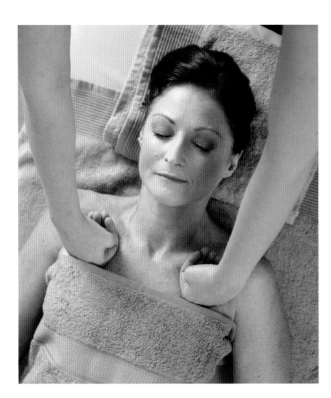

Releasing the chest
Fits of coughing or heavy breathing can make the chest muscles stiffen up. Place your fists just under the collar bone on each shoulder. Ask your partner to take 3 deep breaths in and out while focusing on releasing any tension. Keep your pressure quite gentle but constant, as the breaths will push your hands up.

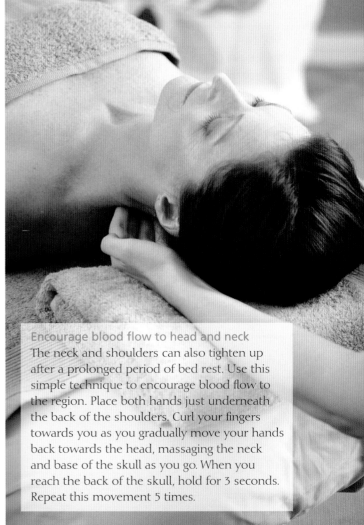

Encourage blood flow to head and neck
The neck and shoulders can also tighten up after a prolonged period of bed rest. Use this simple technique to encourage blood flow to the region. Place both hands just underneath the back of the shoulders. Curl your fingers towards you as you gradually move your hands back towards the head, massaging the neck and base of the skull as you go. When you reach the back of the skull, hold for 3 seconds. Repeat this movement 5 times.

➜ *'Reflexology', page 106*

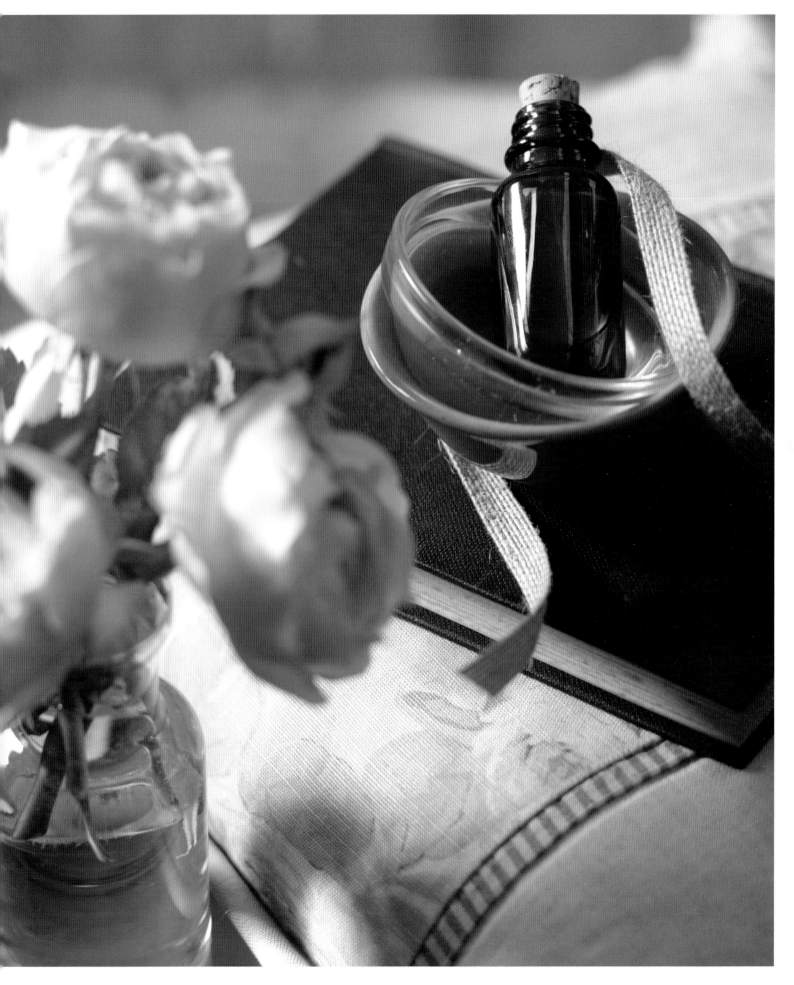

Coughs and colds

A number of massage techniques can help ease the symptoms of coughs and colds, while essential oil blends are fantastic for helping the body recover from some of the symptoms of flu and other respiratory conditions naturally.

Relieving the symptoms

One of the best methods for relieving congestion and helping you breathe more easily is an inhalation. Add boiling water to a bowl, then add a few drops each of eucalyptus, pine and/or thyme essential oil. Tent your head with a towel and inhale the steam for 10 minutes, keeping your face 20 cm away from the water's surface. Breathe in the steam deeply for a couple of minutes.

Another easy remedy if you're having difficulty breathing is to apply a few drops of eucalyptus essential oil to a tissue or hand-kerchief, and inhale it at regular intervals. Alternatively, to help you sleep, place up to 5 drops of eucalyptus or lavender essential oil on your pillow.

By burning eucalyptus and pine essential oils in a vaporiser, you can enjoy a prolonged but subtle therapeutic effect. Add a few drops of the oils to 2 table-spoons of water and burn the blend at night while you sleep.

A chest rub (see step 1) is a great way to facilitate breathing during a cold or a long bout of coughing. You could also try cupping (step 2), or a combination of cupping and rubbing (step 3).

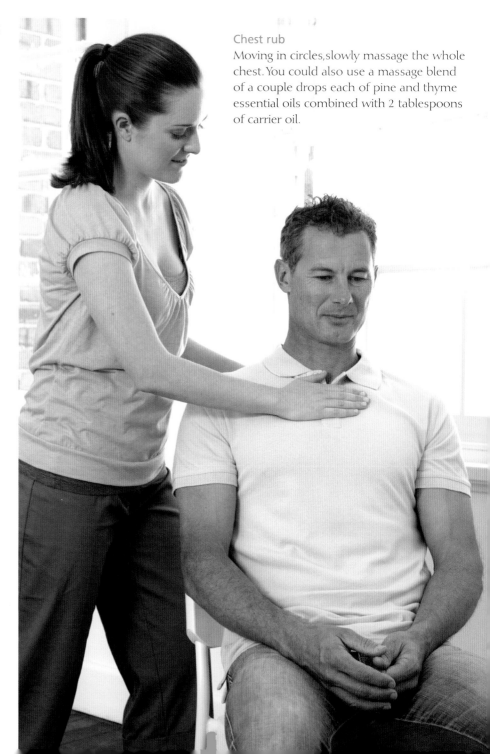

Chest rub
Moving in circles, slowly massage the whole chest. You could also use a massage blend of a couple drops each of pine and thyme essential oils combined with 2 tablespoons of carrier oil.

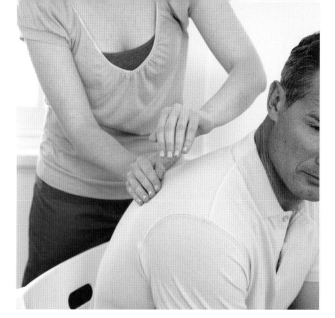

Cupping

Apply cupping to the back to help dislodge the mucous build-up that can occur in the thoracic (lung) area when your partner has a cold. Cup both hands and beat them alternately, one after the other, for up to 40 seconds. It's quite common for the receiver to cough during this movement, but it shouldn't be excessive.

LOOSEN THE BACK AND CHEST MUSCLES

Once you're past the contagious stage of a cold, general Swedish, aromatherapy or remedial massage is wonderful for loosening the muscles of the back and chest that have tightened up as a result of coughing. Apply frictions to the intercostal muscles, located between the ribs, and breathe in deeply as you do so.

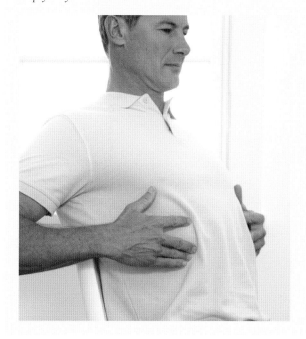

CAUTIONS
- See 'Safety and cautions', page 134.

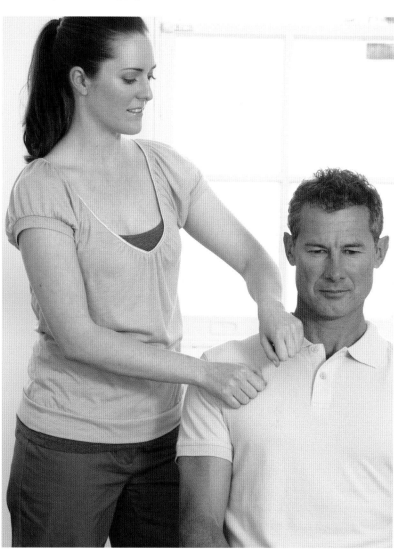

Rubbing and cupping

To help move built up mucus in your partner's lungs, apply rubbing and percussion techniques to the chest. (If your partner is a woman, be careful not to go too hard over the breast tissue.) Start by rubbing your hands back and forth over the chest. Then use gentle striking or cupping techniques over the chest area while your partner breathes in and out.

➜ 'Aromatherapy blends', page 70
- 'Lymphatic massage', page 104
- 'Lymphatic system', page 132

Cramps

The essential oils black pepper, Roman chamomile, clary sage, lavender, sweet marjoram and thyme are great for easing muscular cramps, while regular massage can keep muscle tissue healthy, reducing the risk of further cramps.

What causes cramps

Cramps are painful and sustained muscle contractions or spasms that can occur in both skeletal muscle and the smooth muscle of the internal organs.

Muscle cramps often occur when the muscle is fatigued, or if the diet is deficient in essential minerals such as magnesium, calcium, sodium and potassium. They can also result from a lot of sweating, when the body becomes dehydrated and loses electrolytes, which are essential for healthy muscle function.

Cramps usually occur in the muscles that cross two joints – that is, the larger muscles of the body, such as the gastrocnemius and the hamstring. Stretching and massage may relieve some cramps, but if they are persistent, consult your doctor.

To avoid cramping, be sure to eat a well balanced diet and drink plenty of water, especially on hot and humid days. Finally, to keep your muscles in good condition, use any of the techniques in the Swedish massage routine (see pages 136–53).

Calves and hamstrings

Apply this four-step self-massage sequence to one leg at a time.

PREVENTATIVE STRETCHES

Having good flexibility can help to maintain your muscle health.

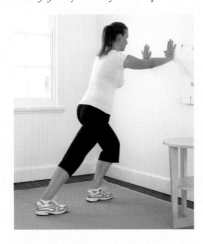

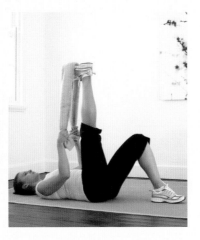

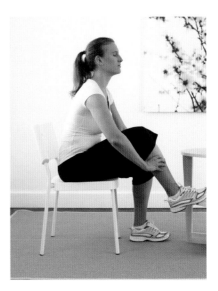

1 **Calf stretch**
Stand about 1 m away from a wall, place both hands against it and step one foot forwards. Keeping the back leg straight, lean against the wall, bending the front knee. You should feel a nice stretch along the length of the calf muscle. Hold for 15–20 seconds. Perform 3 times on both sides.

2 **Hamstring stretch**
Lie on the floor or the bed with one leg bent at the knee. Place a towel around the other foot and lift the leg into the air until you feel a stretch to your hamstrings. Hold the stretch for 15–20 seconds. Perform 3 times on both sides.

1 Sit on a chair and, with your knee bent, place your leg up on another chair in front of you. Begin by grasping your calf muscle with both hands, so that your thumbs meet in the centre of the calf muscle. Move the calf muscle from one side to another. This begins to release the muscle fibres.

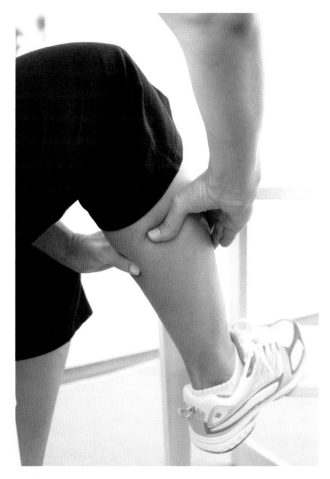

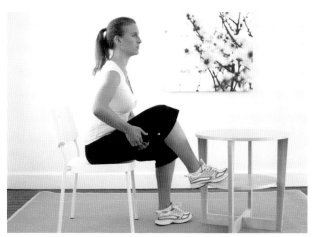

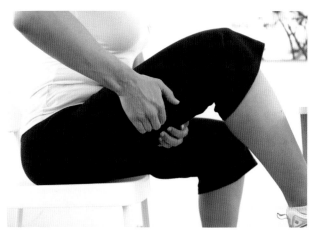

2 With your hands in the same position, use your thumbs to perform circular frictions along the length of the calf muscle. Repeat this 3–5 times.

3 While you are in this seated position, move your hands up to the back of your thigh, this time with your fingers meeting in the middle of the hamstrings. Working your way up and down the thigh, use your hands to pull the hamstrings from one side to the other.

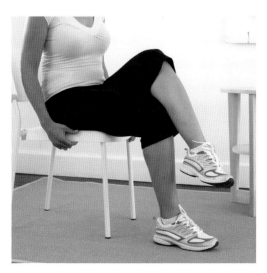

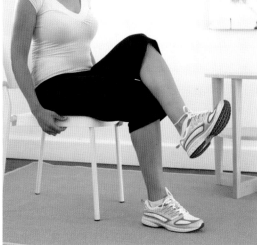

4 Cross your legs so that the calf muscle of one leg is on the kneecap of the other. Press your leg into the kneecap to feel a deep release to the calf muscle. Point your toes up towards the knee, then downwards to the floor. Repeat 3 times.

CAUTIONS
• See 'Safety and cautions', page 134.

➡ 'Aromatherapy blends', page 68
• 'Digestive disorders', page 198
• 'Premenstrual syndrome (PMS)', page 220

Detox

If your body is feeling sluggish, or you're retaining some extra fluid in your arms or legs, try applying some of these simple detox massage techniques in combination with essential oils, but first check with your doctor.

Lymphatic massage

Lymphatic massage is specially designed to assist with detoxing. To move around the body, lymph flow relies mainly on muscle movement, so this style of massage is perfect for a detox treatment.

Apply the movements lightly, as too much pressure will not be as effective. First stimulate the areas where large groups of lymph nodes are found, then use the techniques shown on page 104. Always massage towards the heart, as this helps to move the lymph flow back towards the veins that carry it to the heart.

Skin brushing

Best applied when the skin is warm, skin brushing is a preliminary move that can be used in a lymphatic treatment before the massage is applied, or even in the shower at home. It clears the dead skin cells on the surface and also assists in moving the lymph flow through the body. With the skin brush or glove in your hand, and using repetitive movements, brush over the affected areas, always working back towards the heart.

Other modalities

Swedish, remedial and aromatherapy massage all help improve the circulation, thus assisting in the removal of toxins and lactic acid from the body. Any of these modalities are recommended, with Swedish and aromatherapy being especially effective during convalescence.

Massaging the abdomen can help move toxins or waste that might be lodged in the intestines. Add a few drops each of lemon, grapefruit, cypress and juniper berry essential oils to a carrier oil, diluted 1:10, and massage the abdominal area in a slow clockwise direction.

Detoxifying essential oils

Having a warm shower softens the skin and makes it easier to apply detoxifying essential oils to the body. After the shower, add a few drops each of lemon, grapefruit, cypress and juniper essential oils to a carrier oil, diluted 1:10, to help eliminate toxins. Rub them in slowly, covering the desired area.

Reflexology

Most of the body's organs can be located in their corresponding points in the middle of both sides of the foot; for more information, refer to the chart on page 107. Apply pressure with your thumbs or fingers, especially to the reflexology point of the liver, massaging the points slowly and feeling for any tightness.

CAUTIONS ● See 'Safety and cautions', page 134.

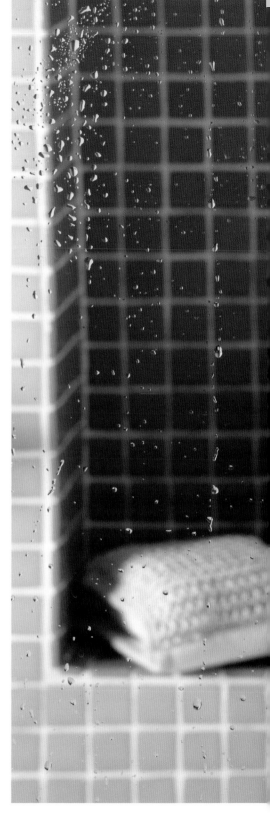

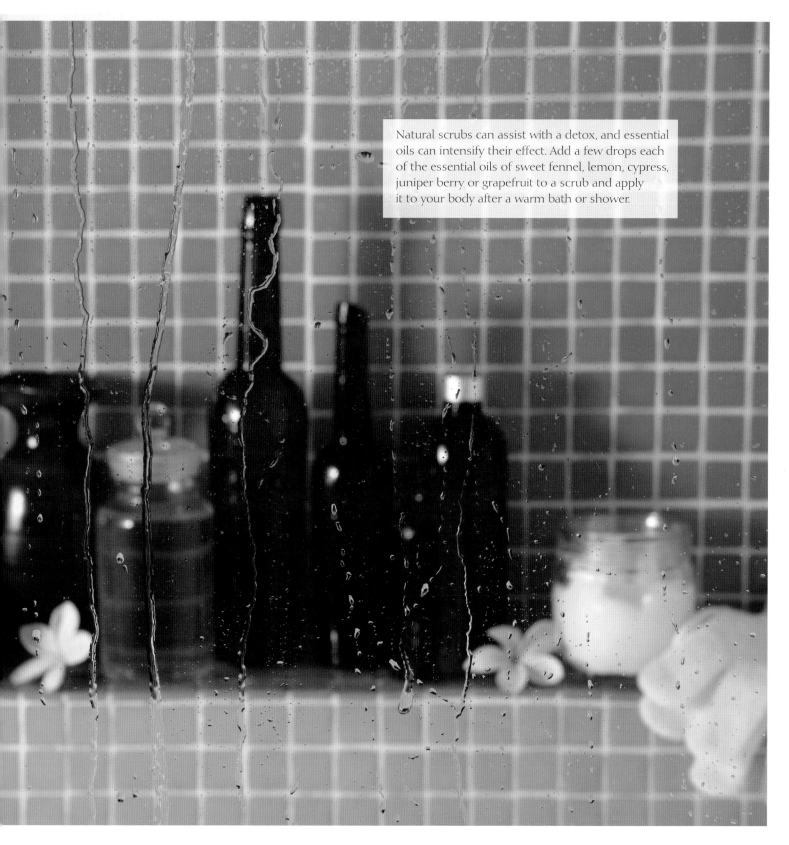

Natural scrubs can assist with a detox, and essential oils can intensify their effect. Add a few drops each of the essential oils of sweet fennel, lemon, cypress, juniper berry or grapefruit to a scrub and apply it to your body after a warm bath or shower.

If you stand all day, try to do a regular stretch, as your calf muscles act like pumps.

➜ *'Aromatherapy blends', page 78*
● *'Lymphatic massage', page 104*
● *'Reflexology', page 106*
● *'Lymphatic system', page 132*

Digestive disorders

Digestive disorders include conditions such as flatulence and vomiting. Stress and emotional tension can both be contributory factors, but massage, deep breathing and aromatherapy can all help ease a stressed digestive system.

Suitable essential oils

Aromatherapy oils can be used for a range of digestive disorders. Combine the appropriate oils – a few drops each in 3 tablespoons of a carrier oil – with the massage techniques described below or, alternatively, use any of the abdominal techniques in aromatherapy or Swedish massage.

- Stomach upsets, including vomiting – ginger and peppermint.
- Constipation – black pepper, sweet fennel, peppermint and sweet orange.
- Flatulence – black pepper, German and Roman chamomile, sweet marjoram, sweet orange and peppermint.
- Diarrhoea – black pepper, German and Roman chamomile, cypress, sweet fennel, ginger, mandarin and peppermint.

CAUTIONS ● See 'Safety and cautions', page 134.

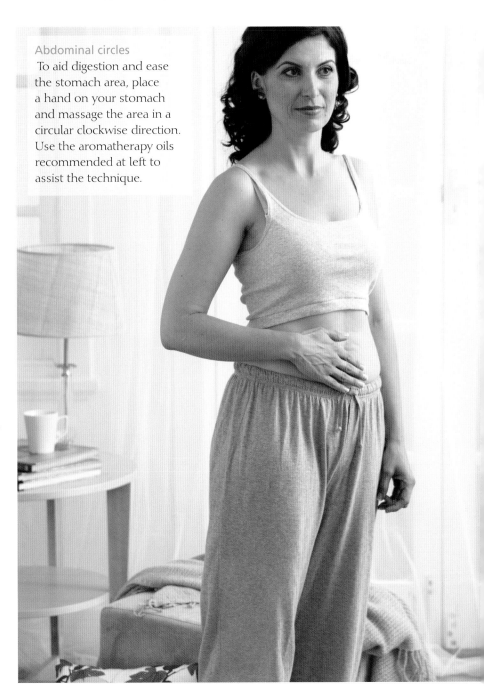

Abdominal circles
To aid digestion and ease the stomach area, place a hand on your stomach and massage the area in a circular clockwise direction. Use the aromatherapy oils recommended at left to assist the technique.

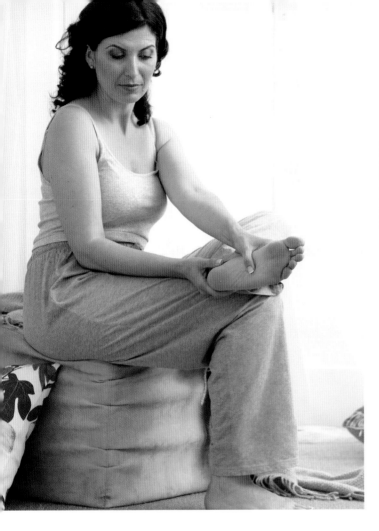

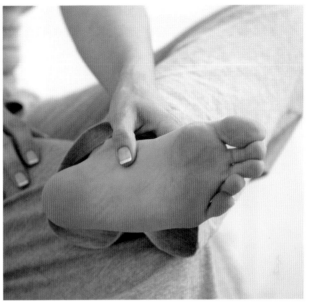

Reflex points for the stomach
With your left foot on your right knee, place your thumb on the stomach reflex point, working it in a diagonal direction along the stomach reflex area of the foot.

Self-stretch/abdominal massage
Lie on your back and bring your knees in to your chest. To massage your digestive system, rest your hands on your knees and rotate your knees in a clockwise circle.

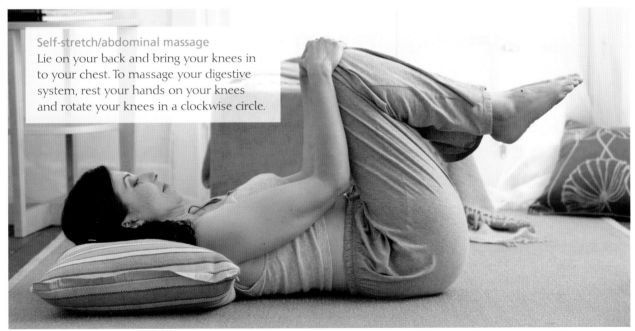

➔ 'Aromatherapy blends', page 66
● 'Abdomen and chest sequence', page 148 ● 'Abdomen', page 162

Eye strain

If you stare at a computer at work all day, your eyes will become tired, as does any area that is being used too much, but there are ways to help prevent this. Following some simple tips and doing a massage sequence will help.

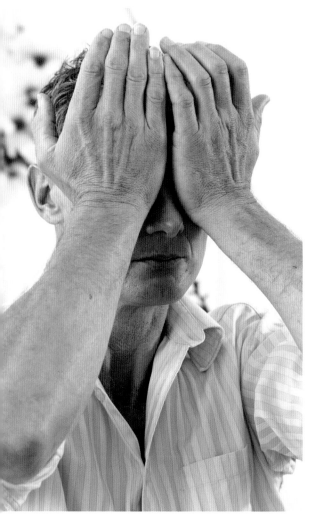

Eye relief
Of course, if your eyes are constantly sore, you may need to have them checked by your doctor or optometrist. But there are other preventative measures you can take.

- Take regular breaks. These will not only rest your eyes but will also give them something else to focus on and stop you staring at the same spot.

- Try to work under natural lighting, if possible. Fluorescent lighting can make your eyes sore during the day.

- Eye strain can be exacerbated by dehydrated air. If you work in an air-conditioned office, try using a humidifier, or use a spray bottle to spray water regularly.

- Check that you're blinking often enough. Blinking maintains moisture in your eyes so they don't dry out.

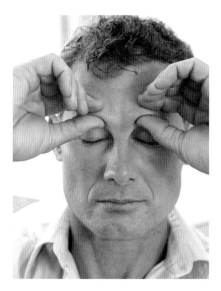

1 To give your eyes some relief, close them, then gently place your hands over your eye sockets and enjoy the break from the light. Hold as long as necessary. Slowly bring your palms out to the sides of your face, lightly massaging the muscles around the eyes as you do so.

2 Place your thumbs on the sides of your nose and slide them up until you get to the hollow between the eyes and the nose, an acupressure point that can assist with tired eyes. Being careful not to push into the eyes, hold for up to 15–20 seconds. Repeat a few times.

3 Place your index fingers and thumbs along each eyebrow, which covers the ridge of the eye socket. Start at the inside and gently roll your finger and thumb together, moving outwards as you go. When you get to the middle, hold for 5 seconds, then continue. Repeat on both sides 3 times.

Eye exercises

Like all muscles, eyes need some exercise. If you do the same exercises all the time, then only certain muscles are used and developed. It's the same for the eyes. If you mainly look at objects in front of you, then you're training your eyes to focus only on objects a certain distance away.

So it's a good idea to give your eyes regular little exercises that force them to move around, thus exercising the muscles responsible for their movement. You should also make yourself focus on objects at different distances.

However, these exercises are preventative measures, and you will find it difficult to do them if your eyes are already feeling tired or strained.

EYE COMPRESS

Soothe tired and strained eyes with a cold compress. Wet a cloth or towel, squeeze it so it's not dripping, and place it over your closed eyes. Lie back in your chair and take a few minutes to chill out. Try adding a few drops of lavender oil to the compress to help relieve the eye strain.

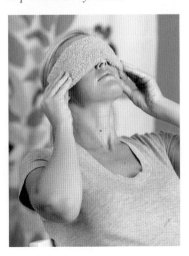

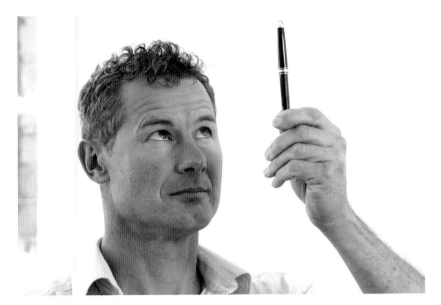

1 Try this exercise regularly in the morning. Hold a pen or small object about 20 cm away from your eyes and focus on it, then slowly move the object to the left. Move it around so that you have to move your eyes to each side as well as up and down. Finish on the starting position and repeat on the other side.

CAUTIONS ● See 'Safety and cautions', page 134.

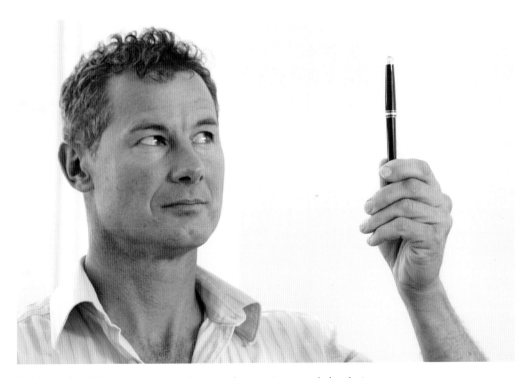

2 Move the object out another 5 cm and move it around slowly in a clockwise circle, following it with your eyes as you do so. Complete 3 circles, then do the same thing anticlockwise 3 times. Next, try doing the same move with one eye closed, forcing the other eye to work a little harder. Repeat with the other eye.

➔ *'Aromatherapy blends', page 64*

Face and scalp

Your face and scalp are constantly exposed to the elements as well as air pollutants, cosmetics and detergents. A facial and scalp massage helps to stimulate the blood flow, removing toxins and keeping the skin healthy and toned.

Scalp massage
You can treat yourself to this blissful head massage at home.

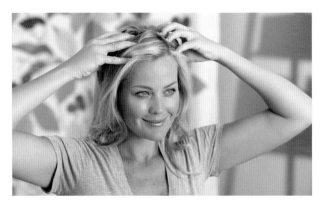

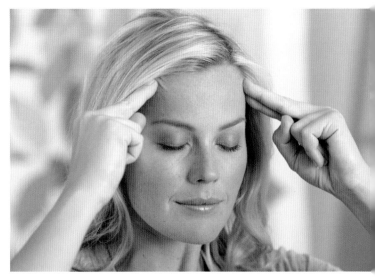

1 'Shampooing' the hair
Begin this sequence by massaging the scalp all over as if you were shampooing your hair. Spend extra time on the base of the skull, as this will help to relax the neck and head muscles.

2 Circular frictions to the forehead
Apply circular frictions with your index and middle fingers to the hairline, starting at the front of the ears and working until your fingers meet in the middle at the top of the head.

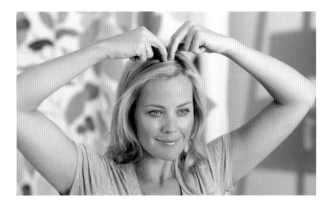

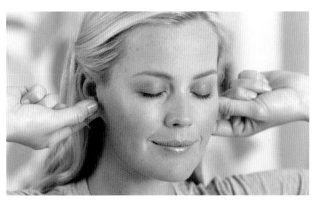

3 Pressure points
Use your fingers to apply pressure to points along the centre line of the head. Depending on the size of your head, there should be 6 or 7 points spread about 2–3 cm apart.

4 Kneading the ear
Like your hands and feet, the ears have reflex points corresponding to different parts of the body. Use the sides of your index fingers and thumbs to knead along the cartilage of the ear, from the top towards the ear lobe.

Natural facelift

By boosting your blood supply and encouraging the flow of oxygen and the removal of toxins, massage can help keep your skin glowing – naturally! You can apply this four-step sequence to your partner, or perform it on yourself, but remember to remove any makeup before applying the essential oils.

ANTI-WRINKLE TREATMENT

The oils of frankincense, myrrh, neroli, rose and sandalwood are known for their anti-wrinkle properties. Mix 2 drops of each of these essential oils with about 5 ml of jojoba oil and, working from the outside of the eyes towards the nose, gently massage around the eyes.

CAUTIONS ● See 'Safety and cautions', page 134.

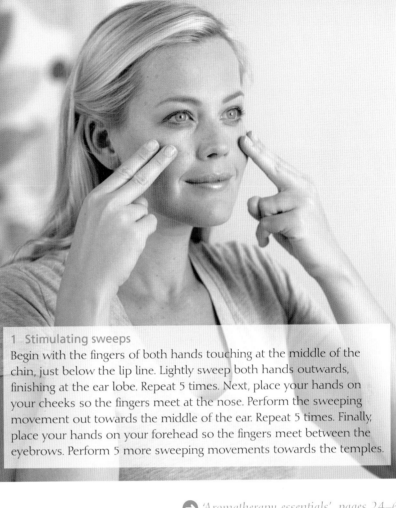

1 Stimulating sweeps
Begin with the fingers of both hands touching at the middle of the chin, just below the lip line. Lightly sweep both hands outwards, finishing at the ear lobe. Repeat 5 times. Next, place your hands on your cheeks so the fingers meet at the nose. Perform the sweeping movement out towards the middle of the ear. Repeat 5 times. Finally, place your hands on your forehead so the fingers meet between the eyebrows. Perform 5 more sweeping movements towards the temples.

➡ *'Aromatherapy essentials', pages 24–6*
● *'Face sequence', page 152*
● *'Scalp, face and chest', page 160*

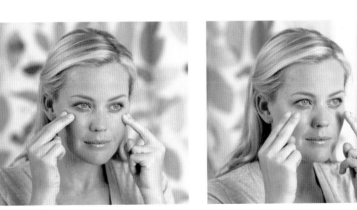

2 Circular frictions
Using your index and middle fingers, perform circular frictions to the temple area, then work down along the cheekbones under the eye sockets. This stimulates blood flow to the areas prone to wrinkles and crow's feet.

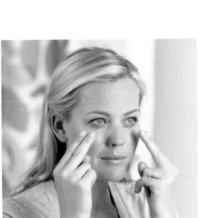

3 Tapping
To further stimulate blood flow, use your index and middle fingers to tap lightly along the cheekbones under the eye sockets. Move backwards and forwards along the cheekbones for 20–30 seconds.

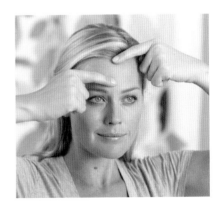

4 Vertical strokes to the forehead
To relax any tension in the brow region, use your index fingers to perform upward strokes from the eyebrows to the hairline. Alternating the index fingers of both hands, gradually move out towards the sides of the head.

Fatigue

Massage is great for treating fatigue, as it stimulates your circulation and moves toxins and wastes that might be lying stagnant in the muscles, making you feel lethargic. For a real boost, combine it with exercise and essential oils.

Energising spray

These days overwork and the general stresses of modern life make fatigue a rather common complaint. Diet is often a factor, as is lack of sleep and insufficient good-quality rest. For a bit of an energy kick, at work or at home, make a blend of essential oils for a room spray. To a spray bottle, add a few drops each of lemon, sweet orange, rosemary and geranium essential oils, diluted in a 1:10 solution of water, and use it when you're feeling a bit low in energy or the air around you is a little stale.

Self-massage to the legs

Sitting or standing for long periods of time can make your legs tired or lazy, but you can get the blood moving again with this simple self-massage routine.

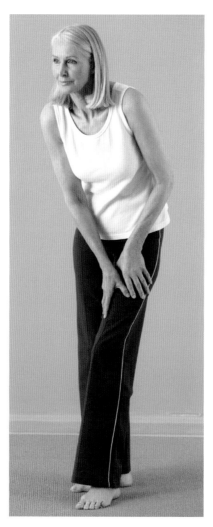

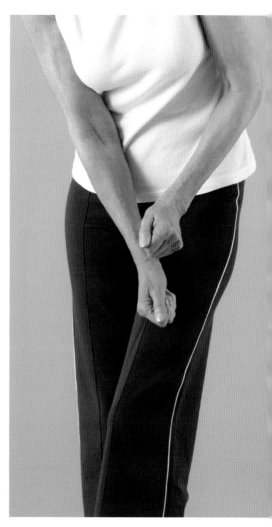

1 Either sitting down or standing, place your palms on the fronts of your thighs. Rub up and down the length of your legs, warming the muscles and stimulating the blood flow. As the quadriceps muscles begin to warm up, slowly increase your pressure and start to use your palms.

2 Once the muscles are warmed up, stimulate the nerve endings of the skin by applying percussion. With loose wrists, bring your fingers together to form a fist, then apply a rhythmic pummelling move up and down the leg. Cover each leg for up to 2 minutes.

Stretching routine

Stretching is great for stimulating fatigued muscles and also for helping with general fatigue. If you're feeling tired at work, boost your energy levels with some stretching. The following 5–10 minute routine is good for tired legs.

CAUTIONS
● See 'Safety and cautions', page 134.

ENERGISE YOURSELF

If you're feeling fatigued, it might be because you're working too hard, or not getting enough sleep. To help you enhance your energy levels, try adding a few drops each of some energising essential oils – such as rosemary, basil, lemon and sweet orange – to a bath, and allow them to soak into your body as you relax. You can also add any of these oils to an oil burner during the day. Add the drops with or without water and enjoy the subtle therapeutic effects of the oils.

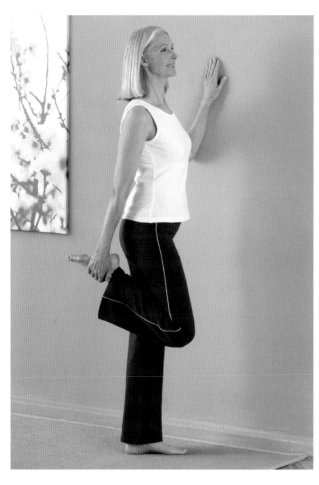

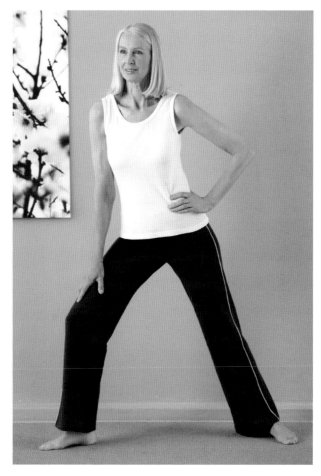

1 With your left hand on a wall for balance, bend your right leg at the knee and grasp your ankle with your right hand, then stretch the front of the leg and the very strong quadriceps muscle. Hold for at least 30 seconds. Repeat twice, then repeat with your left leg.

2 Stand with your legs apart but slightly bent at the knees. Slowly lean to one side, bending the knee on that side while straightening the leg on the other. This stretches the insides of the thighs. Hold for up to 30 seconds, relax and repeat. Then go back to the start position and repeat on the other side.

➜ *'Aromatherapy blends', pages 64 and 74*

Hangover

The effects of overindulging in alcohol can make you feel as if the world has come to an end. If you have had too many drinks, there are some simple techniques for the head and scalp that can assist you the following day.

Rehydrate your body

There are two important reasons why you shouldn't undergo a massage while you're inebriated or intoxicated – you won't have a good sense of pressure, as your senses will be numbed, and, as massage boosts the circulation and moves blood and nutrients around the body, it can also move the alcohol and cause stronger or more sustained effects.

If you've had too much alcohol to drink, you can help reduce the effects of a hangover by drinking plenty of water between alcoholic drinks and also before going to bed. This will help your body to eliminate the alcohol in your bloodstream by regulating it and filtering it through the kidneys. It will also probably make you get up and go to the toilet and release this filtered fluid, but in that case you can drink more water before going back to bed.

Remember, there is no magic cure for a hangover. You will only feel better with time, although drinking plenty of water the next day will also help, as a hangover headache is partly caused by dehydration.

Headache

To help ease the effects of a headache, follow the three-step massage sequence below for the scalp and head, using 1–2 drops each of lavender and rosemary essential oils with 3 tablespoons of a carrier oil.

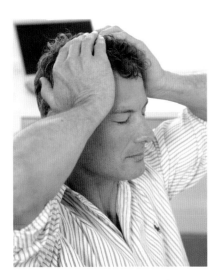

1 With your hands on top of your head, slowly move them in little circles, trying to gently move the scalp. Gently apply more pressure, making the circles broader and bigger, until you cover the entire top of your head. Repeat these moves for a few minutes.

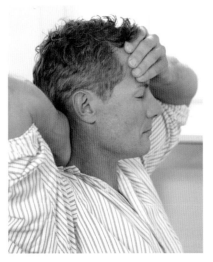

2 For the emotional release move, place one hand on your forehead and the other at the back of your head, below the base of the skull. This move integrates both the past and present aspects of the brain, allowing them to integrate. Hold for a couple of minutes.

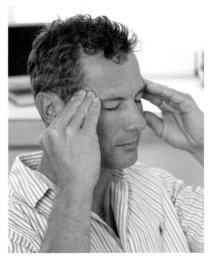

3 Massaging the temples can help alleviate some of the pain. Place three fingers at the outside edge of each eyebrow, then use slow circles to massage over the temples. Use the same move to massage parts of the forehead. Continue for a few minutes.

*To help a hangover headache, apply 1–2 drops
of lavender and rosemary essential oils to the temples.*

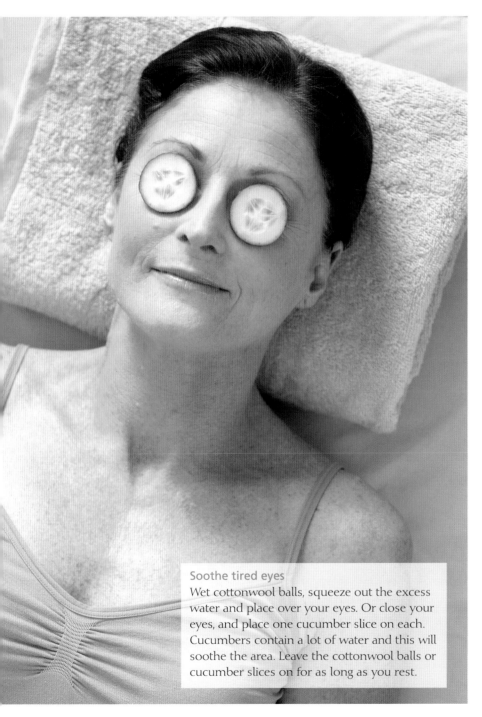

Detox your body

Apply one drop each of juniper berry, grapefruit and/or rosemary essential oils to a face washer, and while you're in the shower, rub it over your body. Or add 10 drops combined of the same detoxifying essential oils to a warm bath, and enjoy a good soak.

COLD COMPRESS

Placing a cold compress over your eyes or forehead helps ease the effects of a sore head. Wet a small towel or face washer with cold water, then add 1–2 drops each of lavender and rosemary essential oils to it. Sit or lie down, and place the compress over the throbbing area. Leave the compress on for as long as you feel comfortable.

CAUTIONS
● See 'Safety and cautions', page 134.

Soothe tired eyes

Wet cottonwool balls, squeeze out the excess water and place over your eyes. Or close your eyes, and place one cucumber slice on each. Cucumbers contain a lot of water and this will soothe the area. Leave the cottonwool balls or cucumber slices on for as long as you rest.

➜ *'Aromatherapy blends', page 78*

Headaches

Headaches can be caused by many factors, such as stress, allergies and eye strain, but massage with a few drops of the essential oils of Roman chamomile, eucalyptus, lavender, peppermint and rosemary can help to relieve them.

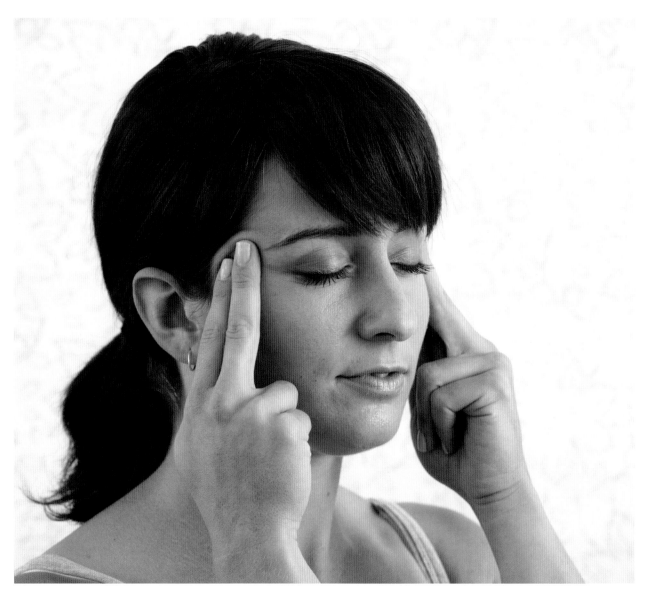

1 Releasing a tension headache
Shut your eyes, and place an index and middle finger on the edge of each temple. Perform slow, circular frictions, moving slowly around the area. As you do so, take deep breaths and let go of any emotional tension. For added benefit, use the essential oils recommended above.

➔ *'Aromatherapy blends', page 64*
• *'Eye strain', page 200*
• *'Sinus congestion', page 224*

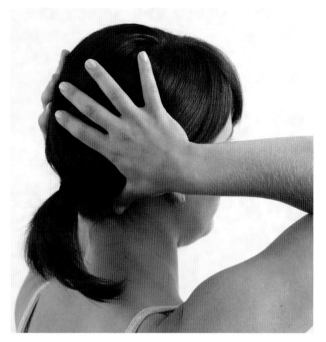

2 The base of the skull

Place your hands at the back of your head with your thumbs positioned at the base of the skull. Press in with your thumbs and perform circular frictions to the muscles at the base of the skull. These muscles can be very sensitive.

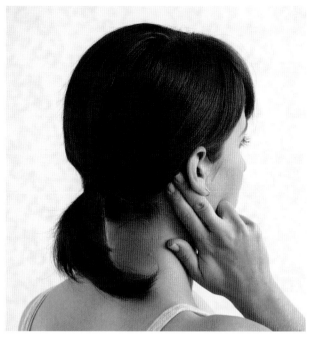

3 Behind the ears

Place your fingers on the bony prominence located just behind your ear lobes. Focusing on any tender areas, perform slow circular frictions to this area.

CAUTIONS ● See 'Safety and cautions', page 134.

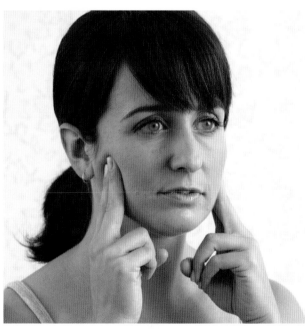

4 Frictions to the jaw

Place your index and middle fingers just in front of your ear lobes, where the jaw bone meets the cheek bones. Focusing on any tender areas, perform slow, circular frictions.

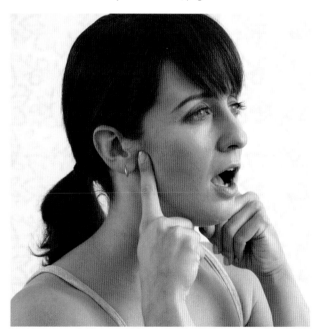

5 Massaging the cheek and jaw muscles

Press into the centre of each cheek with your index fingers, just below the cheek bones. Open your mouth slowly and feel these muscles stretch under your finger pressure. Shut your mouth again. Repeat 5 times for an effective release. These muscles may be very tender, so adjust your pressure accordingly.

Insomnia

Insomnia is often caused by stress and overstimulation, so massage is the perfect way to help you relax and calm your mind. Combined with soothing and sedative essential oils, these techniques will help you enjoy a good night's sleep.

Relaxing massage

Giving your partner a foot massage is a wonderful way to help him relax. Ask him to have a bath or shower, then lie down on the bed. Place a towel over his head, then massage the whole of one foot, slowly and rhythmically, up and down, paying special attention to the toes. If possible, avoid talking. Repeat on the other foot.

If you're having problems sleeping, or going back to sleep after waking, add a few drops of lavender essential oil to your pillow. Slowly breathing in the beautiful smell will help you stay relaxed and keep your mind quiet.

Add a couple of drops each of lavender, bergamot and sweet marjoram essential oil with 1 cup of Epsom salts to a hot bath. This will help your muscles to release tension. If you only have a shower at home, pour 1–2 drops of each of the oils onto a face washer or loofah and rub it over your body.

Alternatively, make a blend to spray in the air above your bed, either before you go to sleep or when you wake during the night. The essential oils of lavender, neroli and bergamot are known for their sedative and relaxing qualities – put a few drops of each in a spray bottle filled with water, and spray the mix in the air so you can breathe it in slowly, which enhances their effect.

SELF-MASSAGE

An overactive mind – thinking about the day's events and worrying about the future – can prevent you from relaxing and sleeping. Try massaging your head at night to assist with calming your mind. Your thoughts will then begin to focus on your hands and the effect on your scalp. Try slow, circular movements and running both hands down your head.

CAUTIONS ● See 'Safety and cautions', page 134.

All the massage modalities are aimed at relaxing your mind and the muscles of your body, but Swedish, aromatherapy, Hawaiian, Shiatsu and hot stone are especially suited to treating insomnia. Have one of these professional treatments towards the end of the day so you can go straight home and relax with a cup of herbal tea before bedtime.

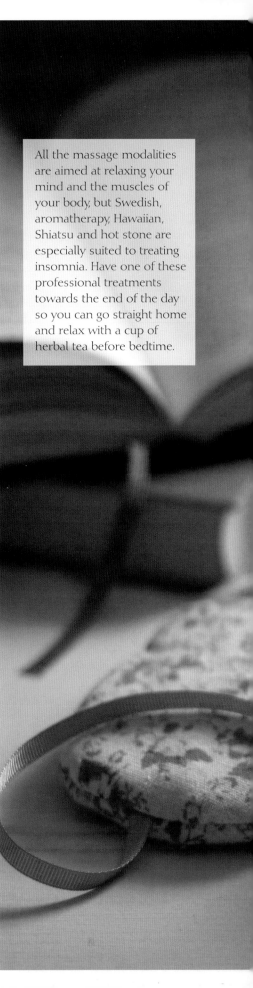

To help you sleep, try drinking a relaxing herbal tea, such as chamomile or valerian, before going to bed.

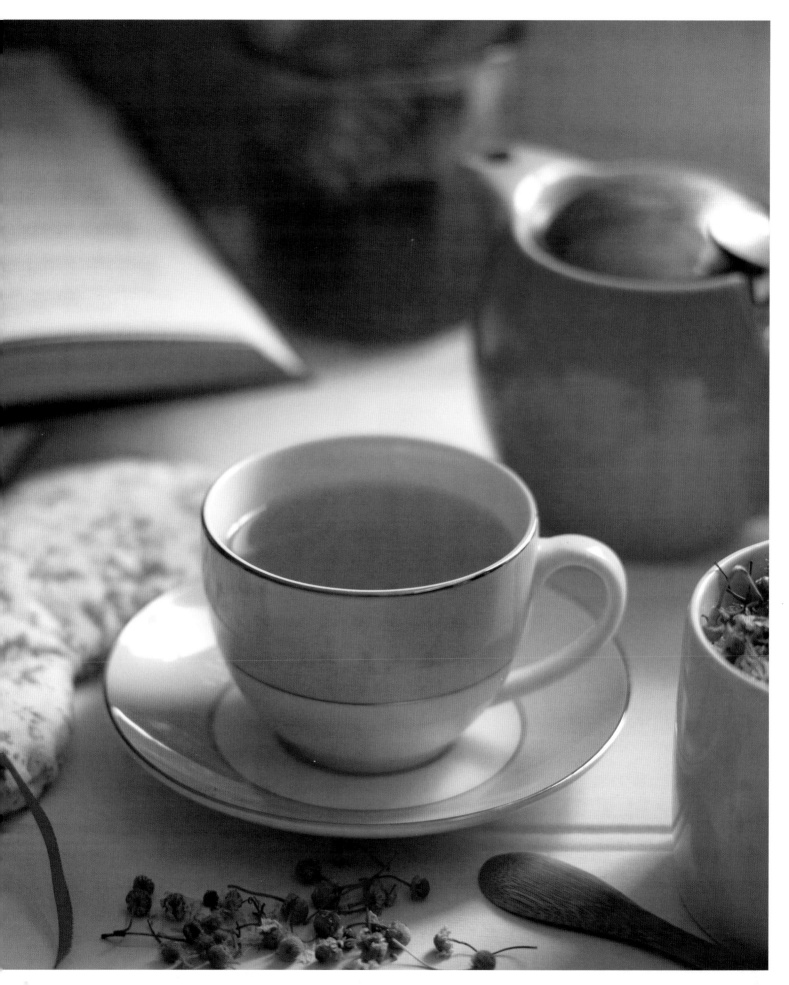

Joint pain

Joint pain can be due to a number of causes, including arthritis. Black pepper, German chamomile, ginger, lavender, pine, rosemary and thyme essential oils all help to reduce joint pain, so try combining them with these techniques.

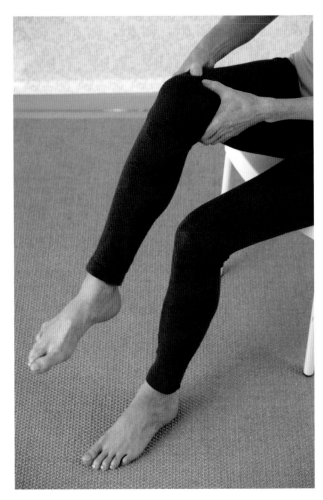

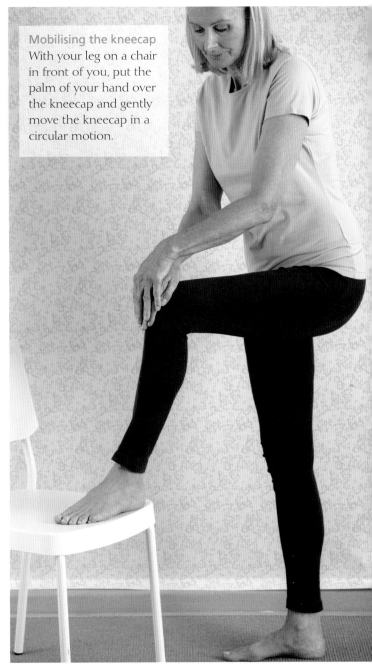

Mobilising the kneecap
With your leg on a chair in front of you, put the palm of your hand over the kneecap and gently move the kneecap in a circular motion.

Massaging the knee
Use your thumbs to apply pressure to the muscle just above the kneecap. Keeping the pressure stable with your thumbs, lift your leg and slightly extend the knee by kicking forwards with your foot (as if you were kicking a ball). Return the leg to the ground. Repeat the move 3–5 times, then repeat on the other leg, if required.

CAUTIONS
● See 'Safety and cautions', page 134.

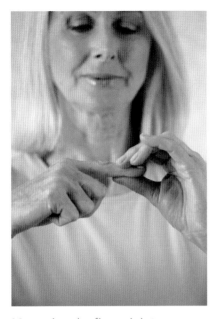
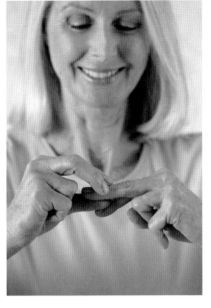

Massaging the finger joints
Move the thumb and fingers of one hand backwards and forwards over all 14 finger joints of the other hand. For added benefit, use a few drops of some of the suggested aromatherapy oils in a carrier oil. Repeat on the other side of the hand, then repeat the whole sequence on the other hand.

To keep joints healthy, eat a well-balanced diet and try to avoid using them excessively.

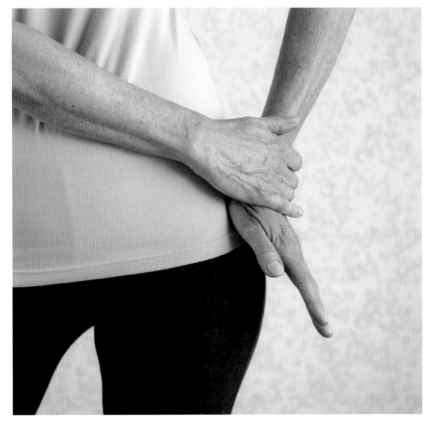

Hip circles
Place the palm of one hand over your hip joint and press inwards. Use your other hand to support the wrist joint. Massage in large circles around the hip joint to promote blood flow to the area.

FIBROMYALGIA

Fibromyalgia is a condition that leads to pain, fatigue and sometimes sensations of pulling or burning in the muscle tissue of the body. Rather than being one problem, fibromyalgia is a group of symptoms that include sleep problems and widespread pain or tenderness in the muscles. People with fibromyalgia have trouble falling into the deepest level of sleep, when the hormones that help with growth, recovery and pain relief are released.

Those suffering from fibromyalgia can be very sensitive, so it's important to use light touch and seek feedback when massaging. To assist with this condition, the essential oils of clove bud, eucalyptus, ginger, lavender, peppermint, rosemary and thyme can all be used with the Swedish or aromatherapy massage sequences.

➔ *'Aromatherapy blends', page 68*

Legs and feet

Many of us tend to neglect our feet and lower legs, but there is a range of different essential oils and massage techniques that can alleviate or ease the various ailments and conditions affecting this part of our bodies.

Stretching the calf muscles

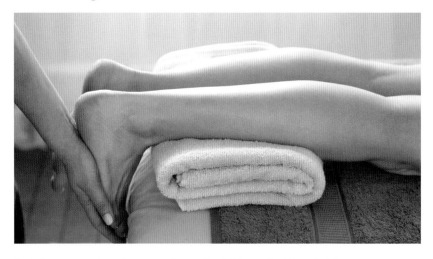

1   Ask your partner to move down the table so that her feet hang over the end, then apply direct pressure to the sole of one foot, pushing it towards the table. This will stretch the gastrocnemius muscle, loosening tension in the calves. Repeat with the other leg.

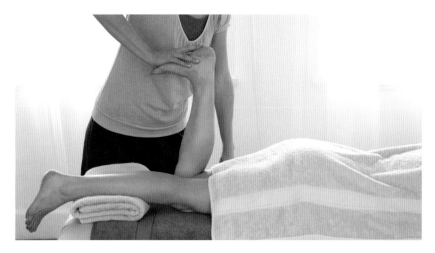

2   This stretch greatly assists in maintaining relaxed leg muscles. Start by bending the leg at the knee joint, then apply pressure on the sole of the foot, thereby stretching the strong postural muscles of the leg. Repeat with the other leg.

Dosage

When using the recommended essential oils for these conditions, dilute up to 10 drops of essential oil, whether it's one or several, with 20–30 ml of a carrier oil.

Tightness in legs and feet

Always massage towards the heart to assist blood return, and use an essential oil such as black pepper, German chamomile, ginger, thyme, lavender, rosemary or sweet marjoram – all known for their analgesic properties. Make up a massage blend, or add a few drops to your bath.

Lymphoedema

Obstruction of the lymph vessels causes swelling of the feet, ankles and legs. Oils that stimulate the lymph flow include cypress and juniper berry, while grapefruit, lime, orange, peppermint and rosemary reduce swelling. Also recommended are lymphatic massage techniques and cold compresses with essential oils.

Achilles tendonitis

This is a painful inflammation of the Achilles tendon that is often due to tight leg muscles, a possible overstrain while exercising or walking or, sometimes, flat feet. Apply ice and cold compresses in the acute stage, then massage the area with oils such as German chamomile or lavender.

Achilles tendon

A restricted, sore or inflamed Achilles tendon, a common problem for athletes, can be due to wearing inadequate footwear, a poor running style, lack of stretching or running on hard surfaces. Relieve this condition by massaging the calf muscles and Achilles tendon, and gently stretching the Achilles tendon.

Corns and warts

These ailments of the feet can be extremely painful, making it difficult to walk comfortably. Ease the pain by massaging around the area with a calendula-infused oil. Lavender and tea tree can also assist with healing.

Bunions

Often the result of the development of arthritis on the joint or wearing poor-quality footwear, bunions cause painful swelling and inflammation around the outside of the big toe. If the ailment is not in the acute stage, gently massage the bunion with lavender, sweet marjoram and peppermint oils to relieve the pain and reduce the swelling.

Tinea

This infectious fungal condition usually appears on the skin between the toes. Oils with antifungal properties — such as myrrh, patchouli and tea tree — are considered the most effective. Add a few drops of one of these oils to a footbath, or massage a blend directly into the affected area. You can also use cypress, lavender and rosemary to help combat foot odour.

Varicose veins

Varicose veins are usually contra-indicated to massage; however, you can assist the treatment of the condition by applying essential oils. Cypress, juniper berry, geranium, lemon and rosemary are among those highly recommended. When applying them, use only gentle, superficial upward movements above the vein. Alternatively, add them to your bath water.

Massaging the Achilles tendon

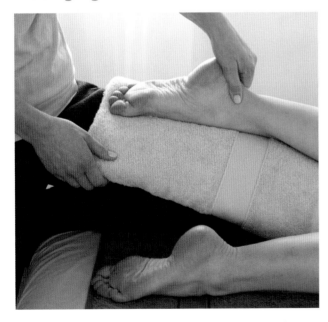

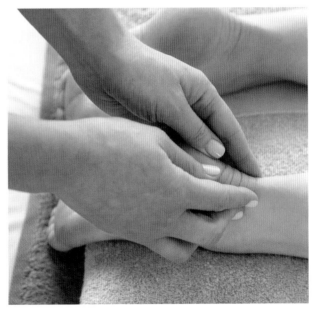

1 Bending your partner's leg at the knee, position his foot over your thigh, covered with a towel. With your thumb and index finger, slowly scoop down the Achilles tendon towards the heel. After 5 passes, apply gentle pressure on the sole of the foot with your other hand, holding for 10 seconds. Repeat on the other side.

2 Place your partner's leg on the table. Starting at the heel and working up, use your thumbs and fingers to gently massage and move the Achilles tendon. Repeat up and down on both sides of the foot.

Mood swings and menopause

Menopause can mean a big change for a woman's system as hormonal imbalances lead to symptoms such as mood swings, hot flushes, cold hands and headaches. Diet, herbs and exercise can help ease this natural process.

Hot flushes

Here are some tips for minimising the discomfort of hot flushes.
- Eat foods containing antioxidants such as Vitamins A, C and E.
- Take evening primrose oil in capsule form, or rub it directly into your body.
- Whenever you go out, wear more light layers of clothing, so if you experience a hot flush, you can remove as many layers as necessary.
- Use layers of blankets on your bed at night, when hot flushes are most common.
- Avoid excessive amounts of caffeine, alcohol, sugar, spicy foods and hot soups or drinks, as they can trigger hot flushes and make mood swings worse.

Cooling blend

Make a cooling blend of essential oils to rub over your body. Pour 2–3 tablespoons of jojoba oil, which is good for the skin, into a small container, then add a couple of drops each of peppermint essential oil for cooling and lavender essential oil for relaxing. Rub this mix over your body, concentrating on any areas that feel flushed.

Perfumed rollette

To assist with mood swings, headaches and insomnia, try applying a perfume rollete. To 8 ml of jojoba oil, add 5–10 drops of each of the following essential oils – geranium, sweet marjoram, rosemary, clary sage and lavender. Whenever you're feeling a little blue, rub this blend onto your neck or face.

Energy-boosting stretch

Stretching is a great way to boost your energy levels and change your outlook. Follow the three-step routine opposite.

Women who eat a lot of soy, particularly tofu and soy milk, may experience fewer hot flushes and mood swings.

CAUTIONS ● See 'Safety and cautions', page 134.

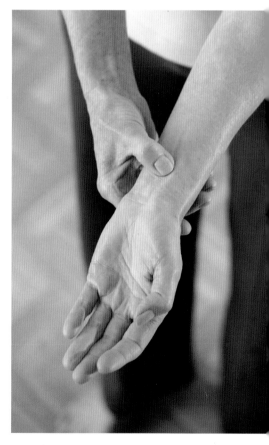

Pressure point
If you're feeling a little irritable or stressed, try pressing this point for some relief. Locate it just below the wrist in a little hollow on the inside of the arm. Press with your thumb and hold for as long as needed.

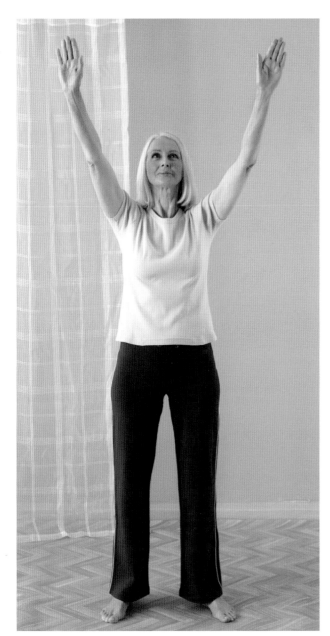

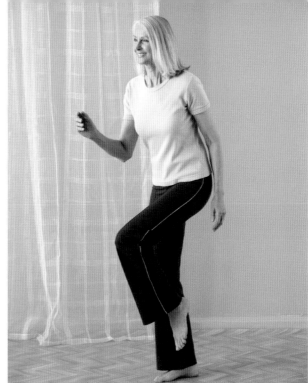

2 Slowly bring up your left knee and at the same time bring your right elbow down towards the knee. You can then swap and bring your right knee towards your left elbow. As you get the hang of this, increase the speed so that it feels as if you're marching or running on the spot. Do this for up to a couple of minutes.

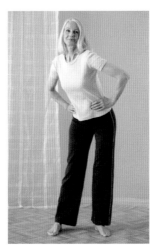 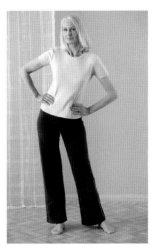

1 Stand with your legs apart, flat on the ground. Then raise your hands up, stretching them as far as you can so that your lower back is being stretched. Hold this for 15 seconds or for as long as is comfortable.

HORMONE-BALANCING OILS

Essential oils combined together offer a great way to help lift a mood and cool down a hot flush. The essential oils of bergamot, German and Roman chamomile, geranium, lavender and neroli will all help you to deal with mood swings and general stress. Use them in the bath, burn them in an oil burner or even sprinkle them on a tissue. Add clary sage and sweet fennel, which have hormone-balancing properties, to the bath, or dilute them in a carrier oil and massage them into your body.

3 Stand with your hands on your hips, then slowly roll your hips in a clockwise direction. As you move, try to make the circles bigger and bigger. After 10 circles, move your hips in the opposite direction. This is great for moving the pelvic joints and releasing some feel-good endorphins.

➡ *'Aromatherapy blends', page 76*
• *'Arms and hands', page 178*

Neck and shoulders

Follow this easy 10-minute sequence of massage and self-massage techniques for shoulder and neck pain at work or at home. Stretching, heat packs and hot baths also help keep the shoulders and neck muscles loose and warm.

Self-massage to the shoulders

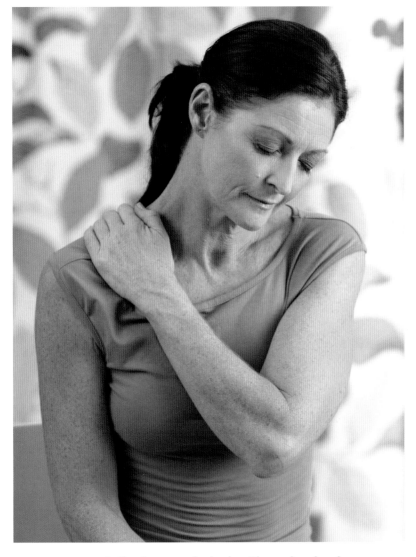

Seated massage is easy to apply and can be given anywhere.

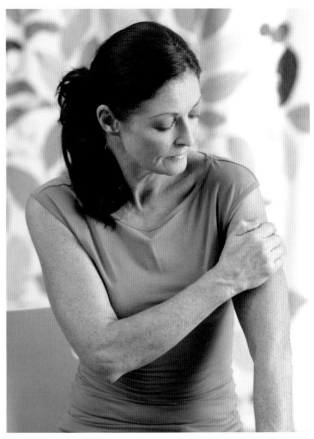

1 Reach across the body with one hand and squeeze the trapezius muscle on the opposite side. Hold the pressure for 10–15 seconds, release and repeat. This pumps blood into the tired shoulder muscles. Repeat the sequence twice, then repeat on the other side.

2 Continue by using your whole hand to knead into the deltoid muscle, which covers the shoulder joint. Gently squeeze, then release. Massage your way up and down, rubbing the shoulder for up to a minute. Repeat on the other side.

Self-massage for the neck

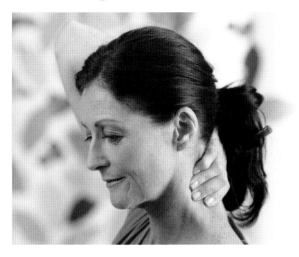

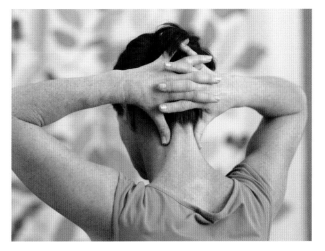

1   To take the edge off your stiff neck, place your hand face down in a C-shape over the neck area and massage into the muscles, up and down. Repeat a few times. You can also gently squeeze and release, then massage into the neck with your thumb for up to 1 minute. Swap hands if necessary.

2   Lock your hands together on the back of the head and use both your thumbs to massage along the base or ridge of your head in a slow, easy manner. This is particularly good for headaches or neck tightness. Work your way along, back and forth, for a few minutes.

Self-stretching

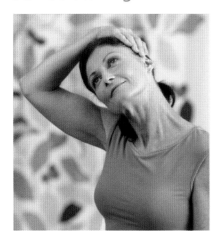

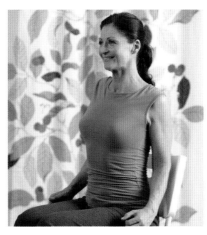

1   Sit in a chair and take hold of the seat with your left hand. Place your right hand on the left side of your head and pull your head to the right, stretching the left side of the neck as far as is comfortable. Hold for up to 30 seconds, if possible. Repeat on the other side. Do this regularly.

2   Sitting or standing comfortably, take a couple of big deep breaths in and out, then roll your shoulders forwards so that they move in a circular fashion. After a few rolls, stop and then roll them backwards. Shoulder rolls are great ways to stretch and loosen the shoulders.

CAUTIONS
• See 'Safety and cautions', page 134.

MAGNESIUM BATH

A therapeutic way to relieve shoulder and neck stiffness is to soak in a bath containing Epsom salts and lavender essential oil. Epsom salts contain magnesium, which muscles require for optimal functioning. Combine a few drops of the oil with 1 tablespoon of the salts before adding the mix to a hot bath. For maximum effect, soak your shoulders and neck.

Alternatively, ask your nutritionist if you can take magnesium tablets. These are good to take at night as they relax the muscles, helping you sleep.

➔ *'Aromatherapy blends', page 69*
• *'Travel ailments', page 228*

Premenstrual syndrome (PMS)

Also known as premenstrual tension (PMT), PMS affects many women during the second stage of the menstrual cycle with a range of symptoms, but massage can help to relieve both the emotional and physical symptoms.

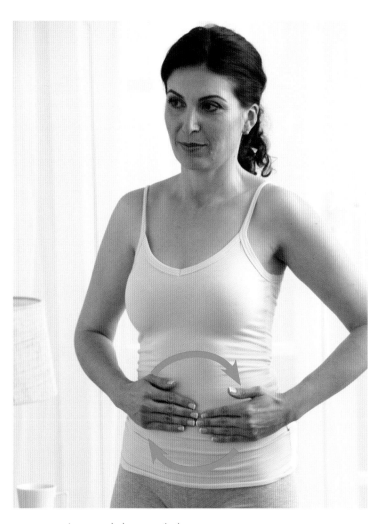

Lower abdomen circles
Begin by placing both hands on your abdomen, then gently massage in large clockwise circles around the belly button. Using the essential oils recommended above will also assist this technique.

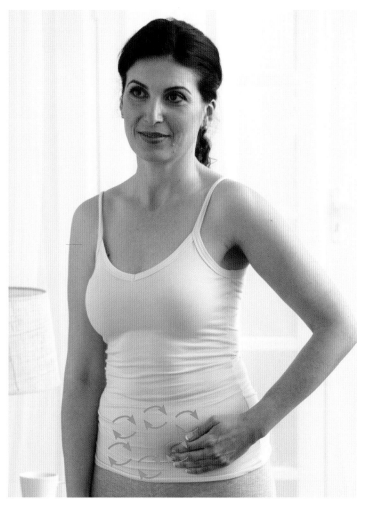

Abdomen massage
Often the pain and cramping is focused on the lower abdomen. With one hand on this region, perform smaller circles in a clockwise direction from one side to the other. Repeat 5 times.

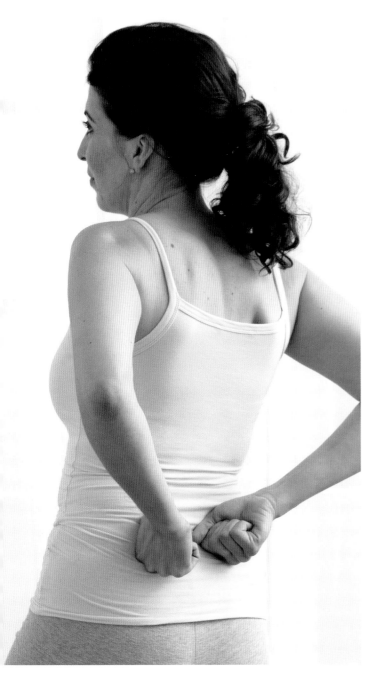

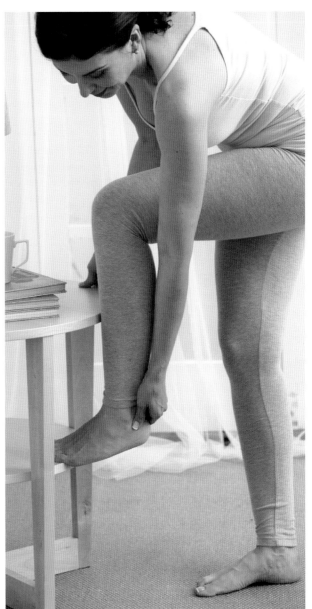

Lower back massage
Place both your fists on your lower back and press in to the muscles of the spine. Begin with 5 deep breaths, focusing on releasing all the tension on each out-breath. Next, rotate your fists, kneading the lower back muscles. If you require more pressure, you can use your thumbs instead of your fists.

Reflex point for the ovaries
Rest your foot on a stool in front of you, then place your thumb or finger on the outside of your right foot, just below the ankle, and use it to work this reflex point for the ovaries.

➡ *'Aromatherapy blends', page 76*

PREMENSTRUAL SYNDROME (PMS) **221**

Posture

Good posture allows your muscles and joints to move efficiently, reducing the risk of muscular imbalance. Always try to sit or stand with your head erect, spine upright, shoulders set back, tummy tucked in and knees unlocked.

Front posture check

It can often be hard to maintain correct posture, so it's important to do a regular posture check. To understand the characteristics of your posture, check it in front of a full-length mirror, and feel the difference between 'good' posture and 'bad' posture. Once you understand the difference, close your eyes and notice how your neck, shoulders, lower back and legs feel in the 'good' posture and then in the 'bad' posture. Recognising the difference will help you to self-correct your posture, whether you're at work or on the go.

To do a posture check front on, stand in front of the mirror and check for the following.

1   Are your shoulders level? Your shoulders should be balanced, but one shoulder may be higher than the other. This is usually due to favouring the use of one side over the other or carrying heavy bags on one shoulder only.

2   Are your arms hanging the same way? This may sound odd, but often one arm will be rotated in further than the other due to tight shoulder muscles on one side. You can usually tell by looking at your hands. How much of the back of the hand is showing compared to the other?

3   Are your hips level? The best way to check this is to locate the bony prominences at the front of your hips and place an index finger on each. If they're not level, it may be that one hip is tilted up compared to the other.

4   Are your kneecaps pointing forwards in the same direction? The kneecaps should point evenly to the front.

5   Are both your feet pointing forwards in the same direction? If there are differences in the hip, knee or ankle, your feet may point in different directions.

Side posture check

You can also check your posture from the side. It may be useful to have someone else perform this check so you don't change your stance as you look sideways into the mirror.

1   Is your head set back? Your head should not be too far forward of your shoulders.

2   Are your shoulders in line with your ears? Rounded

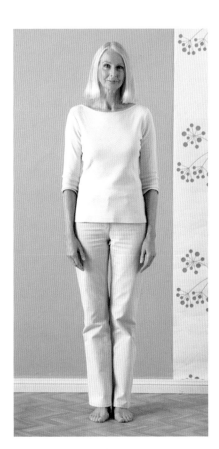

Correct posture, front on

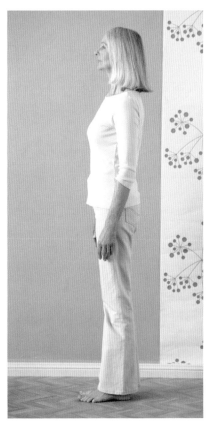

Correct posture, side on

Your posture often reflects your mood. Think of how you sit or stand when you're upset – it's probably with your shoulders forward, head down and back rounded. When you're happy, alert and excited, you're likely to stand with your chest open, your back upright and your chin up. If you're feeling gloomy, change your posture and see what effect it has!

shoulders, due to muscle imbalance between the front and back of the chest, are very common. Your shoulders should be roughly in line with your ears.
3   Is the curve in your lower back normal? Often people with weaker core muscles have an excessive sway back. Activating your core muscles, pulling your tummy in and standing up straight can help reduce this.
4   Are your knees unlocked? Locking your kneecaps can put excessive strain on these joints. Your knees should always be very slightly flexed.

Self-massage and stretching routine

If you slouch, your diaphragm can't move to its full capacity, and consequently you tend to take faster and shallower breaths, which can cause unnecessary strain in the neck muscles. Sitting and standing correctly allows the diaphragm to expand completely so you can take deep, slow and full breaths.

Follow this three-step self-massage and stretching routine.

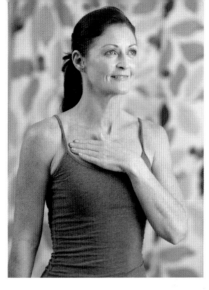

1   Self-massage to pectoral region
Using the fingers of one hand, massage the pectoral muscles on the opposite side of the chest by performing slow circular frictions. Starting near the sternum, work along the collarbone towards your shoulder.

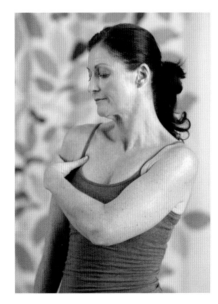

2   Self-massage to pectoral region with breaths
Press your thumbs into the pectoral muscles and breathe in deeply. You'll feel the muscle press into your thumb. Keep the pressure constant as you slowly breathe in and out. After 2–3 breaths, move your thumbs slightly. Repeat this move until you have covered the whole pectoral region.

CAUTIONS ● See 'Safety and cautions', page 134.

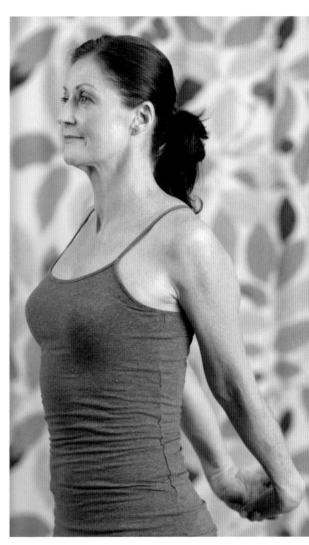

3 Stretching your pectoral region
First, join your hands behind your back, then push forwards through your chest.

Sinus congestion

Minor sinus congestion can clog up your nose and head, making you feel miserable. Massaging specific acupressure points on the face and feet stimulate energy points, helping to alleviate the congestion, and you can also try inhalations.

Easing congestion

For safe and effective relief, try this easy four-step sequence, which can be repeated up to 3 times or as necessary.

1 Put your hands together and lean into your thumbs so that the top of your nose presses into them. Then use your index fingers to press and massage into the sides of the nose, moving down as you go. Do this for up to a minute.

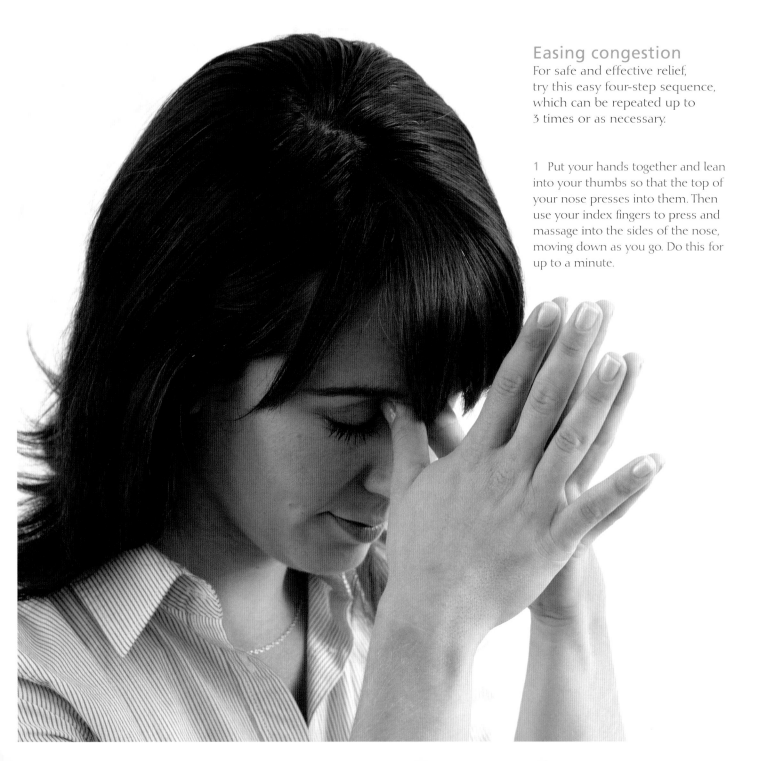

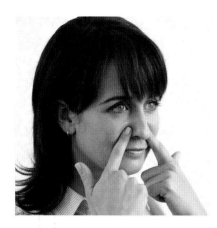

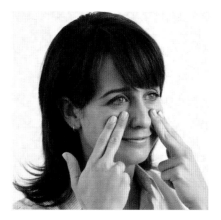

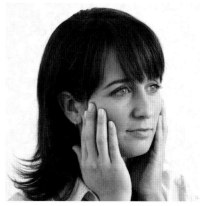

2 Move down to the next acupressure point, which is located at the top of each nostril in a little indent. To further stimulate the sinus congestion points, press and hold this point with each index finger for up to 30 seconds. Remove your fingers, pause briefly and repeat.

3 Place the index and middle fingers of both hands on either side of your nose. With slow pressure, pull them down the nose so they drain away any fluid or mucus that would have been dislodged by the previous move. Continue this movement across both cheekbones. Repeat as many times as necessary.

4 Massage with stroking movements down the sides of the face to move the lymph down to the lymph nodes to be filtered. Starting at the eyebrows, use slow sweeping movements, massaging gently down to the jaw and neck.

INHALATION WITH ESSENTIAL OILS

This is a traditional and useful method for unblocking annoying sinus congestion. The essential oils of eucalyptus, pine and thyme are known for their therapeutic properties, so add a few drops of one of them to a bowl of steaming water and place your face over it. Then cover your face with a towel and breathe deeply into the steam for up to 5 minutes.

In the case of sinusitis or severe flu, always consult your doctor first.

CAUTIONS
● See 'Safety and cautions', page 134.

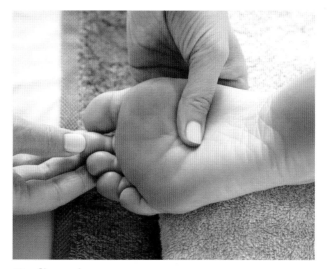

Sniffer stick

Add up to 10 drops combined of eucalyptus, peppermint and tea tree essential oils to an empty sniffer stick, available from aromatherapy suppliers. Insert the stick a little way into your nostril and gently sniff, or spread a few drops of the oils onto a tissue and inhale.

Reflexology

Massaging the tops of the backs of the toes assists with sinus congestion. Grasp your foot and use your thumb to massage into the toes. Stimulate each toe for about 30 seconds.

➔ *'Aromatherapy blends', page 71*

Sports injuries

Sports injuries, such as sprains and strains, are not only common but also need proper attention if you're to avoid the risk of long-term damage to your muscles, bones and joints. If you have been injured, consult your doctor first.

Keep fit

Sprains and strains occur when excessive forces cause muscles and tendons to stretch beyond their normal range, resulting in pain and inflammation. The key to avoiding a sports injury is to be fit enough and strong enough to carry out your sport at the level required.

The essential oils of arnica, black pepper, ginger, thyme and sweet marjoram are excellent for aiding repair of sprains and strains – just add a few drops of each to 3 tablespoons of carrier oil and rub into the affected area.

Regular Swedish massage can also assist in keeping muscle tissue healthy.

Arnica for bruising

Bruising occurs as a result of internal bleeding below the skin, usually caused by an external blow. To help reduce bruising, use small circular frictions to massage a few drops of arnica essential oil into the area.

CAUTIONS ● See 'Safety and cautions', page 134.

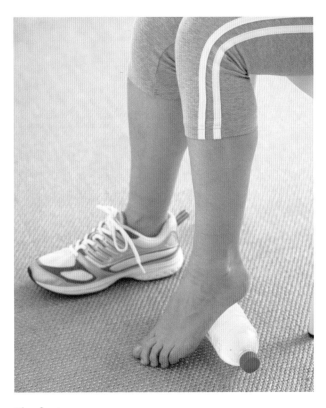

The foot
For a sore or damaged foot arch, place a frozen water bottle under your foot and slowly roll it backwards and forwards.

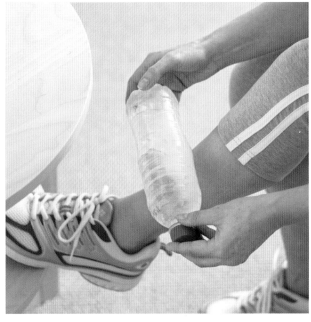

The shin
For a sore shin, place your leg up on a chair in front of you and use your hands to roll a frozen water bottle up and down your shin.

Once the swelling and inflammation have gone, massage can help reduce the build-up of scar tissue to the injured muscle.

ICE MASSAGE DO'S AND DON'TS

Ice massage helps to reduce the inflammation and pain of injured tissue.

- *Do use a frozen water bottle or frozen water in a foam cup to relieve damaged tissue if you don't have an ice pack.*
- *Don't apply an ice pack for more than 20 minutes at any one time.*
- *Don't apply an ice pack directly to the skin, unless it's constantly moving (see below). Wrap it in a layer of cloth.*

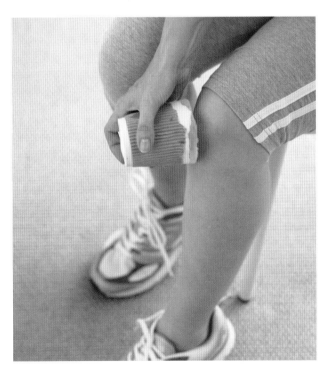

The knee
Freeze some water in a foam cup, then rip a small edge from the cup. Place the now exposed ice section on the sore parts of the knee and perform slow circular frictions along the kneecap.

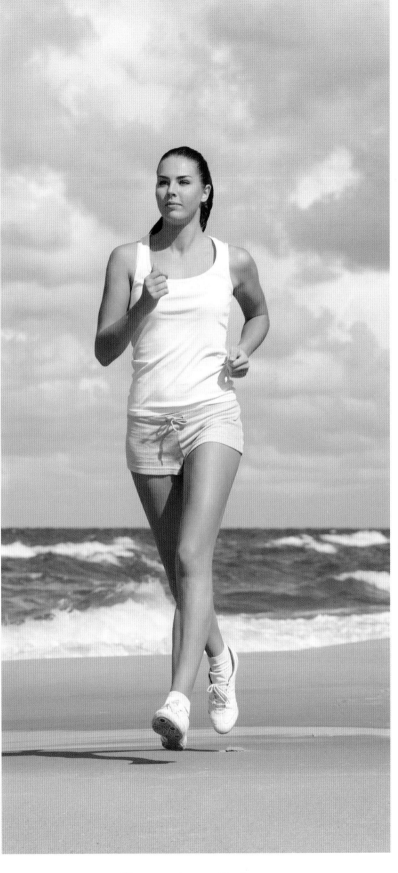

'Aromatherapy blends', page 68

Travel ailments

When you're sitting still in a confined space on a long flight, you can suffer from nausea and serious conditions, such as deep vein thrombosis (DVT), but massage and aromatherapy combined with stretching can help.

Travel sickness and nausea

During your travels you might pick up an upset stomach from eating unusual foods. If you're feeling a bit nauseous, try these two simple ideas. One remedy is to add a few drops of either ginger or peppermint essential oil to a tissue or handkerchief and inhale it repeatedly, while the other is to slowly rub a few drops of either of these oils into your lower abdomen in a clockwise direction.

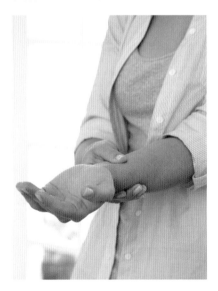

To help calm your nerves or alleviate the symptoms of travel nausea, press the point of Pericardium 6 on the arm, located about three thumbs' width above the wrist. Hold the point in the middle of the arm between the tendons for as long as necessary.

Too much walking while sightseeing can result in blisters and sore feet.
* *Soothe blisters by combining a few drops of calendula essential oil with a few drops of either lavender or tea tree essential oil, mixed with 3 tablespoons of carrier oil, then lightly rubbing it near the affected area.*
* *For sore feet, try massaging the whole foot with a few drops each of German chamomile, lavender and sweet marjoram essential oils mixed with 3 tablespoons of carrier oil.*

Deep vein thrombosis (DVT)

DVT, a blood clot in the veins of the leg, results from the restricted circulation of blood back to the heart. Of course there are other risk factors that contribute to this, including obesity and smoking, but when you're flying long distances, the cabin pressure constricts the passage of blood and lymph back through both the circulatory and lymphatic systems towards the heart.

To help encourage better circulation in your legs, do this simple four-step routine. The calf muscles act like pumps for the lower leg, and the contraction of these muscles aids circulation. Movement and stretching will also help, so make sure you get up regularly and move around the plane.

CAUTIONS
* See 'Safety and cautions', page 134.

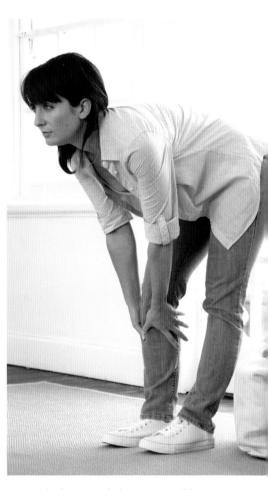

1   Reach down and clasp your calf muscles with both hands, then massage up and down the muscles by rubbing slowly. Work in with your fingertips as well, gently massaging in slow circles.

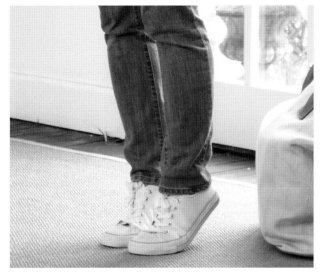

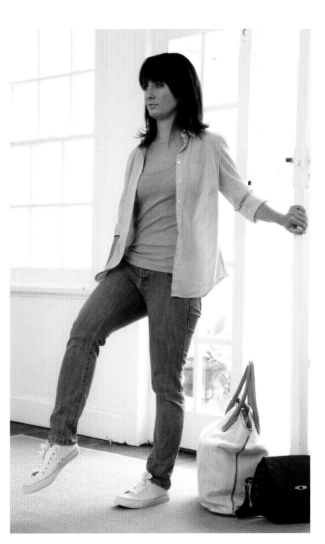

Dehydration is a problem due to the low levels of oxygen on planes, so drink plenty of water and avoid alcohol and caffeine.

2 Stand comfortably, with both feet flat on the ground. Slowly roll yourself forwards so you are standing on your tiptoes. Hold for a few seconds. This will stretch the front leg muscles.

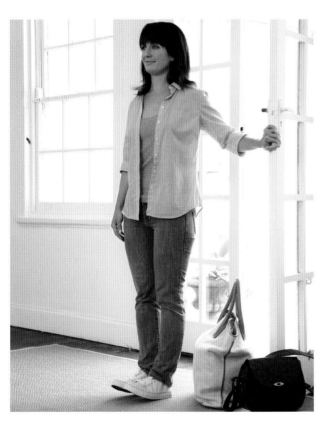

3 Slowly roll yourself back down until you end up on your heels. Try to stretch the back of your calves as you do so. Hold for 10 seconds, then repeat the move, rolling back and forth up to 10 times. This will improve the circulation in your lower legs.

4 To complete this sequence, stand on one leg, then shake the other in the air. Start with the foot, shaking it slowly and moving it in circles. Continue by shaking the lower leg, then progress up to the upper thigh. Do 3 sets of shaking. Repeat on the other leg.

➜ *'Aromatherapy blends', page 64–7* ● *'Digestive disorders', page 198*

Getting older

As you get older, living a healthy and balanced lifestyle becomes an extremely important factor in reducing lifestyle-related diseases, such as cardiovascular disease. Massage and aromatherapy are extremely beneficial for this age group.

Stay active

When you're older, eating well and being active are essential for preventing a decline in your mobility and ability to carry out daily activities. Many elderly people complain of stiff and aching muscles, so massage is a wonderful way to improve their quality of life and help maintain muscle function. However, you should consider age-related conditions such as arthritis and osteoporosis – for example, if a joint is inflamed, do not massage the area, and if bones are osteoporotic, always keep the pressure light.

Massage also plays a social role, as older people may feel isolated if friends and family live far away. Always be gentle when massaging the elderly, and make sure they are in a comfortable position – seated massage may be a viable option.

CAUTIONS ● See 'Safety and cautions', page 134.

SEATED MASSAGE TO THE NECK, HEAD AND SHOULDERS

For a general muscle and tension release, sit your massage partner on a comfortable chair and follow this three-step sequence.

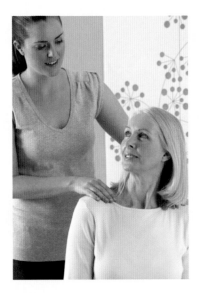

1 Gently knead through your partner's shoulders.

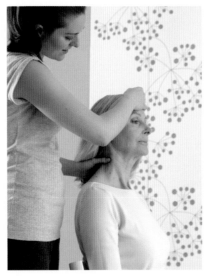

2 Next, support her head with the palm of your hand and knead the neck muscles. Remember to check that the pressure is suitable.

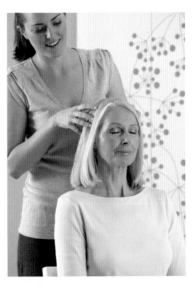

3 Massage the scalp. You can use a few drops of the essential oil rosemary, which is a memory stimulant, in 3 tablespoons of carrier oil.

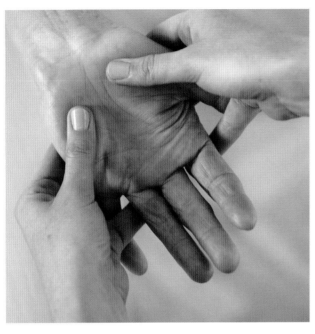

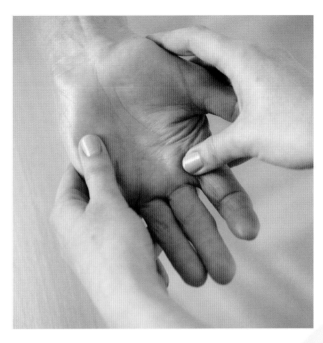

Hand massage

1 Grasp your partner's hands with your own and use your thumbs to strip across the muscles of the hand.

2 Spend time performing slow circular frictions at the base of each finger.

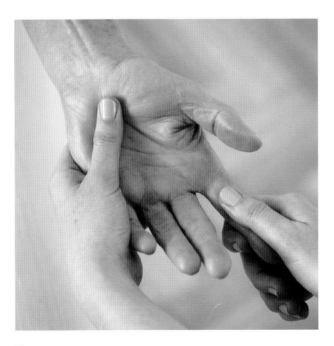

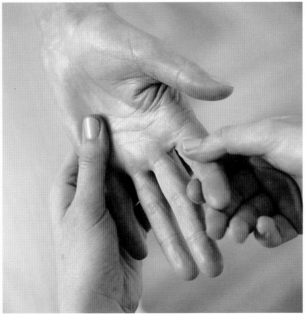

Finger massage

1 Hold each of the recipient's fingers between your hand and thumb and stroke along it.

2 Finish this off with a gentle rotation of the finger joint.

➜ *'Joint pain', page 212*

Pregnancy

As your baby grows inside you, your body will change. Use these simple techniques and movements to assist with any pain in the lower back, arms, legs and back. But first check with your doctor that it's safe for you to have a massage.

The first trimester

Massage is usually contraindicated in the first trimester due to the instability of the new foetus. Certain pressure points must be avoided, as repetitive stimulation of them is said to have an adverse effect. These points are located on and around the foot, the sacrum, the point between the thumb and index finger and the point between the shoulder and neck (see the diagram below).

LOWER BACK PAIN

This often begins to occur in the first trimester. As hormones are released, they begin the slow relaxation of the ligaments that hold the pelvis taut. As a result, you'll often experience pain in the lower back. Massage here greatly assists, as it is very nurturing and warming, and also soothes this area. Take your time doing the moves and enjoy the benefits for yourself and your baby.

PRESSURE POINTS TO AVOID DURING PREGNANCY

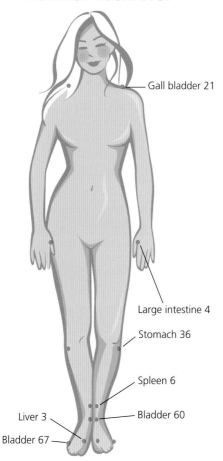

Gall bladder 21

Large intestine 4

Stomach 36

Spleen 6

Liver 3

Bladder 60

Bladder 67

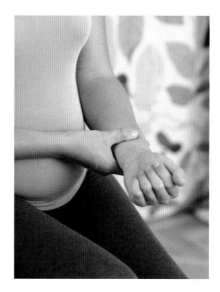

Acupressure
Morning sickness is common, but for some women it can be a significant problem. Use your thumb to press your arm at the point of Pericardium 6, three fingers above the wrist. This technique is especially useful when you're not at home.

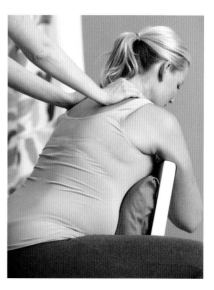

Seated massage
Give your pregnant partner a back massage. Ask her to sit backwards on a comfortable chair and lean on the back. Prop up her stomach with big fluffy pillows so she's not touching the chair back. Massage up and down her back with your hands.

CAUTIONS ● See 'During pregnancy', page 14 ● 'Safety and cautions', page 134.

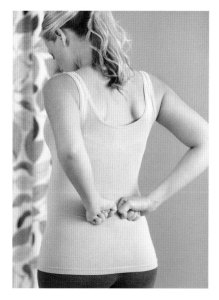

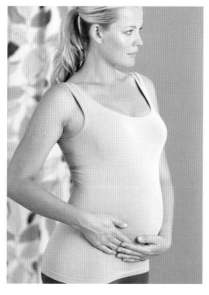

Self-massage

To help ease lower back pain, due to the pelvis beginning to loosen in preparation for birth, massage into your lower back. Place both hands on the lower back, then rub them back and forth, up and down, warming the muscles. Do this for up to 5 minutes, or however long it feels comfortable. This is especially effective in the last trimester.

Abdomen massage

As the baby grows, the stomach muscles stretch. You can assist this process and also bond with your baby by massaging gently over the whole abdomen. Starting at the left side, massage in slow clockwise circles until you reach the other side. Next, start a little higher and do the same thing, covering the whole area. This should take a few minutes.

BENEFITS OF ESSENTIAL OILS IN PREGNANCY

- *Using oils has been known to help prevent stretch marks. Try to massage your body daily with avocado, apricot kernel or wheatgerm oils. From the seventh month, if you wish, add a few drops of mandarin or lavender essential oils.*
- *Spearmint essential oil may help with morning sickness. Add a few drops to a handkerchief or tissue and sniff it when you feel nauseous.*
- *If you're experiencing fluid retention, check with your doctor first. If it's not serious, add a few drops of grapefruit, geranium and/or sweet orange essential oils to 3 tablespoons of carrier oil and use it with lymphatic massage on the feet, legs or arms.*

Side-lying massage

This is a fantastic way to massage your partner, especially in the later stages of pregnancy.

➔ *'Aromatherapy blends', page 76*

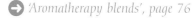

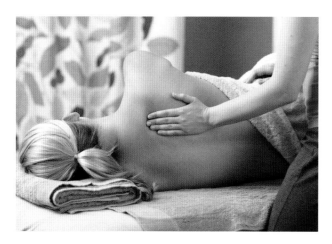

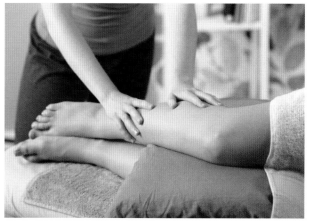

1 Ask her to lie on her side in the foetal position, with a pillow between her legs and another one under her abdomen. Massage one whole side of her body with effleurage and petrissage, allowing her to fully unwind and relax. Help her to turn over, then repeat on the other side.

2 Massaging the legs and feet soothes the muscles that support the extra weight. Starting at the feet, apply oil and gently stroke up, being careful not to stimulate points on the outside of the foot. Then proceed up the legs with soft effleurage and kneading, assisting lymph and tissue flow and helping improve circulation.

Babies and toddlers

Very young children are prone to a range of minor ailments, but you can treat them with massage and a small amount of aromatherapy oil. As always, check with your doctor or paediatrician first.

Colic

It is not known what causes 'colic', although it's traditionally been treated as a digestion problem, and parents often pat their babies on the back. Dilute a couple of drops of mandarin essential oil in 3 tablespoons of carrier oil, and use it as you gently massage your baby's abdomen, working slowly in a clockwise direction.

Tension

A newborn often becomes tense and overtired as he gets used to his new life outside the womb.

For a relaxing bath, mix together 2 drops of lavender essential oil with 3 tablespoons of either sweet almond or apricot kernel oil, and add the blend to the bath water *before* you bathe him.

Sleep

To assist with sleeping, burn a few drops of lavender, neroli or mandarin essential oil in an oil burner. To help baby sleep when he has a cold or bronchitis, add up to 5 drops of eucalyptus essential oil to a vaporiser, either during the day or at night.

Bonding

General Swedish massage is a great way to bond with your child and help him unwind and relax. Add a couple of drops of lavender essential oil to 3 tablespoons of sweet almond or apricot kernel oil, and massage a small amount over his body. Keep the pressure gentle but consistent (uneven pressure may agitate him). Don't force it if he is unhappy.

Common cold

If your baby has a cold, dilute 1 drop of one of the oils recommended in 'Sleep' above, then massage it into the soles of his feet. Its therapeutic effects will travel through the bloodstream to his lungs. Alternatively, apply massage directly onto his chest with little circular movements.

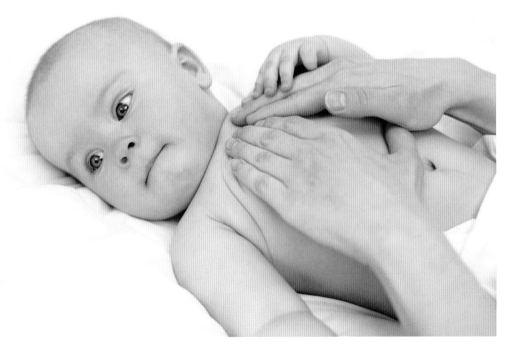

CAUTIONS ● Some practitioners advise against using essential oils on babies under the age of 12 months. ● See 'Babies and children', page 15 ● 'Safety and cautions', page 134.

About the authors

Pamela Allardice BA Communications (Hons)

Pamela is a well-known and respected editor and writer, with special expertise in the areas of health, complementary medicine, nutrition and diet. She is the editor of *Nature & Health*, Australia's leading and original natural health magazine. She is also the author of more than 30 books, including the best-selling *Pamela's Natural Remedies*, *The Body Bible*, *Natural Health Made Easy*, *A Handful of Herbs*, *Essential Oils*, *Making Scents*, *Feel Good*, *Make Time* and *Slow Up*. Her books have been sold in Europe, the United States, Israel, Korea and China. Pamela is also a contributor in *The Complete Book of Herbs* for Reader's Digest, and from 1995 to 2009 she was the 'Naturally Good' columnist for *The Australian Women's Weekly*. She now writes a monthly 'Ask Pamela' column on its website. In addition, her writing credits include the publication of more than 2000 articles in Australian and international print and electronic media.

Ela Bayliss DIBT, DRM, Dip Aroma, Dip Shiatsu

A qualified aromatherapist who runs her own aromatherapy business, Ela currently works as an aromatherapy supervisor at the Australasian College of Natural Therapies, where she has lectured and supervised aromatherapy massage since 2006. She has also worked in private, clinical and corporate environments since 2002, giving remedial, Shiatsu and aromatherapy treatments.

Stephen Bayliss DRM, Dip Sport

Stephen is a qualified remedial massage and sport therapist. He is the Head Massage Supervisor at the Australasian College of Natural Therapies, where he has been supervising and lecturing since 2005. He has worked in private clinical settings alongside chiropractors and physiotherapists, and has also worked extensively within the corporate massage environment. He is currently studying kinesiology.

Shelley Keating DRM, BSc (ExSciRehab), MExSpSci (CliExSci)

Shelley is a remedial massage therapist and an accredited exercise physiologist. She has worked in a private clinical and sport setting since 2004, and in addition to lecturing and supervising, she held the position of Program Director of Manual Therapies at the Australasian College of Natural Therapies from 2008 to 2010. Shelley completed her Masters of Exercise and Sports Science (Clinical Exercise Science) in 2010, and is currently undertaking higher degree research at Sydney University in the field of Exercise Physiology.

Further information

Organic certification

The main organisations for certifying essential oils as organic include:
- Australia: National Association for Sustainable Agriculture, Australia (NASAA; www.nasaa.com.au); Australian Certified Organic/Biological Farmers of Australia (BFA; www.bfa.com.au); and Organic Growers of Australia (OGA; www.organicgrowers.org.au).
- New Zealand: BioGro (www.bio-gro.co.nz); The Bio Dynamic Association (www.biodynamic.org.nz), the New Zealand certifier for Demeter, a world-wide certification system; Organic Farm New Zealand (www.organicfarm.org.nz); and Asure Quality (www.organiccertification.co.nz).
- United States: National Organic Program (USDA; www.ams.usda.gov).
- Canada: There is a national organic standard that covers many different bodies – look for the Canada Organic stamp on packaging.
- Britain: Organic Standard Soil Association (OSSA; www.soilassociation.org).
- Europe: European Union of Organic Farming (http://ec.europa.eu).

To find a qualified therapist

In Australia, you can contact the International Aromatherapy and Aromatic Medicine Association (IAAMA) at www.iaama.org.au. This is the largest independent professional association in this country, and all members are bound to a Code of Ethics and Code of Practice.

You may also find a practitioner near you through the free listing available on either one of the two major natural therapists' associations – the Australian Traditional-Medicine Society at www.atms.com.au or the Australian Natural Therapists Association at www.australiannaturaltherapistsassociation.com.au. Again, you should check any potential practitioner you consult for their professional memberships and qualifications.

In New Zealand, there are three organisations – the New Zealand Register of Holistic Aromatherapists at www.aromatherapy.org.nz, the New Zealand Charter of Health Practitioners at www.healthcharter.org.nz and the New Zealand Natural Medicine Association at www.nznma.com.

In the United Kingdom, you can consult the following organisations – the Federation of Holistic Therapists at www.fht.org.uk, The British Complementary Medicine Association at www.bcma.co.uk and the Institute for Complementary and Natural Medicine at www.icnm.org.uk.

In the United States, there are the following organisations – American Massage Therapy Association at www.amtamassage.org, American Holistic Health Association at www.ahha.org and National Association for Holistic Aromatherapy at www.naha.org.

In Canada, consult the following organisations – Canadian Federation of Aromatherapists at www.cfacanada.com, Natural Health Practitioners of Canada at www.nhpcanada.org and Massage Therapy Canada at www.massage.ca.

References

The following references relate to research findings discussed on the relevant pages of 'Top 30 essential oils', pages 28–59.

Basil
Wei A, Shibamoto T. Antioxidant/lipoxygenase inhibitory activities and chemical compositions of selected essential oils. Journal of Agriculture and Food Chemistry 2010;58(12):8218–25. www.ncbi.nlm.nih.gov/pubmed/20499917

Bergamot
Corasaniti MT, Maiuolo J, Maida S, Fratto V, Navarra M, Russo R, Amantea D, Morrone LA, Bagetta G. Cell signalling pathways in the mechanisms of neuroprotection afforded by bergamot essential oil against NMDA-induced cell death in vitro. British Journal of Pharmacology 2007 June;151(4):518–29. www.ncbi.nlm.nih.gov/sites/pubmed/17401440

Mandalari G, Bennett RN, Bisignano G, Trombetta D, Saija A, Faulds CB, Gasson MJ, Narbad A. Antimicrobial activity of flavonoids extracted from bergamot (*Citrus bergamia* Risso) peel, a byproduct of the essential oil industry. Journal of Applied Microbiology 2007 Dec;103(6):2056–64. www.ncbi.nlm.nih.gov/sites/pubmed/18045389

Rombolà L, Corasaniti MT, Rotiroti D, Tassorelli C, Sakurada S, Bagetta G, Morrone LA. Effects of systemic administration of the essential oil of bergamot (BEO) on gross behaviour and EEG power spectra recorded from the rat hippocampus and cerebral cortex. Functional Neurology 2009 Apr–Jun;24(2):107–12. www.ncbi.nlm.nih.gov/sites/pubmed/19775539

Cedarwood

Asakura K, Kanemasa T, Minagawa K, Kagawa K, Ninomiya M. The nonpeptide alpha-eudexp61 from Juniperus virginiana Linn. (Cupressaceae) inhibits omega-agatoxin IVA-sensitive Ca2+ currents and synaptosomal 45C+ uptake. Brain Research 1999 Mar 27;823(1–2):169–76.
www.ncbi.nlm.nih.gov/sites/pubmed/10095023

Dayawansa S, Umeno K, Takakura H, Hori E, Tabuchi E, Nagashima Y, Oosu H, Yada Y, Suzuki T, Ono T, Nishijo H. Autonomic responses during inhalation of natural fragrance of Cedrol in humans. Autonomic Neuroscience 2003 Oct 31;108(1–2):79–86.
www.ncbi.nlm.nih.gov/sites/pubmed/14614968

Chamomile

Charuluxananan S, Sumethawattana P, Kosawiboonpol R, Somboonviboon W, Werawataganon T. Effectiveness of lubrication of endotracheal tube cuff with chamomile-extract for prevention of postoperative sore throat and hoarseness. Journal of Medical Association of Thailand 2004 Sep;87 Suppl 2:S185–9.
www.ncbi.nlm.nih.gov/pubmed/16083185

Kato A, Minoshima Y, Yamamoto J, Adachi I, Watson AA, Nash RJ. Protective effects of dietary chamomile tea on diabetic complications. Journal of Agricultural and Food Chemistry 2008 Sep 10;56(17);8206–11.
www.ncbi.nlm.nih.gov/sites/pubmed/18681440

Clary sage

Peana AT, Moretti MD, Juliano C. Chemical composition and antimicrobial action of the essential oils of *Salvia desoleana* and *S. sclarea*. Planta Medica 1999 Dec;65(8);752–4.
www.ncbi.nlm.nih.gov/pubmed/10630121

Eucalyptus

Cermelli C, Fabio A, Fabio G, Quaglio P. Effect of eucalyptus essential oil on respiratory bacteria and viruses. Current Microbiology 2008 Jan;56(1):89–92.
www.ncbi.nlm.nih.gov/sites/pubmed/17972131

Frankincense

Frank MB, et al. Frankincense oil derived from *Boswellia carteri* induces tumor cell specific cytotoxicity. BMC Complementary and Alternative Medicine 2009 Mar 18;9:6.
www.ncbi.nlm.nih.gov/sites/pubmed/19296830

Lavender

Buchbauer G, Jirovetz L, et al. Aromatherapy: evidence for sedative effects of the essential oil of lavender after inhalation. Journal of Biosciences 1991 Nov–Dec;46(11–12):1067–72.
www.ncbi.nlm.nih.gov/sites/pubmed/1817516

Hadfield N. The role of aromatherapy massage in reducing anxiety in patients with malignant brain tumours. International Journal of Palliative Nursing 2001 Jun;7(6):279–85.
www.ncbi.nlm.nih.gov/sites/pubmed/12066022

Nakamura A, et al. Stress repression in restrained rats by (R)-(-)-linalool inhalation and gene expression profiling of their whole blood cells. Journal of Agricultural and Food Chemistry 2009 Jun 24;57(12):5480–5.
www.ncbi.nlm.nih.gov/sites/pubmed/19456160

Lemon

Ceccarelli I, et al. Sex differences in the citrus lemon essential oil-induced increase of hippocampal acetylcholine release in rats exposed to a persistent painful stimulation. Neuroscience Letters 2002 Sep 13;330(1):25–8.
www.ncbi.nlm.nih.gov/pubmed/12213626

Lemongrass

Manley CH. Psychophysiological effect of odor. Critical Reviews in Food Science and Nutrition 1993;33(1):57–62.
www.ncbi.nlm.nih.gov/sites/pubmed/8424855

Seth G, et al. Effect of essential oil of cymbopogon citratus stapf. on central nervous system. Indian Journal of Experimental Biology 1976 May;14(3):370–1.
www.ncbi.nlm.nih.gov/sites/pubmed/992793

Marjoram, sweet

Du WX, et al. Antibacterial effects of allspice, garlic and oregano essential oils in tomato films determined by overlay and vapor-phase methods. Journal of Food Science 2009 74(7):M390–7.
www.ncbi.nlm.nih.gov/pubmed/19895486

Orange, sweet

Komori T, et al. Effects of citrus fragrance on immune function and depressive states. Neuroimmunomodulation 1995 May–Jun;2(3);174–80.www.ncbi.nlm.nih.gov/pubmed/8646568

Rose

Umezu T. Anticonflict effects of plant-derived essential oils. Pharmacology Biochemistry & Behavior 1999 Sep;64(1):35–40.
www.ncbi.nlm.nih.gov/pubmed/10494995

Sandalwood

Warnke PH, et al. The battle against multi-resistant strains: Renaissance of antimicrobial essential oils as a promising force to fight hospital-acquired infections. Journal of Craniomaxilo-facial Surgery 2009 Oct;37(7);392–7.
www.ncbi.nlm.nih.gov/pubmed/19473851

Zhu J, et al. Mosquito larvicidal activity of botanical-based mosquito repellents. Journal of the American Mosquito Control Association 2008 Mar;24(1):161–8.
www.ncbi.nlm.nih.gov/pubmed/18437833

Tea tree

Caelli M, et al. Tea tree oil as an alternative topical decolonization agent for methicillin-resistant *Staphylococcus aureus*. Journal of Hospital Infection 2000 Nov;46(3):236–7.
www.ncbi.nlm.nih.gov/pubmed/11073734

Carson CF, et al. Susceptibility of methicillin-resistant *Staphylococcus aureus* to the essential oil of *Melaleuca alternifolia*. Journal of Antimicrobial Chemotherapy 1995 Mar;35(3):421–4.
www.ncbi.nlm.nih.gov/pubmed/7782258

Thyme, sweet

Hotta M. Carvacrol, a component of thyme oil, activates PPARalpha and gamma and suppresses COX-2 expression. Journal of Lipid Research 2010 Jan;51(1):132–9.
www.ncbi.nlm.nih.gov/sites/pubmed19578162

Research paper presented to the Society for General Microbiology, Spring 2010, by the Technological Educational Institute of the Ionian Islands, Greece. Society for General Microbiology (2010, April 4). Essential oils to fight superbugs. ScienceDaily. Retrieved July 5, 2010, from www.sciencedaily.com/releases/2010/03/100330210942.htm

Index

Page numbers in **bold** print refer to main entries

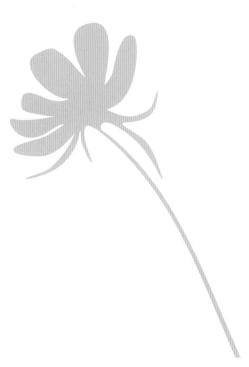

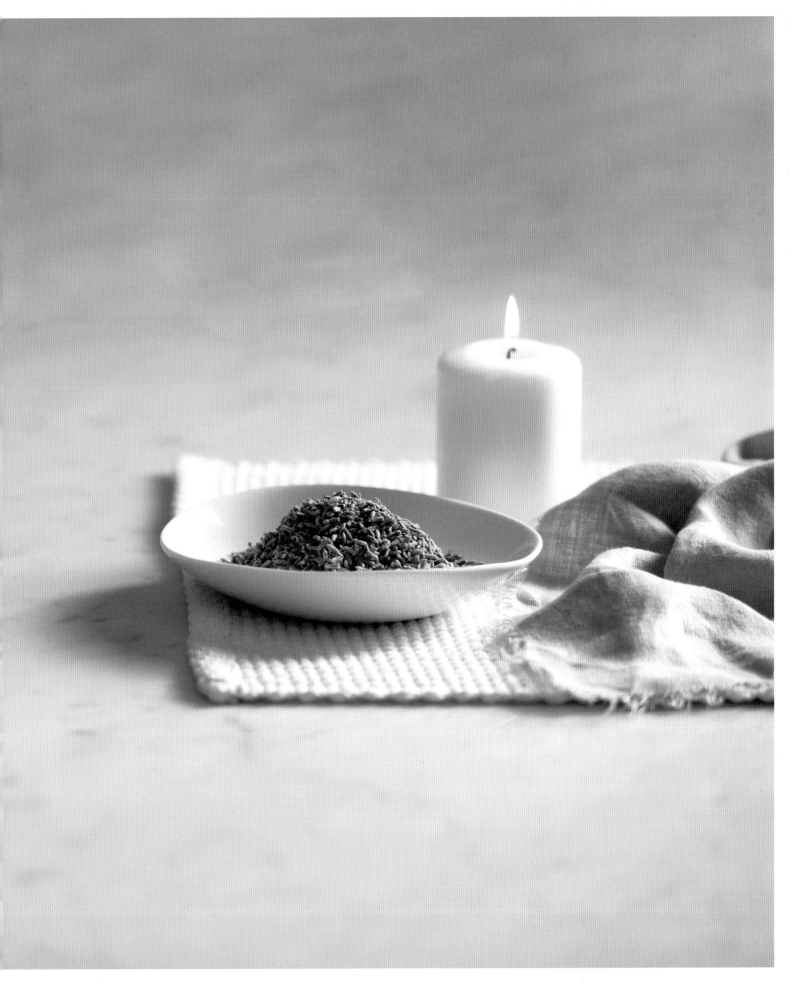

Massage & Aromatherapy

Consultants and Writers:
Shelley Keating DRM, Bsc (ExSciRehab), MExSpSci (CliExSci)
Stephen Bayliss DRM, Dip Sport
Ela Bayliss DIBT, DRM, Dip Aroma, Dip Shiatsu
Pamela Allardice (Aromatherapy, pages 10–81)

Project Editor Sarah Baker
Designer Jacqueline Duncan
Proofreader Christine Eslick
Indexer Diane Harriman
Photographer Andre Martin
Stylists Kate Nixon, Louise Bickle
Illustrators Wendy Blume (pages 91, 93, 107, 232),
    Levent Efe (pages 129, 131, 133)
Picture Rights Coordinator Natalie Zizic
Senior Production Controller Monique Tesoriero
Editorial Project Manager General Books Deborah Nixon

READER'S DIGEST GENERAL BOOKS
Editorial Director Elaine Russell
Managing Editor Rosemary McDonald
Art Director Carole Orbell

Massage & Aromatherapy is published by
Reader's Digest (Australia) Pty Limited
80 Bay Street, Ultimo NSW 2007
www.readersdigest.com.au
www.readersdigest.co.nz
www.readersdigest.co.za
www.rd.com; www.readersdigest.ca

First published 2011.
Copyright © Reader's Digest (Australia) Pty Limited 2011
Copyright © Reader's Digest Association Far East Limited 2011
Philippines Copyright © Reader's Digest Association Far East
Limited 2011

National Library of Australia Cataloguing-in-Publication entry

Title: *Massage & Aromatherapy*
ISBN: 978-1-921743-88-7 (hbk.)
ISBN 978-1-921744-11-2 (pbk.)
Notes: Includes index.
Subjects: Aromatherapy.
Essences and essential oils—Therapeutic use. Massage.
Other Authors/Contributors: Reader's Digest Association.
Dewey Number: 615.3219
ISBN: 978-1-55475-077-1 (North America)
ISBN: 978-1-60652-339-1 (USA)

Prepress by Sinnott Bros, Sydney
Printed and bound by Leo Paper Products, China

We are interested in receiving your comments on the contents
of this book. Write to:
The Editor, General Books Editorial,
Reader's Digest (Australia) Pty Limited,
GPO Box 4353, Sydney, NSW 2001,
or email us at bookeditors.au@readersdigest.com

To order additional copies of *Massage & Aromatherapy*,
please contact us as follows:
www.readersdigest.com.au, 1300 300 030 (Australia);
www.readersdigest.co.nz, 0800 400 060 (New Zealand);
www.readersdigest.co.za, 0800 980 572 (South Africa)
or email us at customerservice@readersdigest.com.au

Acknowledgments

The publishers wish to thank the following individuals, companies and
organisations for their help during the preparation of this book.
Ela Bayliss for the diagram reference for Pressure points to avoid during
pregnancy, page 232; Vanessa Prochowski for kindly providing massage
stones; Jessica Berg and Julia Green for hair and makeup; No Chintz,
Bed Bath N Table and Papier D'Amour for props; Jess Cox, Helen Flint,
Donna Heldon, Nozomi Ikeda, Chantelle Phipps, Krista Smith and
Yoshi Kawahara for modelling assistance.

All images are copyright of Reader's Digest, except for the following.
Photographs: 31 Photolibrary, 33 Photolibrary, 34 Dreamstime,
35 Photolibrary, 36 Photolibrary, 37 Photolibrary, 40 Shutterstock,
41 Photolibrary, 42 iStockphoto, 43 Shutterstock, 44 Shutterstock,
46 Shutterstock, 47 Shutterstock, 49 Photolibrary, 50 Shutterstock,
51 Photolibrary, 52 Getty Images, 53 Shutterstock, 54 Keith McLeod,
55 Shutterstock, 56 Getty Images, 57 Photolibrary, 59 Shutterstock,
227 Shutterstock
Illustrations by Levent Efe: 129, 131, 133

Note to readers

The information in this book is of a general nature. While the
creators of this book have made every effort to be as accurate
and up-to-date as possible, medical and pharmacological
knowledge is constantly changing. Readers are advised to
consult a qualified medical specialist for individual advice. The
writers, researchers, editors and publishers of the book cannot
be held liable for any errors or omissions, or actions that may
be taken as a consequence of the information contained in
this book.

Concept code: AU 0841/IC
Product codes: 041-4392 (hbk)
041-4479 (pbk)